T0228940

Early Arthritis

Guest Editors

KARINA D. TORRALBA, MD, FACR
RICHARD S. PANUSH, MD, MACP, MACR
FRANCISCO P. QUISMORIO Jr, MD, MACR

RHEUMATIC DISEASE CLINICS OF NORTH AMERICA

www.rheumatic.theclinics.com

May 2012 • Volume 38 • Number 2

SAUNDERS an imprint of ELSEVIER, Inc.

W.B. SAUNDERS COMPANY
A Division of Elsevier Inc.
1600 John F. Kennedy Blvd., Suite 1800 • Philadelphia, PA 19103-2899
http://www.theclinics.com

RHEUMATIC DISEASE CLINICS OF NORTH AMERICA Volume 38, Number 2
May 2012 ISSN 0889-857X, ISBN 13: 978-1-4557-3932-5

Editor: Pamela Hetherington
Developmental Editor: Teia Stone

Rheumatic Disease Clinics of North America (ISSN 0889-857X) is published quarterly by Elsevier Inc., 360 Park Avenue South, New York, NY 10010-1710. Months of issue are February, May, August, and November. Business and editorial offices: 1600 John F. Kennedy Boulevard, Suite 1800, Philadelphia, PA 19103-2899. Periodicals postage paid at New York, NY and additional mailing offices. Subscription prices are USD 305.00 per year for US individuals, USD 534.00 per year for US institutions, USD 150.00 per year for US students and residents, USD 360.00 per year for Canadian individuals, USD 659.00 per year for Canadian institutions, USD 427.00 per year for international individuals, USD 659.00 per year for international institutions, and USD 210.00 per year for Canadian and foreign students/residents. To receive student/resident rate, orders must be accompanied by name of affiliated institution, date of term, and the *signature* of program/residency coordinator on institution letterhead. Orders will be billed at individual rate until proof of status received. Foreign air speed delivery is included in all *Clinics* subscription prices. All prices are subject to change without notice. **POSTMASTER:** Send address changes to *Rheumatic Disease Clinics of North America,* Elsevier Health Sciences Division, Subscription Customer Service, 3251 Riverport Lane, Maryland Heights, MO 63043. **Customer Service: 1-800-654-2452 (US and Canada). From outside of the US and Canada: 314-447-8871. Fax: 314-447-8029. For print support, e-mail: JournalsCustomerService-usa@elsevier.com. For online support, e-mail: JournalsOnline Support-usa@elsevier.com.**

Reprints. For copies of 100 or more of articles in this publication, please contact the Commercial Reprints Department, Elsevier Inc., 360 Park Avenue South, New York, New York, 10010-1710; Tel.: (+1) 212-633-3813, Fax: (+1) 212-462-1935, and E-mail: reprints@elsevier.com.

Rheumatic Disease Clinics of North America is covered in *MEDLINE/PubMed (Index Medicus), Current Contents/Clinical Medicine, Science Citation Index, ISI/BIOMED,* and *EMBASE/Excerpta Medica.*

Printed and bound by CPI Group (UK) Ltd, Croydon, CR0 4YY

Transferred to Digital Print 2012

Contributors

GUEST EDITORS

KARINA D. TORRALBA, MD, FACR
Assistant Professor, Division of Rheumatology; Associate Director, USC-LAC
Rheumatology Fellowship Program, Keck School of Medicine University of
Southern California, Los Angeles, California

RICHARD S. PANUSH, MD, MACP, MACR
Professor of Medicine, Division of Rheumatology, Department of Medicine, University
of Southern California Medical Center, Keck School of Medicine, University of Southern
California, Los Angeles, California

FRANCISCO P. QUISMORIO Jr, MD, MACR, FACP
Professor of Medicine and Pathology, Division of Rheumatology, Department of Medicine,
University of Southern California Medical Center, Keck School of Medicine, University of
Southern California, Los Angeles, California

AUTHORS

RICHARD BRASINGTON, MD
Professor, Division of Rheumatology, Department of Medicine, Washington University
School of Medicine, St Louis, Missouri

KEVIN DEANE, MD, PhD
Assistant Professor of Medicine, Division of Rheumatology, Department of Medicine,
University of Colorado School of Medicine, Aurora, Colorado

DAVID A. FOX, MD
Professor and Chief, Division of Rheumatology, Department of Medicine, University of
Michigan School of Medicine, Ann Arbor, Michigan

DAFNA D. GLADMAN, MD, FRCPC
Professor of Medicine, University of Toronto; Senior Scientist Toronto Western Research
Institute; Director, Psoriatic Arthritis Program, University Health Network, Toronto,
Ontario, Canada

ANNA GRAMLING, MD
Division of Rheumatology and Immunology, University of Nebraska Medical Center;
Department of Veterans Affairs Nebraska-Western Iowa Health Care System, Omaha,
Nebraska

CHAIM O. JACOB, MD, PhD
Department of Medicine, Keck School of Medicine, University of Southern California,
Los Angeles, California

NOAM JACOB, MD
Department of Medicine, Keck School of Medicine, University of Southern California, Los Angeles, California

ELIZABETH W. KARLSON, MD
Associate Professor of Medicine, Section of Clinical Sciences, Division of Rheumatology, Allergy and Immunology, Department of Medicine, Brigham and Women's Hospital, Boston, Massachusetts

NASIM A. KHAN, MD
Division of Rheumatology, Department of Internal Medicine, University of Arkansas for Medical Sciences and Central Arkansas Veterans Healthcare System, Little Rock, Arkansas

KATHERINE ANNE B. MARZAN, MD
Division of Rheumatology, Children's Hospital Los Angeles; Assistant Professor of Pediatrics, Keck School of Medicine of University of Southern California, Los Angeles, California

JAMES R. O'DELL, MD
Division of Rheumatology and Immunology, University of Nebraska Medical Center; Department of Veterans Affairs Nebraska-Western Iowa Health Care System, Omaha, Nebraska

EWA OLECH, MD
Associate Professor of Medicine, Division of Rheumatology, Department of Internal Medicine, University of Nevada School of Medicine, Las Vegas, Nevada

ELIZABETH C. ORTIZ, MD
Assistant Professor of Medicine, Division of Rheumatology, Keck School of Medicine, University of Southern California, Los Angeles, California

RICHARD S. PANUSH, MD, MACP, MACR
Professor of Medicine, Division of Rheumatology, Department of Medicine, University of Southern California Medical Center, Keck School of Medicine, University of Southern California, Los Angeles, California

OLGA PIMIENTA, MD
Orrin M. Troum, MD and Medical Associates, Santa Monica, California

DENIS PODDUBNYY, MD
Research Associate, Rheumatology, Medical Department I, Campus Benjamin Franklin, Charité Universitätsmedizin Berlin, Berlin, Germany

FRANCISCO P. QUISMORIO Jr, MD, MACR, FACP
Professor of Medicine and Pathology, Division of Rheumatology, Department of Medicine, University of Southern California Medical Center, Keck School of Medicine, University of Southern California, Los Angeles, California

TUOMAS RANNIO, MD
Department of Rheumatology, Jyväskylä Central Hospital, Jyväskylä, Finland

MARTIN RUDWALEIT, MD
Professor of Rheumatology, Endokrinologikum Berlin, and Charité University Medicine, Berlin, Germany

DEEPALI SEN, MD
Fellow, Division of Rheumatology, Department of Medicine, Washington University School of Medicine, St Louis, Missouri

BRACHA SHAHAM, MD
Assistant Professor of Clinical Pediatrics, Keck School of Medicine, University of Southern California; Division of Rheumatology, Children's Hospital Los Angeles, Los Angeles, California

SHUNTARO SHINADA, MD
Assistant Professor of Medicine, Division of Rheumatology, Keck School of Medicine, University of Southern California, Los Angeles, California

TUULIKKI SOKKA, MD, PhD
Department of Rheumatology, Jyväskylä Central Hospital, Jyväskylä, Finland

RALF THIELE, MD, FACR
Assistant Professor of Medicine, Allergy/Immunology and Rheumatology Division, Department of Medicine, University of Rochester School of Medicine and Dentistry, Rochester, New York

ORRIN M. TROUM, MD
Clinical Professor of Medicine, Keck School of Medicine, University of Southern California, Santa Monica, California

Contents

> Rheumatoid arthritis (RA) is the most common rheumatic disease. The genetic basis of RA is supported through the identification of more than 30 susceptibility genetic variants. Each of these genes individually makes only a slight contribution to the risk of disease. Moreover, there is significant disparity in the genetic variants associated with different RA subgroups and patient ethnicities, which emphasizes the intricate nature of the disease's pathogenesis, and the complexities involved in large-scale genetic studies. This review evaluates critically the recent literature on the genetic contribution to RA and assesses the methodology used to identify these risk alleles.

> Ultrasonography is an elegant tool for the detection of tenosynovitis, synovitis, and erosions very early in rheumatoid arthritis, and the presence of a power Doppler signal is one of the best predictors of joint damage. Although clinical scores remain the mainstay of disease activity assessment, ultrasonography has proved to be a remarkably robust tool for reliable assessment of changes in rheumatoid arthritis. There is no evidence to suggest that problems with operator dependence would be greater than with other imaging modalities or physical examination, if performed by trained providers.

> Early diagnosis and treatment have been recognized as essential for improving clinical outcomes in patients with rheumatoid arthritis (RA). Magnetic resonance imaging (MRI) is a sensitive modality that can assess both inflammatory and structural lesions. MRI can assist in following the disease course in patients treated with traditional disease-modifying antirheumatic drugs and biological therapies both in the clinic and in research trials. Therefore, it is anticipated that MRI becomes the diagnostic imaging modality of choice in RA clinical trials while remaining a useful tool for clinicians evaluating patients with RA.

> Quantitative assessment of disease activity and patient-reported outcomes are recognized as valuable in the management of rheumatoid

arthritis (RA). Complexities of assessment of RA include challenges concerning measures themselves, as a gold standard measure for disease status does not exist. This article discusses the hurdles in the implementation of quantitative assessment of RA in usual clinical care and also provides an example to monitor patients with early RA.

The prognosis for the patient with newly diagnosed rheumatoid arthritis (RA) has dramatically changed over the last two decades. If a patient is diagnosed and treated early by a rheumatologist with the goal of remission or low disease activity, half of patients can expect to achieve remission while taking their disease-modifying antirheumatic drugs. This article discusses the initial therapy in early RA and reviews the studies and trials available in the literature.

The past decade has brought increasing evidence to support aggressive therapeutic intervention in early rheumatoid arthritis (RA). Treat-to-target strategies that focus on frequent monitoring and treatment adjustments to achieve states of low disease activity or clinical remission have shown superior long-term results. Both oral disease-modifying antirheumatic drugs and biologic agents are effective in treating early RA. It remains unclear if initial combination therapy or biologic use is more effective in early active disease as compared with the traditional approach. The authors review various studies on the treatment of early RA with a focus on studies with a treat-to-target approach.

Classification criteria are created in an attempt to produce a homogenous group of subjects with rheumatoid arthritis (RA) who can be used for clinical and basic research. The 1987 revised criteria lead to improved performance and more confidence in correct classification compared with the 1958 criteria. As therapies were introduced and early, aggressive approaches to RA management became common, there was a growing need for clinical trials focusing on early RA. The 2010 criteria were created to facilitate study of subjects at earlier stages in the disease. This article reviews the diagnostic performance of the 2010 criteria.

Early juvenile idiopathic arthritis (JIA) is important to recognize as timely diagnosis and treatment improves prognosis. It is a misconception that complications of JIA arise only from long-standing disease and that children will outgrow it. Early aggressive treatment is the paradigm as early disease activity has long-term consequences. There are predictors of persistent disease and joint erosions that may identify patients at higher risk. Control of disease activity within the first 6 months of onset confers improved clinical course and outcomes. The treatment perspective is thus one of early aggressive treatment for induction of disease control and ultimately remission.

biomarkers will be discussed. We will also examine the incremental consequences of delaying therapy, particularly for 'preclinical' disease. Medical
economic analyses can help us balance benefits and avoid some adverse
outcomes for patients. To conclude, we will discuss the new roles that
need developing for primary care physicians and non-physican providers.

RHEUMATIC DISEASE CLINICS OF NORTH AMERICA

Preface

Early Arthritis

A Race to the Starting Line

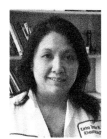
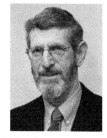
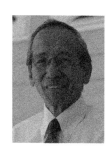

Karina D. Torralba, MD   Richard S. Panush, MD   Francisco P. Quismorio Jr, MD

Guest Editors

Every Friday morning we have our early inflammatory arthritis clinic at the Los Angeles County Medical Center. The patients come almost monthly and describe to us how they are doing; physicians examine the patients and do their joint counts, review laboratory findings, and calculate their disease activity scores. Often, we use the ultrasound machine to quantify synovitis or to detect smoldering and subclinical synovitis.

As all patient care systems go, there are challenges and one of the greatest ones we had (and continue to have) is to capture patients early in their disease course and to prevent disability. This clinic was established in April 2008 to provide improved accessibility to care to a largely indigent population of patients, with the primary objectives of providing closer monitoring and achieving clinical remission of their arthritis. It is a constant reminder of why I became a rheumatologist. Approximately 10 years ago, during one of the American College of Rheumatology meetings, I sat riveted listening to Dr Ravinder Maini describe how tumor necrosis factor causes damage in rheumatoid arthritis. Over the next 15 years, progress into our understanding of the pathophysiology of this disease has greatly altered our treatment of rheumatoid arthritis and has allowed more patients to achieve clinical remission in greater numbers than before. There is an increasing impetus to diagnose inflammatory arthritis earlier and to institute proper treatment in order to reach remission as soon as possible. It involves rethinking old ways of clinical practice to provide innovative approaches to earlier access to care and closer monitoring of disease. In fact there is now increasing focus not only on early rheumatoid arthritis, which is defined as the period of disease 2 years from onset of symptoms, but also on very early rheumatoid arthritis, which is defined as the period of disease 3 months from onset of symptoms.

In a way, we as rheumatologists are in a race, a race where rheumatoid arthritis, or any other kind of inflammatory arthritis, is our opponent. We are propelled by our desire to catch up with the destructive effects of inflammation, with the biggest challenge for us to be present at the starting line.

Rheum Dis Clin N Am 38 (2012) xiii–xv
doi:10.1016/j.rdc.2012.05.002
0889-857X/12/$ – see front matter © 2012 Elsevier Inc. All rights reserved.

rheumatic.theclinics.com

In this edition of *Rheumatic Disease Clinics*, we have brought together a variety of views on approaches to the early diagnosis and treatment of inflammatory arthritis. It is virtually impossible to encompass the entire spectrum of arthritides, and for this purpose we have particularly focused on rheumatoid arthritis, ankylosing spondylitis, psoriatic arthritis, and juvenile idiopathic arthritis.

In order to have a good understanding of the management of rheumatoid arthritis, it is important to look at the past, the present, and the future. Drs Shuntaro Shinada and Elizabeth Ortiz elaborate on the recent changes to the classification criteria of rheumatoid arthritis, comparing its performance to the performance of prior criteria, discussing its utility in selecting out patients with early disease. Various indices are available to monitor patient progress. Drs Tulikki Sokka, Tuomas Rannio, and Nasim Khan delve into the practical role of disease activity measurements and eliciting patient-reported outcomes. There are certainly inherent challenges involved in the use of these measurements. They have graciously lent us their own experiences, describing the solutions they have provided in the implementation of these assessment methods.

Drs Deepali Sen and Richard Brasington examine the evidence embracing the role of aggressive treatment and close monitoring, looking at data that explore the role of "tight control" that use conventional disease-modifying antirheumatic drugs and biologic medications. They remind us that the key target in RA management is remission. Drs Anna Gramling and Jim O'Dell provide convincing data on the role of therapies in tackling the effects of early disease, and in improving outcomes.

Apart from ongoing innovations in the development of medications, many of which are in the pipeline, the future remains bright for the other aspects of the management of rheumatoid arthritis. The role of imaging in the early diagnosis of rheumatoid arthritis is ripe with promise. Dr Ralf Thiele explores the role of ultrasonography in detecting subclinical synovitis and erosions. Ultrasonography is increasingly being used and we are entering an exciting era where this modality can be used to complement our clinical examination of patients in real-time. Drs Orrin Troum, Olga Pimienta, and Ewa Olech give us insight on the usefulness of magnetic resonance imaging (MRI) in detecting inflammatory and structural lesions. MRI distinguishes itself by its ability to detect bone marrow edema, which is a precursor to the development of erosions. Both ultrasound and MRI have demonstrated sensitivity in detecting early and even subclinical disease, even among patients deemed to be in clinical remission. However more studies are needed to establish definitive outcome measures for both modalities.

Is the term "pre-early" even a possibility? Certainly a revolutionary approach to disease management would be to approach it even before it becomes a problem. Drs Elizabeth Karlsson and Kevin Deane provide captivating evidence about the preclinical phases of rheumatoid arthritis where the role of genes and environmental factors trigger immunoregulatory mechanisms in genetically predisposed individuals. Drs Chaim Jacob and Noam Jacob discuss the role of genes that predispose to the development of rheumatoid arthritis. The idea of developing measures to prevent rheumatoid arthritis prior to its clinical phase is certainly an intriguing prospect.

Other inflammatory types of arthritis have also focused on early approaches to management. Dr Dafna Gladman offers us an update on approaches to the management of psoriatic arthritis. Drs Karen Marzan and Bracha Shaham offer us an overview on approaches to the diagnosis and treatment of early juvenile idiopathic arthritis. Drs Denis Poddubnyy and Martin Rudwaleit provide insights on recent advances on the spondyloarthropathies, including insights on the various classification criteria and the key clinical features that should clue us into the presence of this kind of problem.

For the millions of individuals with inflammatory arthritis, there is certainly hope. There is no better way to approach disease but to tackle it head on and strike while it is early, before long-lasting complications settle in. The race against rheumatoid arthritis has certainly been running for a very long time, and trying to win it early on, close to the starting line, is the way to go.

Karina D. Torralba, MD
Division of Rheumatology
Keck School of Medicine of the
University of Southern California
Health Sciences Campus
2011 Zonal Avenue, HMR 711
Los Angeles, CA 90033, USA

Richard S. Panush, MD
Division of Rheumatology
Department of Medicine
Keck School of Medicine of the
University of Southern California
USC Medical Center
IRD 427, 2010 Zonal Avenue
Los Angeles, CA 90033, USA

Francisco P. Quismorio Jr, MD
Division of Rheumatology
Department of Medicine
Keck School of Medicine of the
University of Southern California
USC Medical Center
IRD 427, 2010 Zonal Avenue
Los Angeles, CA 90033, USA

E-mail addresses:
ktorralb@usc.edu (K.D. Torralba)
Panush@usc.edu (R.S. Panush)
quismori@usc.edu (F.P. Quismorio)

Genetics of Rheumatoid Arthritis: An Impressionist Perspective

Noam Jacob, MD, Chaim O. Jacob, MD, PhD*

KEYWORDS

- Rheumatoid arthritis • Anti-citrullinated protein antibodies
- HLA • Risk allele

Key Points

- More than 30 susceptibility gene variants associated with RA were identified, individually most making only slight contribution to the risk of disease.
- Gene variants within the HLA locus account for 30% to 50% of overall genetic susceptibility to RA.[1,2]
- Three main approaches have been used to identify non-HLA susceptibility loci: classical family linkage studies, case-control candidate gene studies, and genome-wide association studies.

INTRODUCTION

In 1913, at the age of 72 years, having produced numerous masterpieces, the great impressionist painter Pierre-Auguste Renoir declared, "I am just learning how to paint." Although suffering from severe rheumatoid arthritis (RA), Renoir went on to produce additional paintings, each subtly beautiful and profound. One might imagine Renoir was hinting that given the advanced stage of his disease, with the ability to paint nimbly across the canvas now constrained by tormented joints, every stroke of his brush had to be planned, deliberately focused, and refined. And with these brush-strokes one might say that Renoir's connection to RA goes beyond his diagnosis. As opposed to previous classical paintings that consisted of subjects illustrated

---

Department of Medicine, Keck School of Medicine, University of Southern California, 2011 Zonal Avenue HMR 703, Los Angeles, CA 90033, USA
* Corresponding author. University of Southern California, Keck School of Medicine, 2011 Zonal Avenue HMR 705, Los Angeles, CA 90033.
E-mail address: jacob@usc.edu

Rheum Dis Clin N Am 38 (2012) 243–257
doi:10.1016/j.rdc.2012.05.001
0889-857X/12/$ – see front matter © 2012 Elsevier Inc. All rights reserved.

with contiguous hard outlines and smooth paint surfaces, Renoir's paintings depict vibrant figures comprising numerous small brush strokes. When the canvas and individual strokes are viewed up-close and analyzed independently of the rest of the painting, the image is blurry and meaningless (**Fig. 1**A). When viewed from a distance, however, it becomes apparent that distinct strokes each contribute to a great masterwork depicting, for example, a hidden path emerging through the woods (see **Fig. 1**B). Decades of research in RA have also seen a path emerge in the disease's complex pathogenesis and mounting evidence has been accumulated to support the genetic basis of RA through the identification of more than 30 susceptibility genetic variants. Thus far, however,each of these genes individually makes only a slight impression on the picture of disease, much like the brush-strokes on the canvas of an impressionist painting. As an artistic movement, impressionism also sought to reassess the previously accepted methods in classical painting, focusing on the evaluation of novel techniques and subjects to create vivid works of art. From this perspective, the aims of the following article are 2-fold: (1) a critical evaluation of the recent literature on the genetic contribution to RA pathogenesis, and (2) an assessment of the methodology used in the studies from which these data are derived.

THE LANDSCAPE

RA is the most common rheumatic disease with a prevalence of 0.5% to 1% in the general population worldwide. Among siblings, the prevalence increases to 2% to 4%.[3] In monozygotic twins, the concordance rate for RA is between 12.3% and 15.4% compared with 3.5% for dizygotic twins.[4] These sibling and twin pair studies demonstrate that genetic factors substantially affect RA susceptibility, resulting in an estimated genetic contribution to RA of approximately 50% to 60%.[3–5] The relatively low concordance rates between monozygotic twins; however, emphasize the importance of environmental factors in RA susceptibility. Among them, long-term

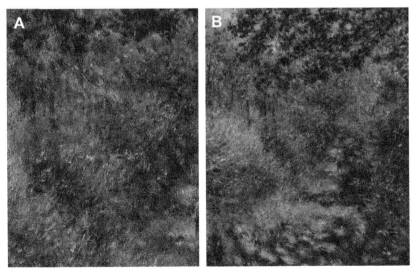

Fig. 1. Pierre-Auguste Renoir, *Path through the woods,* (oil on canvas). An analogy for the genetic contribution to RA pathogenesis. (*A*) Magnified view of a portion of Renoir's painting: *Path through the woods,* which is depicted in its entirety in (*B*).

smoking remains the only validated environmental factor that contributes to an increased risk of developing seropositive RA.[6]

As is the case for other autoimmune diseases, there is growing awareness that RA is not a single disease entity, but rather can be divided into distinct subphenotypes that have disparate clinical outcomes. Such a classification is achieved based on the serologic traits, such as the rheumatoid factor (RF) and anti-citrullinated protein antibodies (ACPA). RF is an autoantibody against the Fc portion of IgG, whereas ACPA are autoantibodies against citrullinated proteins that are formed by the conversion of arginine into citrullin by peptidylarginine deiminase (PADI).[7] Citrullination is a physiologic process that can occur under different conditions including inflammation. Although RF is not unique to RA, ACPA are highly specific for the disease. Indeed, 75% of subjects who present with undifferentiated arthritis and ACPA progress to RA within 3 years of follow-up.[8] The subdivision of RA into ACPA-positive and ACPA-negative subtypes is useful because these distinct groups of patients often differ clinically, with ACPA-positive patients with RA suffering a more aggressive clinical course, higher rates and severity of erosions, and lower rates of remission.[9] Furthermore, they also vary with regard to the genetic risk factors that contribute to their development.

Thus far, more genetic risk alleles have been described for ACPA-positive RA compared with ACPA-negative RA, but this does not imply that genetic factors contribute more to the former than the latter. The heritability of RA among twin pairs for ACPA-positive and ACPA-negative disease was found to be 68% and 66%, respectively,[5] which suggests that the heritability of both serotypes of RA is roughly equivalent. The relative lack of identified risk alleles in ACPA-negative disease might be because most studies to date relied solely on cohorts of ACPA-positive patients with RA.

A DOMINANT THEME: THE HLA RISK FACTOR

The most statistically significant genetic contributor to RA is the HLA locus, which accounts for 30% to 50% of the overall genetic susceptibility to RA.[1,2] Within the HLA, a group of alleles that encode the HLA-class II DRβ chain (HLA-DRB1) seem to be associated most strongly with predisposition to RA. Using HLA-DRB1 genotyping, multiple studies have described a significant association of 8 particular DRB1 alleles with RA: DRB*0401, 0404, 0405, 0408, 0101, 0102, 1001, and DRB*09, with DRB*0401 (odds ratio [OR] = 3.30) and DRB*0405 (OR = 3.84) showing the strongest association.[10] Positions 70 to 74 in the third hypervariable region of the DRβ1 chain of the RA-associated HLA-DRB1 alleles all contain the conserved amino acids QKRAA, QRRAA, or RRRAA. This sequence of amino acids is called the shared epitope (SE), and the risk alleles carrying this sequence are widely known as SE alleles.[11] An individual who carries 2 copies of DRB1 SE alleles increases his/her chances of developing RA with an increase in OR to 11.97.[12] This association between SE-encoding HLA-DRB1 alleles and RA was, however, observed only for ACPA-positive disease.[12]

Despite much progress in understanding the structure and function of HLA-DRB1 molecules, the underlying mechanism by which particular HLA-DRB1 alleles predispose to the development of ACPA-positive RA remains uncertain. The HLA-DR molecule is a heterodimer consisting of an α (DRA) and a β chain (DRB), both anchored in the membrane of antigen-presenting cells. The function of HLA-DR molecules is to present antigenic peptides to T lymphocytes. For efficient antigen presentation to T cells, the T-cell receptor recognizes residues from both the peptide and the HLA-DR molecule itself. The part of HLA-DR that binds to the peptide, denoted as the peptide-binding groove, comprises 2 α-helical walls and a floor of β-pleated sheets.[13] The SE is situated in the α-helix wall of the peptide-binding groove.[11] In this position, the SE may influence both peptide binding to the HLA molecule and T cell presentation. The SE motif itself is directly involved in the pathogenesis of RA by allowing the presentation of an arthritogenic peptide to T cells.[11,14] However, to date, no specific arthritogenic peptides that bind to SE DR molecules have been identified to confirm this hypothesis. Citrullinated peptides, can bind to HLA-SE molecules for presentation to T cells, which alludes to the direct pathogenic involvement of ACPA in RA.[15] Alternative hypotheses to explain the contribution of HLA-SE to RA have been also proposed: the HLA-SE molecules may contribute to RA pathogenesis by shaping the T cell repertoire to permit escape from negative selection and promote survival of autoreactive clones.[16] Furthermore, SE molecules may serve as targets for autoreactive T cells because of the molecular mimicry with a pathogen.[17] Although much indirect evidence to support molecular mimicry in RA (as in other autoimmune processes) has been offered, the hypothesis has not been confirmed directly.

Other studies have suggested additional independent associations to RA within the HLA gene in addition to that at HLA-DRB1.[18,19] However, pinpointing the associated loci has been challenging, in part because of the complexity of complete HLA genotyping and the broad linkage disequilibrium (LD) across the HLA locus. By using genotype imputation to generate very large data sets from previous studies, Raychaudhuri and colleagues[20] refined the association between the HLA region and RA. The investigators used existing genome-wide association studies (GWAS) data sets from 5018 ACPA-positive individuals with RA and 14,974 controls from independent studies. They then used a large reference panel of 2767 individuals to impute classical HLA alleles, single nucleotide polymorphisms (SNPs), and amino acids across the entire HLA region. These imputed data made it possible to use a much larger sample size than would have been possible with classical typing in resolving specific HLA signals among these very highly correlated variants. The investigators subsequently used conditional analyses in an effort to pinpoint the causal variants. Although the association P values at the top signals in the HLA were so infinitesimal as to make comparisons between raw results meaningless, the value of the study became apparent when testing each signal as conditional on the others. For example, amino acid positions 11 and 13 in HLA-DRβ1 (which are encoded by a locus with very high LD) had association P values of 1×10^{-581} and 1×10^{-574}, respectively. However, the conditional analyses for these 2 amino acids showed that, whereas conditioning on amino acid 11 explained the association at amino acid 13 (residual $P = .57$), the reverse was not true (residual $P = 3.5 \times 10^{-8}$). Based on multiple series of conditional analyses, the entire association within the HLA could be explained by 5 independent polymorphic sites in 3 HLA molecules. Two of these 5 residues were within the SE (amino acids 71 and 74). An important causal mutation was found outside the SE at the base of the DRB1 antigen-binding groove at position 11. Amino acids at the base of the groove of the HLA-B and HLA-DPB1 were also found to modulate causally RA risk. In addition to fine mapping the HLA-class II risk loci, the study resurrects the importance of HLA-class I molecules for RA risk, providing genetic evidence that implicates cytotoxic T cells in RA pathogenesis.

In contrast, the HLA association with ACPA-negative RA is clearly different because HLA-DR4 alleles are not associated. ACPA-negative disease has been associated with the HLA-DRB1*0301 allele in European populations[21,22] and the HLA-DRB1*0901 allele in a Japanese population.[23] Also, the non-SE DRB1 alleles DRB1*13 and DRB1*03, in combination, have been strongly associated.[21,24] DRB1*1301 actually confers protection from RA risk in ACPA-positive individuals,[25] possibly by neutralizing the effects of the SE alleles.

BRUSH-STROKES: NON-HLA RISK FACTORS IN ACPA-POSITIVE RA

Three main approaches have been used to identify non-HLA susceptibility loci: classical family linkage studies, case-control candidate gene studies, and GWAS. Associations of new individual genes were discovered by testing *candidate genes* within genomic regions linked to RA susceptibility in previous family linkage studies, analyses of biologic pathways involved in known RA-associated risk loci, or by testing genes known to be associated with other autoimmune diseases. Although these methods of testing candidate genes yielded important information, they have been criticized for potentially limiting their focus to previously identified regions/pathways rather than exploring new avenues in disease pathogenesis. In contrast, because newer methods involving GWAS do not rely on previous data as a starting point, they potentially overcome these limitations. GWAS are wrought with their own problems, however, namely, reductions in statistical power due to multiple testing, which are discussed subsequently. To potentially overcome these limitations, the latest trend is the use of meta-analyses from multiple GWAS, resulting in a very large (>10,000) number of subjects and thus increased statistical power.

Regarding associations discovered via candidate gene studies, the *PTPN22* gene is recognized as the second most important risk loci (after the HLA) in populations of European descent with ACPA-positive RA.[26,27] *PTPN22* encodes the lymphoid-specific tyrosine phosphatase, Lyp, which is a negative regulator of T-cell antigen receptor signal transduction during T-cell activation.[27] The associated risk allele is a nonsynonymous SNP (rs2476601, 1858 C > T) that encodes an arginine to tryptophan substitution at residue 620 (R620W) in the polypeptide chain, thereby disrupting the binding to C-src tyrosine kinase. There is evidence that this change confers a gain-of-function mutation to the PTPN22 protein, with the 620W variant enhancing the inhibitory effect on T-cell receptor signaling during thymic development, resulting in the survival of potentially autoreactive T cells.[28,29] No RA association with *PTPN22* could be demonstrated in Asian RA populations.

Among Asian populations with ACPA-positive RA, the second largest genetic risk factor is *PADI4*.[30,31] The *PADI4* gene encodes a peptidylarginine deiminase enzyme that converts arginine residues to citrulline posttranscriptionally.[30] Therefore, *PADI4* may play a significant role in the development of ACPA by influencing protein citrullination. Together with the finding that ACPA can induce and aggravate arthritis in mouse models,[32,33] these results suggest that ACPA are actually involved in human disease pathogenesis, as opposed to just serving as a serologic marker for RA subtype classification.[8,34] With the exception of the *PTPN22* gene, other non-HLA RA risk factors identified (mainly by GWAS) have a very modest effect size. **Table 1** illustrates all identified, and subsequently validated, risk factors for RA with their heritability estimates.

GWAS have been appreciated for representing an agnostic approach that is unbiased by assumptions regarding genetic association with the disease. However, such approaches typically ignore all valuable prior information collected over decades about the pathogenesis and genetic basis of the disease. This oversight inevitably leads to the inclusion of regions (and numerous additional SNPs) that have little to no possibility of being associated with RA, and thereby increases the number of tests performed. The massive number of statistical tests presents an unprecedented potential for false-positive results, leading to multiple test correction to control levels of

Table 1
Non-HLA genetic risk factors for RA

Genetic Risk Factor	Chromosomal Location	Heritability est (OR)	Association with Other Autoimmune Diseases	References
PTPN22	1p13	1.94	GD, HT, MG, SLE, DM1, SSc, UC	26,35–38
TNFRSF14	1p36	1.12		39
CD2, CD58	1p13	1.13	MS	40
FCGR2A	1q23	1.13	SLE	40,41
PTPRC	1q31	1.14		40
REL	2p16	1.13		42
AFF3	2q11	1.12		43
STAT4	2q32	1.16	SLE, GD, DM1, UC, CD, SS	44–49
CD28	2q33	1.12	DM1	40
CTLA4	2q33	1.11	HT, SS, DM1	38,43,50
IL-2, IL-21	4q27	1.09	DM1	43,51
PRDM1	6q21	1.1	CD	40
TNFAIP3	6q23	1.4	JIA, PsA, SLE, SSc, DM1	40,47,52,53
TAGAP	6q25	1.1	DM1, CD	40
BLK	8p23	1.12		42,54
CCL21	9p13	1.13		39
TRAF-1, C5	9q33	1.13	JIA, SLE	55
IL-2RA	10p15	0.92	JIA, MS, DM1	38,56
PRKCQ	10p15	1.14		39
TRAF6	11p12	0.88		40
KIF5A, PIP4K2C	12q13	1.12		39,56
CD40	20q13	1.11	GD, MS	39,56–58
IL-2RB	22q12	1.09		54
SPRED2	2p14	1.13		54
ANKRD55, IL-6ST	5q11	1.23		54
C5orf30	5q21	1.11		54
PXK	3p14	1.13		54
RBPJ	4p15	1.18		54
CCR6	6q27	1.11		59
IRF5	7q32	1.21		54,60
PADI4	1p36	1.12		30,31,61,62
CDK6	7q21	1.11		39
FCRL3	1q22	2.15	SLE, HT, GD	63,64
CD244	1q22	1.09		65
KLF12	13q22	N/A		66

All identified, and subsequently validated, non-HLA risk factors for RA with their chromosomal location, heritability estimates (OR), and associations with other autoimmune diseases are illustrated.

Abbreviations: CD, Crohn disease; DM1, type 1 diabetes mellitus; GD, Graves disease; HT, Hashimoto thyroiditis; JIA, juvenile idiopathic arthritis; MG, myasthenia gravis; MS, multiple sclerosis; N/A, not available; OR, odds ratio; PsA, psoriatic arthritis; SLE, systemic lupus erythematosus; SSc, systemic sclerosis; SS, Sjogren syndrome; UC, ulcerative colitis.

statistical significance, and an increased need for replicating findings. When performed appropriately, correction for multiple testing renders most of the findings insignificant because of the large number of tests (>300,000, typically). Moreover, because the case-control samples for GWAS usually number in the thousands, it might be supposed that such studies are well powered. However, several investigators have shown that given the strict genome-wide significance criteria that these studies must fulfill, their power is significantly lower than might have been imagined a priori.[67,68] There is also an additional limitation to the overall size of these large population-based studies because of constraints, such as budget, time, and the physical number of cases in the population (ie, prevalence of the disease).

Two main approaches have been undertaken to overcome the reduced power associated with GWAS. One approach uses imputation of SNP data in GWAS meta-analyses so that a much larger sample size is available for analysis, as has been successfully demonstrated regarding HLA fine mapping (see Raychaudhuri and colleagues[20]). The other approach, applies a type of Bayesian method of prioritizing genes or SNPs using prior information from the known pathogenetics of the disease as a starting point for candidate gene validation studies. This method significantly reduces the number of SNPs and genes to be tested to an amount commensurate with available samples and resources, as well as maintains appropriate power. Indeed, the authors have presented such a program to select and order genes by their prior likelihood of association with the disease[69] and applied it successfully to identify systemic lupus erythematosus (SLE) -associated risk factors.[70] Gene relationships across implicated loci (GRAIL) developed by Raychaudhuri and colleagues[71] is another method of prioritizing SNPs for evaluation in a candidate gene validation study. This method was applied to identify new susceptibility genes in RA. Accordingly, 370 SNPs were selected from 179 loci that reached a P-value of less than .001 in a previous independent GWAS meta-analysis and were investigated by GRAIL. A genomic region in LD with each candidate SNP was defined and all genes within these regions were selected. The literature was then mined to assess and score the relatedness of the implicated loci with genomic regions already known to be associated with disease. High GRAIL scores implicated 22 loci with functional connectivity. SNPs representing these candidate loci were then genotyped in an independent study of 8096 cases and 11,822 matched controls. Three of these loci, CD28, CD2/CD58, and PRDM1 were convincingly replicated.[40] PRDM1 functions as a regulator of gene expression of B and T lymphocytes' maturation and differentiation. CD28 is a molecule expressed on T cells that provides co-stimulatory signals, which are required for T cell activation. CD58 is a cell adhesion molecule expressed on antigen-presenting cells (APCs) and binds CD2 on T cells, strengthening the adhesion between T cells and APCs before T-cell activation. The CD2 protein is a co-stimulatory molecule on the surface of T cells, and CD2 signaling is mediated by directly binding PTPRC, also known as CD45. PTPRC (encoding protein tyrosine phosphatase, receptor type C), has been identified as a genetic factor involved in predisposition to RA, as well (**Table 1**).

These studies have begun to elucidate the complex genetic profile of RA with identification of over 30 risk loci. However, for almost all of these risk loci, the significant SNPs identified are within introns, or noncoding regions of the genes, and do not seem to have functional significance. It is thus, most likely that these SNPs are not causal, but rather in LD with other (not yet discovered) polymorphisms that need to be identified. Large-scale sequencing of selected patients and controls is the method most likely to result in identifying the causal variants in each of these risk genes that leads to RA susceptibility. Furthermore, as pointed out by de Vries,[72] it is remarkable how few *functional* studies have been undertaken to evaluate the risk factors identified and to understand the potential mechanisms of the known associations in disease. *TNFAIP3* is one of the few RA risk genes in which some functional studies have been undertaken.[52] These studies have determined that TNFAIP3 inhibits NF-kappa B activation as well as TNF-mediated apoptosis.[73] Knockout studies of this gene in mice suggest that this gene is critical for limiting inflammation by terminating TNF-induced NF-kappa B responses.[74–76]

BRUSH-STROKES: NON-HLA RISK FACTORS IN ACPA-NEGATIVE RA

The paucity of validated genetic factors involved in the predisposition to ACPA-negative RA is primarily because of the significantly lesser number of studies performed to date. The differences in HLA risk factors between ACPA-positive and ACPA-negative RA have already been discussed. Among non-HLA genes, variants in C-type lectinlike domain family 16, member A (*CLEC16A*) have been shown to confer susceptibility to ACPA-negative but not ACPA-positive RA.[77,78] Similarly, a variation in the promoter region of interferon regulatory factor 5 (*IRF5*), a transcription factor that controls macrophage-promoted inflammation or regulation, was associated with ACPA-negative RA only.[60] A neuropeptide S receptor gene polymorphism has likewise been implicated in ACPA-negative RA susceptibility and its clinical manifestations.[79] In a recent meta-analysis, the signal transducer and activator of transcription 4 gene (*STAT4*), which is involved in Th1 immune responses, was identified as a risk factor for both subgroups of RA.[44]

However, a GWAS that involved massive imputation to evaluate more than 1,700,000 SNPs[80] in 774 Swedish ACPA-negative patients with RA, 1147-ACPA-positive patients with RA, and 1079 controls, failed to achieve genome-wide significance when comparing ACPA-negative patients with RA to controls. This result does not imply the lack of genetic risk factors in ACPA-negative RA, but rather the lack of power in conventional GWAS studies of moderate size (as discussed earlier). A meta-analysis of 14 well-established variations for association with ACPA-positive RA in combined material from Sweden, the United States, and the United Kingdom was compared with ACPA-negative RA in the Swedish cohort. Most previously detected genetic variations (9/14) were associated only with ACPA-positive RA; 3 genes, *STAT4*, *IRF5*, and *CCL2* seemed to be associated with both subgroups; and 1 gene, *HTR2A* seemed to be specific for ACPA-negative disease.[80] CCL2 is a cytokine belonging to the CC chemokine family involved in recruiting monocytes, memory T cells, and dendritic cells to sites of tissue injury and inflammation. The *HTR2A* gene encodes one of the receptors for serotonin; its role in RA is unclear at present. The C-type lectin and the neuropeptide S receptor polymorphisms (mentioned above) were not evaluated in this study.

BACKGROUND IMPRESSIONS: ETHNIC VARIATION IN RA RISK FACTORS

Evidence pointing to the genetic heterogeneity in RA is based on the fact that whereas some risk alleles such as *TNFAIP3* and *STAT4* are common across multiple ethnic groups, other risk polymorphisms are restricted to specific ethnic populations. On the one hand, although the causal mutation R620W of the *PTPN22* gene has been repeatedly replicated in Caucasian populations, this polymorphism is rarely seen in Asian populations.[81] On the other hand, *PADI4* is an important risk factor in East Asian populations,[31,81] but its importance in the European population is marginal, at best.[61,62] Similarly, an SNP in the regulatory region of the *FCRL3* gene has been associated with susceptibility to RA in East Asian populations,[63,64] but showed minimal association in Caucasian patients with RA. The *FCRL3* gene encodes a member of the immunoglobulin receptor superfamily that may play a role in the regulation of the immune system. *CD244*, which encodes a membrane receptor expressed on natural killer cells that modulate non-HLA–restricted killing, was found to be a risk factor in 2 Japanese cohorts, but not in European populations of RA.[65]

Although the HLA-DRB1 is the major risk factor in both European and Asian populations, there are significant differences in the details of the HLA genotypes between these populations. HLA-DRB1*0401 and HLA-DRB1*0404 are the most frequent alleles identified in patients with RA in populations of European ancestry,[82] whereas HLA-DRB1*0405 represents the most prominent allele observed in East Asian populations.[81,83] Similarly, the HLA-DRB1*0901 allele is common in Asian populations,[83,84] but much less common in European patients with RA. It should be emphasized; however, that most studies have been performed in subjects of European ancestry, thus many of the risk factors identified are still awaiting validation in non-European populations.

SHARED MOTIFS ACROSS GENRES: COMMON AUTOIMMUNE RISK FACTORS

By comparing the identified risk alleles in different autoimmune diseases, one notices that there is overlap in the predisposing genes; namely, genes implicated in one disease also show association with other diseases (summarized in **Table 1**). For example, *PTPN22*, discussed above, is also associated with Graves disease, Hashimoto thyroiditis, myasthenia gravis, SLE, Type 1 diabetes mellitus (DM1), systemic sclerosis, and ulcerative colitis.[35–37,85] Similarly, *STAT4*, which has been established as a risk factor for RA, is also a risk factor in SLE, Graves disease, DM1, ulcerative colitis, and Crohn disease.[45–47,49] Another RA risk factor, *CD40* (encoding a co-stimulatory receptor expressed on APCs) has also been implicated in Graves disease and multiple sclerosis.[57,58]

Reviewing the genetic literature of autoimmune diseases by Zhernakova and colleagues[86] revealed that shared genetic risk factors between different autoimmune diseases may indicate common etiology and pathogenesis. This view is supported by familial clustering of RA with other autoimmune diseases and by several reports of several autoimmune conditions coexisting in the same individual.[87] These findings led to the notion that the genes predisposing to autoimmunity may be divided into 2 major groups: (1) autoimmune genes, which serve in the regulation and function of the immune system, thus providing the genetic background and common pathways predisposing to multiple autoimmune conditions; (2) disease-specific genes that determine the organ or tissues targeted by the autoimmune response, which may differ between the various diseases. However, one should be cautious in interpreting the ramifications of these genetic associations because sharing a predisposing gene does not necessarily imply that the risk factor functions identically in the 2 conditions in which it appears. Thus, although *STAT4* is a risk factor in both RA and SLE, deletion of the *STAT4* gene in lupus mice results in exacerbation of the autoimmune process,[88] whereas deficiency of the same gene in an arthritis model promotes a significantly reduced disease phenotype.[89] These findings allude to the real possibility that the causal *STAT4* polymorphisms in RA and SLE may differ from each other.

CLINICAL RELEVANCE AND CONCLUDING REMARKS

A recent study assessed whether cumulative genetic profiles can help identify individuals at high-risk for developing RA. Chibnik and colleagues[10] examined the impact of 39 validated genetic risk alleles (including 31 SNPs in non-HLA risk loci and 8 HLA alleles) on the risk of RA phenotypes characterized by serologic and erosive status, among 542 Caucasian patients with RA and 551 Caucasian controls. A weighted genetic risk score (GRS) was designed and evaluated as 7 ordinal groups using logistic regression (adjusting for age and smoking) to assess the relationship between GRS group and odds of developing seronegative (RF− and ACPA−), seropositive (RF+ or ACPA+), erosive, and seropositive-erosive RA phenotypes. Comparing the highest GRS risk group to the median group yielded an OR of 1.2 (95% confidence interval [CI] = 0.8–2.1) for seronegative RA, 3.0 (95% CI = 1.9–4.7) for seropositive RA, 3.2 (95% CI = 1.8–5.6) for erosive RA, and 7.6 (95% CI = 3.6–16.3) for seropositive-erosive RA. This finding likely represents the relative weight of HLA and PTPN22 in calculating the GRS, as these 2 genes have been shown to have the most attributable risk; the effect of most other risk alleles was modest, at best. In addition, the GRS showed no significant ability to discriminate between seronegative RA and controls.

Given the very modest effect size of the most established RA risk factors, it is likely that more than 50% of the genetic risk to RA remains unknown. Thus, considering that the sibling risk ratio (λs) is somewhere between 5 and 10, it is estimated that all established risk loci contribute only 33% to 47% of total heritability to RA.[90] In a most recent paper, Stahl and colleagues[91] have modeled the genetic profile underlying GWAS data for RA and developed a method to deduce the total liability variance explained by associated GWAS SNPs. The method was applied to published GWAS data on greater than 28,000 samples from RA case-control studies.[54,92] Using this method, it is estimated that an additional 20% of disease risk (excluding all known associated loci) can be explained by thousands of additional SNPs embedded in RA GWAS.

Aside from possibly HLA and PTPN22, genotyping of relevant risk polymorphisms in other validated genes is unlikely to become practical for predicting RA diagnosis, severity, or progression because, as has already become painfully evident, each gene individually confers narrow attributable risk. Thus most susceptibility alleles would seem to have limited current practical implication for the clinical rheumatologist. Based on the authors' knowledge to date; however, RA is a pathway disease: it is primarily driven by pathologic changes or dysregulation of some intracellular pathways, rather than a specific gene, or a small set of genes. Accordingly, RA can be triggered by genetic changes at many points in the pathway leading to a weak dependence on any specific gene in association studies. For example, the following risk genes C-REL, TNFAIP3, TRAF-1, STAT4, CD40, and TNFSF14 are all involved in the NFkB pathway. The CD2/CD58, PTPRC connection, discussed above, points also to the pathway character of RA regarding T-cell activation and costimulation. There is a long list of risk factors that are involved in T-cell stimulation, activation, and functional differentiation, including the HLA risk factors, PTPN22, AFF3, CD28, CD40, CTLA4, IL-2RA, IL-2, IL-21, PRKCP, TAGNAP, PRDM1, STAT4, and CD244. Although, at present, the identification of these individual genes might not be useful for predicting clinical outcomes or attributing risk toward RA diagnosis, it can provide valuable insight into the pathogenesis of disease and thus serve to elucidate potential therapeutic targets.

REFERENCES

1. Bowes J, Barton A. Recent advances in the genetics of RA susceptibility. Rheumatology 2008;47:399–402.
2. Imboden JB. The immunopathogenesis of rheumatoid arthritis. Annu Rev Pathol 2009;4:417–34.

3. Seldin MF, Amos CI, Ward R, et al. The genetics revolution and the assault on rheumatoid arthritis. Arthritis Rheum 1999;42:1071–9.
4. MacGregor AJ, Snieder H, Rigby AS, et al. Characterizing the quantitative genetic contribution to rheumatoid arthritis using data from twins. Arthritis Rheum 2000;43:30–7.
5. van der Woude D, Houwing-Duistermaat JJ, Toes RE, et al. Quantitative heritability of anti-citrullinated protein antibody-positive and anti-citrullinated protein antibody-negative rheumatoid arthritis. Arthritis Rheum 2009;60:916–23.
6. Stolt P, Bengtsson C, Nordmark B, et al. Quantification of the influence of cigarette smoking on rheumatoid arthritis: results from a population based case-control study, using incident cases. Ann Rheum Dis 2003;62:835–41.
7. Makrygiannakis D, af Klint E, Lundberg IE, et al. Citrullination is an inflammation dependent process. Ann Rheum Dis 2006;65:1219–22.
8. van Gaalen FA, Linn-Rasker SP, van Venrooij WJ, et al. Autoantibodies to cyclic citrullinated peptides predict progression to rheumatoid arthritis in patients with undifferentiated arthritis: a prospective cohort study. Arthritis Rheum 2004;50:709–15.
9. van der Helm-van Mil AH, Verpoort KN, Breedveld FC, et al. Antibodies to citrullinated proteins and differences in clinical progression of rheumatoid arthritis. Arthritis Res Ther 2005;7:R949–58.
10. Chibnik LB, Keenan BT, Cui J, et al. Genetic risk score predicting risk of rheumatoid arthritis phenotypes and age of symptom onset. PLoS One 2011;6(9):e24380.
11. Gregersen PK, Silver J, Winchester RJ. The shared epitope hypothesis. An approach to understanding the molecular genetics of susceptibility to rheumatoid arthritis. Arthritis Rheum 1987;30:1205–13.
12. Huizinga TW, Amos CI, van der Helm-van Mil AH, et al. Refining the complex rheumatoid arthritis phenotype based on specificity of the HLA-DRB1 shared epitope for antibodies to citrullinated proteins. Arthritis Rheum 2005;52:3433–8.
13. Brown JH, Jardetzky TS, Gorga JC, et al. Three-dimensional structure of the human class II histocompatibility antigen HLA-DR1. Nature 1993;364:33–9.
14. van der Helm-van Mil AH, Huizinga TW, de Vries RR, et al. Emerging patterns of risk factor make-up enable subclassification of rheumatoid arthritis. Arthritis Rheum 2007;56:1728–35.
15. Feitsma AL, van der Voort EI, Franken KL, et al. Identification of citrullinated vimentin peptides as T cell epitopes in HLA-DR4-positive patients with rheumatoid arthritis. Arthritis Rheum 2010;62:117–25.
16. Firestein GS. Evolving concepts of rheumatoid arthritis. Nature 2003;423:356–61.
17. Kohm AP, Fuller KG, Miller SD. Mimicking the way to autoimmunity: an evolving theory of sequence and structural homology. Trends Microbiol 2003;11:101–5.
18. Lee HS, Lee AT, Criswell LA, et al. Several regions in the major histocompatibility complex confer risk for anti-CCP-antibody positive rheumatoid arthritis, independent of the DRB1 locus. Mol Med 2008;14:293–300.
19. Vignal C, Bansal AT, Balding DJ, et al. Genetic association of the major histocompatibility complex with rheumatoid arthritis implicates two non-DRB1 loci. Arthritis Rheum 2009;60:53–62.
20. Raychaudhuri S, Sandor C, Stahl EA, et al. Five amino acids in three HLA proteins explain most of the association between MHC and seropositive rheumatoid arthritis. Nat Genet 2012;44:291–6.

21. Irigoyen P, Lee AT, Wener MH, et al. Regulation of anti-cyclic citrullinated peptide antibodies in rheumatoid arthritis: contrasting effects of HLA-DR3 and the shared epitope alleles. Arthritis Rheum 2005;52:3813–8.

22. Verpoort KN, van Gaalen FA, van der Helm-van Mil AH, et al. Association of HLA-DR3 with anti-cyclic citrullinated peptide antibodynegative rheumatoid arthritis. Arthritis Rheum 2005;52:3058–62.

23. Furuya T, Hakoda M, Ichikawa N, et al. Differential association of HLA-DRB1 alleles in Japanese patients with early rheumatoid arthritis in relationship to auto-antibodies to cyclic citrullinated peptide. Clin Exp Rheumatol 2007;25:219–24.

24. Lundström E, Källberg H, Smolnikova M, et al. Opposing effects of HLA-DRB1*13 alleles on the risk of developing anti-citrullinated protein antibody-positive and anti-citrullinated protein antibody-negative rheumatoid arthritis. Arthritis Rheum 2009;60:924–30.

25. van der Woude D, Lie BA, Lundström E, et al. Protection against anti-citrullinated protein antibody-positive rheumatoid arthritis is predominantly associated with HLA-DRB1*1301: a meta-analysis of HLA-DRB1 associations with anti-citrullinated protein antibody-positive and anti-citrullinated protein antibody-negative rheumatoid arthritis in four European populations. Arthritis Rheum 2010;62(5):1236–45.

26. Begovich AB, Carlton VE, Honigberg LA, et al. A missense single nucleotide polymorphism in a gene encoding a protein tyrosine phosphatase (PTPN22) is associated with rheumatoid arthritis. Am J Hum Genet 2004;75:330–7.

27. Michou L, Lasbleiz S, Rat AC, et al. Linkage proof for PTPN22, a rheumatoid arthritis susceptibility gene and a human autoimmunity gene. Proc Natl Acad Sci U S A 2007;104:1649–54.

28. Vang T, Congia M, Macis MD, et al. Autoimmune-associated lymphoid tyrosine phosphatase is a gain-of-function variant. Nat Genet 2005;37:1317–9.

29. Bottini N, Vang T, Cucca F, et al. Role of PTPN22 in type 1 diabetes and other autoimmune diseases. Semin Immunol 2006;18:207–13.

30. Suzuki A, Yamada X, Chang S, et al. Functional haplotypes of PADI4, encoding citrullinating enzyme peptidylarginine deiminase 4, are associated with rheumatoid arthritis. Nat Genet 2003;34:395–402.

31. Ikari K, Kuwahara M, Nakamura T, et al. Association between PADI4 and rheumatoid arthritis: a replication study. Arthritis Rheum 2005;52:3054–7.

32. Kuhn KA, Kulik L, Tomooka B, et al. Antibodies against citrullinated proteins enhance tissue injury in experimental autoimmune arthritis. J Clin Invest 2006;116:961–73.

33. Uysal H, Bockermann R, Nandakumar KS, et al. Structure and pathogenicity of antibodies specific for citrullinated collagen type II in experimental arthritis. J Exp Med 2009;206:449–62.

34. van Gaalen FA, van Aken J, Huizinga TW, et al. Association between HLA class II genes and autoantibodies to cyclic citrullinated peptides (CCPs) influences the severity of rheumatoid arthritis. Arthritis Rheum 2004;50:2113–21.

35. Criswell LA, Pfeiffer KA, Lum RF, et al. Analysis of families in the multiple autoimmune disease genetics consortium (MADGC) collection: the PTPN22 620W allele associates with multiple autoimmune phenotypes. Am J Hum Genet 2005;76:561–71.

36. Orozco G, Sanchez E, Gonzalez-Gay MA, et al. Association of a functional single-nucleotide polymorphism of PTPN22, encoding lymphoid protein phosphatase, with rheumatoid arthritis and systemic lupus erythematosus. Arthritis Rheum 2005;52:219–24.

37. Dieude P, Guedj M, Wipff J, et al. The PTPN22 620W allele confers susceptibility to systemic sclerosis: findings of a large case-control study of European Caucasians and a meta-analysis. Arthritis Rheum 2008;58:2183–8.

38. Wellcome Trust Case Control Consortium. Genome-wide association study of 14,000 cases of seven common diseases and 3,000 shared controls. Nature 2007;447:661–78.

39. Raychaudhuri S, Remmers EF, Lee AT, et al. Common variants at CD40 and other loci confer risk of rheumatoid arthritis. Nat Genet 2008;40:1216–23.

40. Raychaudhuri S, Thomson BP, Remmers EF, et al. Genetic variants at CD28, PRDM1 and D2/CD58 are associated with rheumatoid arthritis risk. Nat Genet 2009;41:1313–8.

41. Harley JB, Alarcon-Riquelme ME, Criswell LA, et al. Genome-wide association scan in women with systemic lupus erythematosus identifies susceptibility variants in ITGAM, PXK, KIAA1542 and other loci. Nat Genet 2008; 40:204–10.

42. Gregersen PK, Amos CI, Lee AT, et al. REL, encoding a member of the NF-kappaB family of transcription factors, is a newly defined risk locus for rheumatoid arthritis. Nat Genet 2009;41:820–3.

43. Barton A, Eyre S, Ke X, et al. Identification of AF4/FMR2 family, member 3 (AFF3) as a novel rheumatoid arthritis susceptibility locus and confirmation of two further pan-autoimmune susceptibility genes. Hum Mol Genet 2009;18:2518–22.

44. Lee YH, Woo JH, Choi SJ, et al. Association between the rs7574865 polymorphism of STAT4 and rheumatoid arthritis: a meta-analysis. Rheumatol Int 2010; 30:661–6.

45. Martinez A, Varade J, Marquez A, et al. Association of the STAT4 gene with increased susceptibility for some immune-mediated diseases. Arthritis Rheum 2008;58:2598–602.

46. Glas J, Seiderer J, Nagy M, et al. Evidence for STAT4 as a common autoimmune gene: rs7574865 is associated with colonic Crohn's disease and early disease onset. PLoS One 2010;5:e10373.

47. Prahalad S, Hansen S, Whiting A, et al. Variants in TNFAIP3, STAT4, and C12 or f30 loci associated with multiple autoimmune diseases are also associated with juvenile idiopathic arthritis. Arthritis Rheum 2009;60:2124–30.

48. Remmers EF, Plenge RM, Lee AT, et al. STAT4 and the risk of rheumatoid arthritis and systemic lupus erythematosus. N Engl J Med 2007;357:977–86.

49. Namjou B, Sestak AL, Armstrong DL, et al. High density genotyping of STAT4 gene reveals multiple haplotypic associations with systemic lupus erythematosus in different racial groups. Arthritis Rheum 2009;60:1085–95.

50. Plenge RM, Padyukov L, Remmers EF, et al. Replication of putative candidate-gene associations with rheumatoid arthritis in >4,000 samples from North America and Sweden: association of susceptibility with PTPN22, CTLA4, and PADI4. Am J Hum Genet 2005;77:1044–60.

51. Zhernakova A, Alizadeh BZ, Bevova M, et al. Novel association in chromosome 4q27 region with rheumatoid arthritis and confirmation of type 1 diabetes point to a general risk locus for autoimmune diseases. Am J Hum Genet 2007;81: 1284–8.

52. Plenge RM, Cotsapas C, Davies L, et al. Two independent alleles at 6q23 associated with risk of rheumatoid arthritis. Nat Genet 2007;39:1477–82.

53. Orozco G, Hinks A, Eyre S, et al. Combined effects of three independent SNPs greatly increase the risk estimate for RA at 6q23. Hum Mol Genet 2009;18: 2693–9.

54. Stahl EA, Raychaudhuri S, Remmers EF, et al. Genome-wide association study meta-analysis identifies seven new rheumatoid arthritis risk loci. Nat Genet 2010;42:508–14.
55. Plenge RM, Seielstad M, Padyukov L, et al. TRAF1-C5 as a risk locus for rheumatoid arthritis–a genomewide study. N Engl J Med 2007;357:1199–209.
56. Barton A, Thomson W, Ke X, et al. Rheumatoid arthritis susceptibility loci at chromosomes 10p15, 12q13 and 22q13. Nat Genet 2008;40:1156–9.
57. Tomer Y, Concepcion E, Greenberg DA. A C/T single-nucleotide polymorphism in the region of the CD40 gene is associated with Graves' disease. Thyroid 2002;12:1129–35.
58. Blanco-Kelly F, Matesanz F, Alcina A, et al. CD40: novel association with Crohn's disease and replication in multiple sclerosis susceptibility. PLoS One 2010;5:e11520.
59. Kochi Y, Okada Y, Suzuki A, et al. A regulatory variant in CCR6 is associated with rheumatoid arthritis susceptibility. Nat Genet 2010;42:515–9.
60. Sigurdsson S, Padyukov L, Kurreeman FA, et al. Association of a haplotype in the promoter region of the interferon regulatory factor 5 gene with rheumatoid arthritis. Arthritis Rheum 2007;56:2202–10.
61. Harney SM, Meisel C, Sims AM, et al. Genetic and genomic studies of PADI4 in rheumatoid arthritis. Rheumatology 2005;44:869–72.
62. Burr ML, Naseem H, Hinks A, et al. PADI4 genotype is not associated with rheumatoid arthritis in a large UK Caucasian population. Ann Rheum Dis 2010;69:666–70.
63. Kochi Y, Yamada R, Suzuki A, et al. A functional variant in FCRL3, encoding Fc receptor-like 3, is associated with rheumatoid arthritis and several autoimmunities. Nat Genet 2005;37:478–85.
64. Ikari K, Momohara S, Nakamura T, et al. Supportive evidence for a genetic association of the FCRL3 promoter polymorphism with rheumatoid arthritis. Ann Rheum Dis 2006;65:671–3.
65. Suzuki A, Yamada R, Kochi Y, et al. Functional SNPs in CD244 increase the risk of rheumatoid arthritis in a Japanese population. Nat Genet 2008;40:1224–9.
66. Julià A, Ballina J, Cañete JD, et al. Genome-wide association study of rheumatoid arthritis in the Spanish population: KLF12 as a risk locus for rheumatoid arthritis susceptibility. Arthritis Rheum 2008;58:2275–86.
67. Wang WY, Barratt BJ, Clayton DG, et al. Genome-wide association studies: theoretical and practical concerns. Nat Rev Genet 2005;6:109–18.
68. Jorgenson E, Witte JS. Coverage and power in genomewide association studies. Am J Hum Genet 2006;78:884–8.
69. Armstrong DL, Jacob CO, Zidovetzki R. Function2Gene: a gene selection tool to increase the power of genetic association studies by utilizing public databases and expert knowledge. BMC Bioinformatics 2008;9:311–7.
70. Armstrong DL, Reiff A, Myones BL, et al. Identification of new SLE-associated genes with a two-step Bayesian study design. Genes Immun 2009;10:446–56.
71. Raychaudhuri S, Plenge RM, Rossin EJ, et al. Identifying relationships among genomic disease regions: predicting genes at pathogenic SNP associations and rare deletions. PLoS Genet 2009;5:e1000534.
72. de Vries R. Genetics of rheumatoid arthritis: time for a change. Curr Opin Rhematol 2011;23:227–32.
73. Vereecke L, Beyaert R, van Loo G. Genetic relationships between A20/TNFAIP3, chronic inflammation and autoimmune disease. Biochem Soc Trans 2011;39:1086–91.

74. Tavares RM, Turer EE, Liu CL, et al. The ubiquitin modifying enzyme A20 restricts B cell survival and prevents autoimmunity. Immunity 2010;33:181–91.
75. Chu Y, Vahl JC, Kumar D, et al. B cells lacking the tumor suppressor TNFAIP3/A20 display impaired differentiation, hyperactivation, cause inflammation and autoimmunity in aged mice. Blood 2011;117:2227–36.
76. Hovelmeyer N, Reissig S, Thi Xuan N, et al. A20 deficiency in B cells enhances B-cell proliferation and results in the development of autoantibodies. Eur J Immunol 2011;41:595–601.
77. Lorentzen JC, Flornes L, Eklöw C, et al. Association of arthritis with a gene complex encoding C-type lectin-like receptors. Arthritis Rheum 2007;56: 2620–32.
78. Skinningsrud B, Lie BA, Husebye ES, et al. A CLEC16A variant confers risk for juvenile idiopathic arthritis and anti-cyclic citrullinated peptide antibody negative rheumatoid arthritis. Ann Rheum Dis 2010;69:1471–4.
79. D'Amato M, Zucchelli M, Seddighzadeh M, et al. Analysis of neuropeptide S receptor gene (NPSR1) polymorphism in rheumatoid arthritis. PLoS One 2010; 5:e9315.
80. Padyukov L, Seielstad M, Ong RT, et al. A genome-wide association study suggests contrasting associations in ACPA-positive versus ACPA-negative rheumatoid arthritis. Ann Rheum Dis 2011;70:259–65.
81. Kochi Y, Suzuki A, Yamada R, et al. Ethnogenetic heterogeneity of rheumatoid arthritis-implications for pathogenesis. Nat Rev Rheumatol 2010;6:290–5.
82. Jawaheer D, Li W, Graham RR, et al. Dissecting the genetic complexity of the association between human leukocyte antigens and rheumatoid arthritis. Am J Hum Genet 2002;71:585–94.
83. Lee HS, Lee KW, Song GG, et al. Increased susceptibility to rheumatoid arthritis in Koreans heterozygous for HLA-DRB1*0405 and *0901. Arthritis Rheum 2004; 50:3468–75.
84. Kochi Y, Yamada R, Kobayashi K, et al. Analysis of single-nucleotide polymorphisms in Japanese rheumatoid arthritis patients shows additional susceptibility markers besides the classic shared epitope susceptibility sequences. Arthritis Rheum 2004;50:63–71.
85. Vang T, Miletic AV, Bottini N, et al. Protein tyrosine phosphatase PTPN22 in human autoimmunity. Autoimmunity 2007;40:453–61.
86. Zhernakova A, van Diemen CC, Wijmenga C. Detecting shared pathogenesis from the shared genetics of immune-related diseases. Nat Rev Genet 2009;10: 43–55.
87. Lin JP, Cash JM, Doyle SZ, et al. Familial clustering of rheumatoid arthritis with other autoimmune diseases. Hum Genet 1998;103:475–82.
88. Jacob CO, Zang S, Li L, et al. Pivotal role of Stat4 and Stat6 in the pathogenesis of the lupus-like disease in the New Zealand mixed 2328 mice. J Immunol 2003; 171:1564–71.
89. Finnegan A, Grusby MJ, Kaplan CD, et al. IL-4 and IL-12 regulate proteoglycan-induced arthritis through Stat-dependent mechanisms. J Immunol 2002;169: 3345–52.
90. McAllister K, Eyre S, Orozco G. Genetics of rheumatoid arthritis: GWAS and beyond. Open Access Rheumatol Res Rev 2011;3:31–46.
91. Stahl EA, Wegmann D, Trynka G, et al. Bayesian inference analyses of the polygenic architecture of rheumatoid arthritis. Nat Genet 2012;44(5):483–9.
92. Chen R, Stahl EA, Kurreeman FA, et al. Fine mapping the TAGAP locus in rheumatoid arthritis. Genes Immun 2011;12:314–8.

Ultrasonography Applications in Diagnosis and Management of Early Rheumatoid Arthritis

Ralf G. Thiele, MD

KEYWORDS

- Early-onset rheumatoid arthritis • Synovitis • Power Doppler
- Ultrasonography • Ultrasound

Key Points

- High-frequency ultrasonography allows detailed assessment of superficial structures including tendons, tendon sheaths, joint capsule, cartilage, and cortical surface of bone.

- Gray-scale ultrasonography can visualize proliferative synovial tissue, fluid collections in tendon sheaths or joints, and bony erosions.

- Doppler ultrasonography can visualize synovial hyperemia, the strongest predictor of future joint damage in rheumatoid arthritis.

- Change in synovial thickening and hyperemia in response to treatment can be documented with serial ultrasonography.

As arthritis is so common, new imaging modalities have often been used for its assessment shortly after they have become available. Only a few months after Konrad Roentgen began lecturing on his "X-rays," the first articles on imaging features of arthritis were published in 1896.[1] The first articles on the use of ultrasonography in rheumatoid arthritis (RA) came from the University of California at Los Angeles, and were published in 1975.[2] It was not until the 1980s and 1990s that the potential of ultrasonography to assess typical changes of RA became apparent. At that time, ultrasound equipment with higher frequencies became more readily available. Higher ultrasound

---

Allergy/Immunology and Rheumatology Division, Department of Medicine, University of Rochester School of Medicine and Dentistry, 601 Elmwood Avenue, Box 695, Rochester, NY 14642, USA
E-mail address: Ralf_Thiele@URMC.Rochester.edu

Rheum Dis Clin N Am 38 (2012) 259–275
doi:10.1016/j.rdc.2012.05.006
0889-857X/12/$ – see front matter © 2012 Elsevier Inc. All rights reserved.

frequencies allow better resolution of structures at shallow locations. These probes were initially developed for the assessment of thyroid glands, but were soon used by providers in musculoskeletal medicine. Since then, annual numbers of publications on musculoskeletal ultrasonography have increased almost exponentially (**Fig. 1**).

Ultrasonography can now be a point-of-care modality: The provider performs the examination in the office, with no referral needed. Findings can be addressed immediately, and necessary adjustments of treatment can be made at the same visit. If a fluid collection is detected and an aspiration is indicated, ultrasound guidance can help improve the accuracy of the aspiration and injection.[3]

RATIONALE FOR USING ULTRASONOGRAPHY IN THE ASSESSMENT OF EARLY RHEUMATOID ARTHRITIS

Without imaging of soft tissues, providers in rheumatology have to rely on surrogate markers of joint inflammation. It is assumed that tenderness and swelling over joints are due to synovitis. If serologic markers of inflammation are abnormal, this is taken as an additional indicator of joint inflammation. However, fullness and pain on examination may have causes other than synovitis, and elevated sedimentation rates or levels of C-reactive protein may not always be due to RA. Even fibromyalgia patients may complain about morning stiffness and swollen hands.

Assessment of Early Rheumatoid Arthritis: Ultrasonography Versus Clinical Scores

Clinical scores remain the mainstay of assessment of disease activity. These scores, alone or in combination with measurement of acute-phase reactants, give no actual information about presence or absence of features of RA such as synovitis,

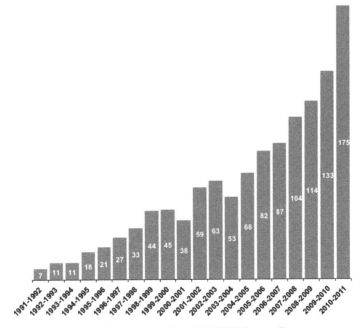

OVID search terms "musculoskeletal" AND "ultrasound"

Fig. 1. Publications on musculoskeletal ultrasonography, 1991 to 2011. OVID search terms "musculoskeletal" and "ultrasound."

tenosynovitis, or erosive disease, but serve as surrogate markers to help guide treatment recommendations. With ultrasonography or magnetic resonance imaging (MRI), synovial inflammation can often be detected in patients assumed to be in remission based on clinical scores alone.[4,5] There thus appears to be a disconnect between Disease Activity Score (DAS) remission and imaging remission.[6]

Interobserver and intraobserver reliability of ultrasonography and clinical scores have been compared in several studies. Ultrasonography was found to be at least as good, or better, for repeatability (intraobserver) and reproducibility (interobserver) of findings than was assessment of disease activity with surrogate clinical scores.[7,8] When ultrasonography assessment is added to clinical scores, such a composite index (US-DAS) may be a better predictor of future joint damage than a standard DAS28 alone.[9]

Assessment of Early Rheumatoid Arthritis: Ultrasonography Versus Conventional Radiography

In a world where conventional radiography is the only readily available imaging modality, the features of RA that can be assessed with this modality assume great importance. Erosions, joint-space narrowing, and periarticular osteopenia are the classic features. However, even though conventional radiography is the historical gold standard of erosion assessment, it is insensitive when compared with ultrasonography.[10]

When ultrasonography was compared with conventional radiography in a study of patients with RA, sonography detected 6.5-fold more erosions in early disease, in 7.5-fold the number of patients (**Fig. 2**). Two independent operators performed scans of metacarpophalangeal (MCP) joints sequentially for this study, and reached good interobserver reliability (Cohen κ = 0.75).[11]

Is there such a thing as "operator dependence" when obtaining conventional radiographs? As radiography projects 3-dimensional structures on 2-dimensional planes, breaks in the bony cortex need to be seen in profile to be characterized as erosions (lesions that are not seen in profile may be either cysts or erosions). To help detect erosions of the cortex in RA, extremities are assessed in different views, for example,

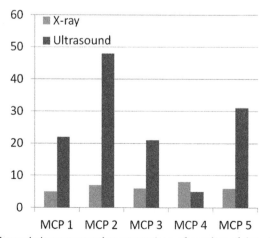

Fig. 2. Radiography and ultrasonography: comparison of number of detected bony erosions in early rheumatoid arthritis by joint. (*Data from* Wakefield RJ, Gibbon WW, Conaghan PG, et al. The value of sonography in the detection of bone erosions in patients with rheumatoid arthritis: a comparison with conventional radiography. Arthritis Rheum 2000;43(12):2762–70.)

anterior-posterior, lateral and oblique, or "ball-catcher's" views of the hands. Detection of cortical breaks will vary with positioning of the extremity. The radiology technician, and the patient, will make an effort to standardize the position of the extremity as much as possible. Nevertheless, a few degrees in difference of rotation can render an erosion impossible to detect. Furthermore, for an assessment at a different time point, for example, to evaluate progression of erosions, the exact same position would need to be assumed, which is problematic in a free-hand approach (**Fig. 3**). Once radiographs are obtained, will different readers come to the same conclusions? John T. Sharp found that "the variability in scoring radiographic abnormalities is considerable among this group of 11 expert readers" in a study with standard data sets of patients with RA.[12]

Synovitis or tenosynovitis, both very early findings in RA, cannot be assessed radiographically.

Assessment of Early Rheumatoid Arthritis: Ultrasonography Versus MRI

For the image assessment of RA, ultrasonography is often compared with MR imaging. Both are cross-sectional modalities that evaluate similar features of RA. It is therefore of considerable interest to identify the modality that is more sensitive, specific, reproducible, and repeatable. Both modalities can assess bony erosions, synovial tissue proliferation, synovial fluid collections, tenosynovitis, enthesitis, and synovial hyperemia. MRI can identify bone marrow edema, which ultrasonography cannot. Ultrasonography can be a dynamic, real-time examination, which MRI is not (dynamic cardiac MRI would be the exception). Displaceability of synovial fluid and compressibility of synovial tissue can only be assessed sonographically. Synovial hyperemia can be seen in real time with ultrasonography. The greatest extent of hyperemia during systole can safely be appreciated and used for scoring of disease. It has not been studied well if MRI assessment of hyperemia is subject to variation during systole and diastole, and if an MR image taken during diastole could lead to inaccurate assessment of synovial hyperemia. It is frequently mentioned that operator dependence could be a discriminating factor between MRI and ultrasonography. The operator dependence of MRI assessment of rheumatic disease has not been systematically studied. For such a study, 2 or more operators (radiology technicians or physician providers) would need to separately perform MRI studies of the same patients to assess predefined features of RA, using 2 or more different MRI coils.

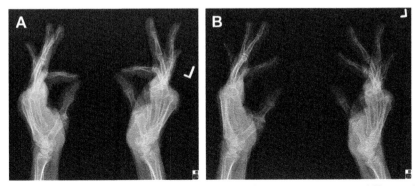

Fig. 3. (*A, B*) Lateral radiographs of hands and wrists of the same patient at 2 different time points. The slight variation as 2 different poses are assumed makes comparison of specific details more difficult.

The resulting images would need to be read by 2 or more radiologists. If the agreement were 100% at all times, MRI could be called operator independent—an unlikely scenario at best. Unsurprisingly, the diagnostic accuracy of MRI interpretations varies between readers and depends on the experience of the provider.[13] In a study of 21,482 consecutive computed tomography (CT), MRI, and ultrasonography studies, MRI and CT interpretations had significantly higher rates of discrepancy among readers than ultrasonography.[14]

MRI and ultrasonography: erosions
A recent systematic literature review found no statistical difference in the efficacy of MRI and ultrasonography in detecting erosions in RA.[10] In early RA, ultrasonography tended to detect more erosions than MRI, whereas MRI tended to detect more erosions in late disease. Good reproducibility of ultrasonography findings for erosion detection was found. Ultrasonography assessment of erosions may therefore be regarded more cost effective than MRI for this indication.

MRI and ultrasonography: synovitis and tenosynovitis
For a reliable assessment of RA, an imaging modality must depict the anatomic reality as faithfully as possible. Ultrasonography findings of synovial hyperplasia and hyperemia correlate well with histopathological findings after surgery.[15,16] In a recent study, findings of power Doppler ultrasonography were closely associated with all "pathologic compartments" of synovitis, including inflammatory cell infiltrates, synovial lining layer thickness, and vascularity. Ultrasonography findings more faithfully illustrated active synovitis than those of MRI.[17]

Small fluid collections and tenosynovitis in patients with RA are more readily detected by ultrasonography when compared with MRI.[18,19]

ULTRASONOGRAPHIC FEATURES OF RHEUMATOID ARTHRITIS
Tenosynovitis

There is some evidence that tenosynovitis is a very early feature of RA.[20–22] It may precede synovial proliferation within the joints. Tenosynovitis can, by definition, only occur at sites where tendon sheaths encase the tendons. Tendon sheaths around the wrists particularly are affected early on but also later in the disease process. Tendon sheaths of the extensor carpi ulnaris tendon (extensor compartment 6) and extensor digitorum together with extensor indicis tendon (extensor compartment 4) are typical tendon sheaths affected by tenosynovitis in RA.

Sonoanatomy of tendon and sheath
Tendons with their sheaths share anatomic characteristics with joints. The tendon fibers are encased by a layer of synovial tissue, the inner lining or visceral layer. The fibrous tendon sheath connects to the adjacent periosteum and is lined by the outer or parietal synovial layer. The 2 synovial layers connect through a duplication along the mesotendineum, or mesotenon, a vascularized suspensory ligament that connects the tendon with its environment. In RA, synovial tissue can proliferate from both layers, as well as from the lining of the mesotendineum, the "third layer" (**Fig. 4**).

Tenosynovial effusions
Fluid collections, or tenosynovial effusions, will distend the layers. Synovial fluid is usually anechoic. It will provide contrast to better appreciate the anatomic structures. In RA, effusions of the tendon sheath are often associated with synovial proliferation. By contrast, effusions caused by mechanically induced tenosynovitis will have only little coexisting synovial thickening.

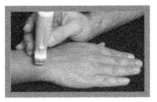

Tenosynovitis
short axis

Mesotendineum:
Tendon tethered through
duplication of sheath

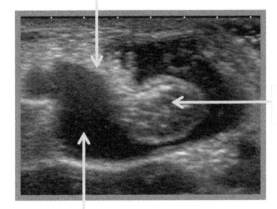

Tendon
on-end

Increased fluid
collection
surrounding tendon

Fig. 4. Wrist tendon, short-axis view. A hyperechoic tendon is seen surrounded by anechoic fluid and hyperechoic fibrous tendon sheath. Proliferative synovial tissue is seen adjacent to mesotenon and tendon.

Synovial proliferation

The delicate synovial lining of tendon and sheath can usually not be seen sonographically in healthy individuals. Detection of synovial tissue is an abnormal finding. Synovial tissue will appear as hypoechoic, gray-appearing tissue interposed between the fibrous and bright, or hyperechoic-appearing tendon sheath and the bright, hyperechoic tendon fibers. If synovial fluid is present, it will usually appear as dark or anechoic, and will accentuate the anatomy of tendon, sheath, and synovial tissue. With transducer pressure, fluid will be displaceable: it will flow away from the pressure of the transducer. By contrast, synovial tissue is not displaceable and will stay in place. A minimal compressibility of synovial tissue may be seen, due to its often villous structure with sponge-like qualities.

Synovial hyperemia

No significant blood flow is usually detectable sonographically in tendon and sheath of healthy adults. If synovial proliferation is detected or suspected on gray-scale ultrasonography, this tissue must be examined for hyperemia using Doppler ultrasonography.

Paratenonitis

Another concept is the idea of paratenonitis. Inflamed tissue adjacent to tendons without sheath can occasionally be seen by ultrasonography in inflammatory arthritis, including RA. This feature has found its way into the US7 ultrasonography scoring system for RA.[23] It is unclear what precise tissues become edematous and hyperemic adjacent to sheathless tendons, and paratenonitis has not been described elsewhere as a typical feature of RA. It is possible that synovial pannus breaks through the joint capsule and allows for synovitis to distribute along the tendon (**Fig. 5**).

Synovitis

Based on clinical examination alone, it may be difficult to tell if palpable fullness or warmth over a joint, or tenderness on palpation, is due to subcutaneous edema, tenosynovitis, paratenonitis, a joint effusion, or synovial proliferation within the joint. Ultrasonography can help with a more precise assessment.

Joint effusion

Ultrasonography appears to be more sensitive than clinical examination or MRI for the detection of small, supraphysiologic fluid collections in early RA. Synovial fluid has an anechoic, or "black" sonographic appearance. It will distend the more hyperechoic fibrous joint capsule. Early on, synovial fluid will collect in the proximal recesses of the joint capsules of small joints of hands and feet (**Fig. 6**). Later in the disease process, excess synovial fluid can displace the fibroadipose pad that reinforces the dorsal joint capsule in these joints, and eventually lead to a convex elevation of the joint capsule over proximal and distal bony endings. The fibrous volar and plantar plates that prevent overextension of finger and toe joints may be displaced by synovial fluid. In contrast to tissue, synovial fluid moves freely within the joint. Ultrasonography is a dynamic, real-time imaging modality. Transducer pressure on the joints can displace fluid away from the transducer. By contrast, synovial tissue will be just slightly compressible (sponge-like) as in tendon sheaths, but will not be displaced by transducer pressure.

Synovial hypertrophy

Proliferation of synovial-lining tissue will be one of the earliest features of RA that can be detected sonographically. As physiologic synovial lining tissue is only 1 to 3 cell layers strong, any sonographically detectable synovial thickening raises the suspicion of inflammatory arthritis. Sonographically, synovial tissue will appear hypoechoic or gray, in contrast to adjacent hyperechoic, fibrous capsule tissue; anechoic, or black-appearing synovial fluid; anechoic hyaline cartilage; and hyperechoic bony contour.

Synovial hyperemia

Once synovial tissue is detected using gray-scale, or B-mode, ultrasonography, color Doppler or power Doppler can help assess the degree of hyperemia of this tissue (**Fig. 7**).[24]

Doppler signals will represent blood flow rather than artifact if they are seen over an area that was identified as abnormal in the preceding gray-scale assessment, have a pulsatile quality synchronous to the pulse, and are seen persistently in the same area during a real-time examination.

Bony Erosions

Bony erosions can be detected sonographically relatively early in the disease process (**Fig. 8**). Ultrasonography of erosions performs better in joints that are readily

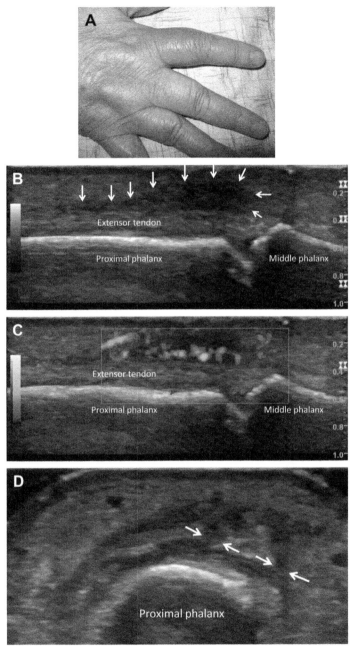

Fig. 5. (*A*) Erythema and swelling of second proximal interphalangeal (PIP) joint of the right hand. (*B*) Dorsal long-axis view of second PIP joint of the right hand. A hypoechoic to anechoic area is seen overlying the extensor tendon (*arrows*). (*C*) Hyperemia is seen over the area of interest. (*D*) Dorsal short-axis view of second PIP joint of the right hand. Breaks in the dorsal joint capsule (*between arrows*) allow synovial pannus tissue to escape the confines of the joint and distribute along the extensor tendon.

Inflammatory arthritis:
Proliferation of synovial lining cells

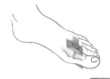
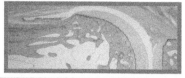

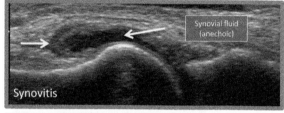

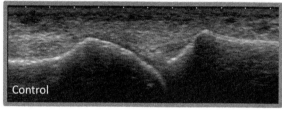

Fig. 6. Inflammatory arthritis. (*Middle*) Dorsal long-axis view of first metatarsophalangeal joint. Distension of hyperechoic joint capsule is seen. Hypoechoic synovial tissue and anechoic synovial fluid are shown (*arrows*). (*Bottom*) Healthy control. (Histologic image *courtesy of* American College of Rheumatology © 2012 American College of Rheumatology. Used with permission.)

accessible to sonographic evaluation, including small joints of hands and feet. It is less strong in deeper-seated bony structures and in bones that will not allow circumferential assessment, such as the carpal bones in wrists or the tarsal bones in feet. Bony erosions are defined as breaks in the bony cortex, seen in 2 perpendicular planes.[25] It is helpful to gain experience with the sonographic appearance of the anatomic neck of the distal metacarpal and metatarsal bones, as it is located near typical sites of erosion in RA.

As the precursors of erosions including synovial pannus formation and synovial hyperemia can be seen sonographically, and these are sensitive to therapeutic intervention, the detection of erosions loses some of its prior importance.

DESCRIBING AND QUANTIFYING ULTRASONOGRAPHIC FINDINGS OF RHEUMATOID ARTHRITIS

Erosions, synovial effusions, and proliferation of synovial tissue seen on gray-scale ultrasonography can be described as present or absent. Similarly, synovial hyperemia seen on Doppler ultrasonography can be described as present or absent. As the mere presence of synovitis and hyperemia indicates the absence of remission, such a dichotomous description can be useful in clinical practice. To create a score that helps describe worsening or improvement of disease in clinical trials, semiquantitative scoring systems are used. The most commonly used systems describe findings on

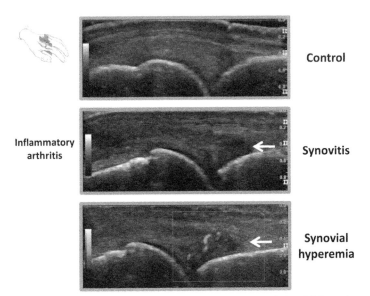

Fig. 7. Dorsal long-axis views of MCP joint. (*Top*) Healthy control. (*Middle*) Displacement of fibrous capsular triangle is seen. The distal recess of the joint is distended by synovitis (*arrow*). (*Bottom*) Hyperemia seen over the area of interest.

a scale from 0 to 3, with 0 representing absence of findings (**Table 1**). Efforts have been undertaken to identify condensed scoring systems that examine a small number of joint areas thought to be representative of the disease on the patient level. The US7 system assesses 7 joints for erosions, synovitis, and tendon involvement.

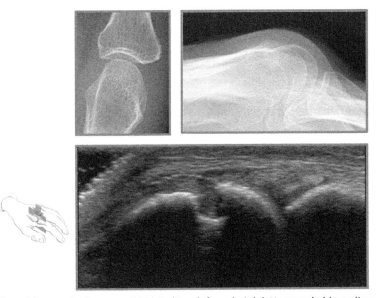

Fig. 8. Dorsal long-axis view over MCP 2. (*Top left* and *right*) Unremarkable radiographs. (*Bottom*) Ultrasonogram of the same patient, taken on the same day as the radiographs. A large bony erosion with invasion of synovial pannus tissue is seen over the metacarpal head.

Table 1
Grades of ultrasonography findings

Grade		Comment
0	No gray-scale change	
1	Mild synovitis	Small anechoic or hyperechoic line beneath hyperechoic fibrous joint capsule
2	Moderate synovitis	Joint capsule is distended. Remains parallel to bony contour up to straightening out of the convexity of joint recesses
3	Severe synovitis	Convex distension of joint capsule

A high-yield examination can be obtained if MCP joints 2 to 4 are evaluated for synovitis from the dorsal aspect, proximal interphalangeal joints 2 to 4 are evaluated from the volar aspect, and the wrist is evaluated from the dorsal aspect in the midline for tenosynovitis of extensor tendons and synovitis in the radiocarpal and midcarpal joints, and for tenosynovitis of the extensor carpi ulnaris tendon from the ulnar aspect.

ULTRASONOGRAPHY IN THE DIFFERENTIAL DIAGNOSIS OF EARLY RHEUMATOID ARTHRITIS

Particularly early in the disease, the diagnosis of RA may not yet be firmly established. Ultrasonography can help distinguish typical features of RA from other inflammatory arthritides, and from noninflammatory musculoskeletal conditions.

Rheumatoid Arthritis Versus Crystal-Associated Arthritis

Both synovial pannus tissue and tophaceous material can distend the joint capsule and lead to a clinical picture of swollen and tender joints. Sonographically, synovial pannus tissue is more hypoechoic than crystal deposition because of its higher water content.[26,27] If conventional radiographs are available, synovial tissue as well as monosodium urate (MSU) crystals will be radiolucent (ie, escape radiographic detection). Calcium-containing crystals will be detected radiographically. Sonographically they may produce a posterior acoustic shadow, that is, they will not permit through-transmission of sound waves once they reach a critical size.

Synovial tissue proliferates from the inner lining of the hyperechoic joint capsule: it is attached to the capsule. By contrast, tophaceous material is generally not attached to the joint capsule (with the exception of microtophi). A hypoechoic or anechoic margin separates more hyperechoic tophi from the joint capsule and synovial lining.

Rheumatoid nodules appear sonographically as more hypoechoic, or darker than hyperechoic crystalline tophi.

Rheumatoid Arthritis Versus Spondyloarthritis

Few sonographic features truly discriminate between RA and the spondyloarthropathies. Inflammatory changes at the interface of tendons or ligaments and bone are characteristic of spondyloarthritis, but enthesitis can also be seen in RA. Sonographic features of the entheseal involvement in spondyloarthritis include edematous thickening of the tendon or ligament near and at origin or insertion with a loss of the pattern of densely packed, hyperechoic parallel fibers; blood flow at the interface with bone; synovial proliferation in adjacent bursae; erosion formation outside of synovial joints; and new bone formation.[28,29] The combination of these findings would not be a typical sonographic feature of RA. Dactylitis, or "sausage digits" of spondyloarthritis, may be due to enthesitis of ligaments or involvement of tendons rather than joint involvement alone, and ultrasonography can help shed light on this.[30,31]

The extensor tendons over fingers are devoid of a tendon sheath, so that the term tenosynovitis is not applicable here. The term paratenonitis is used to describe extra-articular hyperemia or anechoic fluid collections along the extensor tendons of the fingers. This term has found entrance into one sonographic scoring system of RA, the US7.[23] One study found paratenonitis in patients with spondyloarthritis but not RA, and the investigators have proposed this as a discriminating sonographic feature.[32]

Rheumatoid Arthritis Versus Erosive Osteoarthritis

Distinction of erosive osteoarthritis from RA is generally not a problem, because of the different patterns of distribution of the erosions. Typical central erosions of distal and prox-imal interphalangeal joints in erosive osteoarthritis associated with new bone formation can be readily distinguished on conventional radiographs from more marginal erosions in proximal interphalangeal and metacarpophalangeal joints without new bone formation in RA. The operational term "inflammatory osteoarthritis" has been coined to describe patients with periarticular redness, swelling, or even warmth. However, true synovitis defined as an increased intra-articular fluid collection, synovial proliferation, or synovial hyperemia is rare in osteoarthritis.[33] Minimal fluid collections can be seen sonographically around prominent intra-articular bone spurs. This appearance has been described as a "tent-pole" phenomenon, with the bony spur mechanically expanding the fibrous joint capsule, and adding room for fluid collections (G. Kunkel, personal communication, 2011).

As osteoarthritis is often accompanied by shedding of calcium-containing crystals, a response to these crystals has been postulated as the mechanism for synovitis in osteoarthritis.[34] Small calcific concrements can often be seen both radiographically and sonographically in osteoarthritis.

Synovial pannus tissue invading the subchondral bone seen on ultrasonography is consistent with RA, but clearly not with osteoarthritis. Two very distinct disease mech-anisms are at work forming the erosions.

Rheumatoid Arthritis Versus Fibromyalgia

Patients with fibromyalgia share several symptoms and complaints with patients affected by RA. Patient and caregiver may be concerned that an actual inflammatory arthritis is present. Patients with fibromyalgia may complain about symmetric joint pain and swelling affecting small joints of hands and wrists. Perceived morning stiffness may last for more than 1 hour, and patients may point out a family history of arthritis; they may have difficulty taking off the rings from their fingers. In this situation, an ultrasono-graphic assessment of the small finger joints and wrist joints can be extremely helpful to safely rule out any effusion or synovitis. Joint effusions and synovial hyperemia are not sonographic features seen in painful hands in the fibromyalgia syndrome.

TECHNICAL ASPECTS OF ULTRASONOGRAPHIC ASSESSMENT OF RHEUMATOID ARTHRITIS

Higher ultrasound frequencies provide better resolution of superficial structures, but will not penetrate tissues as deep as will lower frequencies. For the assessment of soft-tissue structures in small joints, ultrasound transducers with frequencies of 12 to 18 MHz are typically used. Lower frequencies may be needed for the deeper-seated hip joint. Details of synovial proliferation and synovial hyperemia can therefore be less well seen in the hip joint, but effusions can be seen as a distension of the joint capsule at the femoral neck. Linear transducers with a straight end are appropriate for most joints. Some examiners may prefer a probe with a small footprint (which can have a "hockey-stick" appearance) to maneuver around metacarpal or metatarsal heads for the assessment of erosions. The following can be helpful for ultrasonographic assessment of early RA:

- Start with a gray-scale assessment and identify structures of interest
- Adjust the frequency to the depth of the examined structure (higher frequencies for more superficial structures)
- Adjust the gray-scale gain so that hyperechoic bony cortex, hyperechoic fibrous joint capsule, as well as hypoechoic synovial tissue and anechoic synovial fluid, if present, can be distinguished
- Place focal point or focal points at the level or slightly deep to the level of the structure of interest
- Adjust the overall depth of the image on the screen so that not more than one-third of the image on the screen is located deep to the bony cortex
- If synovitis is identified with gray-scale ultrasonography, assess this tissue with Doppler ultrasonography
- Decrease Doppler gain until artifacts, particularly signals deep to the bony cortex, just disappear
- Label and save images
- Communicate findings and create a report.

Gauging the Doppler Function for RA Assessment

Sensitivity and specificity of the Doppler signal is variable among different ultrasound machines. Color or power Doppler should be able to detect blood flow in a vessel, and depict this flow within the confines of the vessel. A sensitive Doppler function will detect flow in vessels down to the size of capillaries if they are superficially located, as in small joints of hands and feet. The specificity for intraluminal flow is decreased if the Doppler signal is amplified so that color signals extend beyond the vascular wall. Such "bleeding" of the Doppler signal may potentially lead to an overestimation of hyperemia or vascularization of a given tissue.

Doppler assessment of blood flow in the volar aspect of the fingertip, the pulp, can help to calibrate and assess the quality of the Doppler function. Blood flow should be seen at least in the digital artery that overlies the bone of the distal phalanx. Smaller branches will extend medially and laterally from this artery and turn superficially toward the skin. The caliber of these terminal branches resembles the neovascularization of synovial pannus tissue in RA. Assessment of blood flow in the finger tip of healthy controls can help determine the suitability of the Doppler function for the assessment of synovial blood flow.

ULTRASONOGRAPHIC ASSESSMENT OF TREATMENT RESPONSE

Ultrasonography is safe and inexpensive, and can be repeated at consecutive office visits. Once abnormalities of RA are identified at baseline, they can be followed with serial ultrasonography over time, and a treatment response can be documented (**Fig. 9**).[35] Enlargement or healing of bony erosions can be documented. Changes in synovial thickening can be measured using sonographic calipers. Changes in the degree of synovial hyperemia can be visualized and scored using typical scoring systems. Ultrasonographic findings of RA are sensitive to change.[36]

ULTRASONOGRAPHY OF RHEUMATOID ARTHRITIS IN PERSPECTIVE

Because of initial concerns that the usefulness of ultrasonography to assess RA could be hampered by operator dependence, studies using ultrasonography routinely include assessments of interobserver and intraobserver variability. Ultrasonography

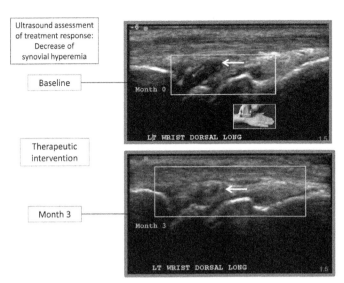

Fig. 9. Dorsal long-axis view over wrist. (*Top*) Baseline image of patient with rheumatoid arthritis shows distension of radiocarpal joint. Color Doppler shows intra-articular synovial hyperemia. (*Bottom*) After therapeutic intervention, the joint recess is physiologically collapsed. No synovial proliferation or hyperemia is appreciated.

has proved to be a remarkably robust tool for reliable assessment of changes in RA.[37–42] No evidence can be gleaned from the literature showing that problems with operator dependence would be greater than with other imaging modalities or physical examination, if performed by trained providers.

Ultrasonography is an elegant tool for the detection of tenosynovitis, synovitis, and erosions very early in RA, and the presence of a power Doppler signal is one of the best predictors of joint damage.[43]

ACKNOWLEDGMENT

The author would like to thank Ms. Jutta Roether, Hamburg, Germany, for the artwork of the anatomic illustrations.

REFERENCES

1. Huber N. Zur Verwerthung der Röntgen-Strahlen im Gebiete der inneren Medicin. Dtsch Med Wochenschr 1896;22(12):182–4 [in German].
2. Moore CP, Sarti DA, Louie JS. Ultrasonographic demonstration of popliteal cysts in rheumatoid arthritis. A noninvasive technique. Arthritis Rheum 1975;18(6):577–80.
3. Khosla S, Thiele R, Baumhauer JF. Ultrasound guidance for intra-articular injections of the foot and ankle. Foot Ankle Int 2009;30(9):886–90.
4. Brown AK, Quinn MA, Karim Z, et al. Presence of significant synovitis in rheumatoid arthritis patients with disease-modifying antirheumatic drug-induced clinical remission: evidence from an imaging study may explain structural progression. Arthritis Rheum 2006;54(12):3761–73.
5. Foltz V, Gandjbakhch F, Etchepare F, et al. Power Doppler ultrasound, but not low-field magnetic resonance imaging, predicts relapse and radiographic disease progression in rheumatoid arthritis patients with low levels of disease activity. Arthritis Rheum 2003;64(1):67–76.

6. van der Heijde D. Remission by imaging in rheumatoid arthritis: should this be the ultimate goal? Ann Rheum Dis 2012;71(Suppl 2):i89–92.
7. Dougados M, Jousse-Joulin S, Mistretta F, et al. Evaluation of several ultrasonography scoring systems for synovitis and comparison to clinical examination: results from a prospective multicentre study of rheumatoid arthritis. Ann Rheum Dis 2010;69(5):828–33.
8. Mandl P, Balint PV, Brault Y, et al. Metrologic properties of ultrasound versus clinical evaluation of synovitis in rheumatoid arthritis: results of a multicenter, randomized study. Arthritis Rheum 2012;64(4):1272–82.
9. Damjanov N, Radunovic G, Prodanovic S, et al. Construct validity and reliability of ultrasound disease activity score in assessing joint inflammation in RA: comparison with DAS-28. Rheumatology (Oxford) 2012;51(1):120–8.
10. Baillet A, Gaujoux-Viala C, Mouterde G, et al. Comparison of the efficacy of sonography, magnetic resonance imaging and conventional radiography for the detection of bone erosions in rheumatoid arthritis patients: a systematic review and meta-analysis. Rheumatology (Oxford) 2011;50(6):1137–47.
11. Wakefield RJ, Gibbon WW, Conaghan PG, et al. The value of sonography in the detection of bone erosions in patients with rheumatoid arthritis: a comparison with conventional radiography. Arthritis Rheum 2000;43(12):2762–70.
12. Sharp JT, Wolfe F, Lassere M, et al. Variability of precision in scoring radiographic abnormalities in rheumatoid arthritis by experienced readers. J Rheumatol 2004; 31(6):1062–72.
13. Theodoropoulos JS, Andreisek G, Harvey EJ, et al. Magnetic resonance imaging and magnetic resonance arthrography of the shoulder: dependence on the level of training of the performing radiologist for diagnostic accuracy. Skeletal Radiol 2010;39(7):661–7.
14. Ruma J, Klein KA, Chong S, et al. Cross-sectional examination interpretation discrepancies between on-call diagnostic radiology residents and subspecialty faculty radiologists: analysis by imaging modality and subspecialty. J Am Coll Radiol 2011;8(6):409–14.
15. Walther M, Harms H, Krenn V, et al. Correlation of power Doppler sonography with vascularity of the synovial tissue of the knee joint in patients with osteoarthritis and rheumatoid arthritis. Arthritis Rheum 2001;44(2):331–8.
16. Koski JM, Saarakkala S, Helle M, et al. Power Doppler ultrasonography and synovitis: correlating ultrasound imaging with histopathological findings and evaluating the performance of ultrasound equipments. Ann Rheum Dis 2006;65(12): 1590–5.
17. Takase K, Ohno S, Takeno M, et al. Simultaneous evaluation of long-lasting knee synovitis in patients undergoing arthroplasty by power Doppler ultrasonography and contrast-enhanced MRI in comparison with histopathology. Clin Exp Rheumatol 2012;30(1):85–92.
18. Hoving JL, Buchbinder R, Hall S, et al. A comparison of magnetic resonance imaging, sonography, and radiography of the hand in patients with early rheumatoid arthritis. J Rheumatol 2004;31(4):663–75.
19. Szkudlarek M, Narvestad E, Klarlund M, et al. Ultrasonography of the metatarsophalangeal joints in rheumatoid arthritis: comparison with magnetic resonance imaging, conventional radiography, and clinical examination. Arthritis Rheum 2004;50(7):2103–12.
20. Thiele RG, Tabechian D, Anandarajah AP. Ultrasonographic demonstration of tenosynovitis preceding joint involvement in early seropositive rheumatoid arthritis. Arthritis Rheum 2008;58(Suppl 9):S407.

21. Eshed I, Feist E, Althoff CE, et al. Tenosynovitis of the flexor tendons of the hand detected by MRI: an early indicator of rheumatoid arthritis. Rheumatology (Oxford) 2009;48(8):887–91.
22. Filippucci E, Gabba A, Di Geso L, et al. Hand tendon involvement in rheumatoid arthritis: an ultrasound study. Semin Arthritis Rheum 2012;41(6):752–60.
23. Backhaus M, Ohrndorf S, Kellner H, et al. Evaluation of a novel 7-joint ultrasound score in daily rheumatologic practice: a pilot project. Arthritis Rheum 2009;61(9): 1194–201.
24. Thiele R. Doppler ultrasonography in rheumatology: adding color to the picture. J Rheumatol 2008;35(1):8–10.
25. Wakefield RJ, Balint PV, Szkudlarek M, et al. Musculoskeletal ultrasound including definitions for ultrasonographic pathology. J Rheumatol 2005;32(12):2485–7.
26. Thiele RG, Schlesinger N. Diagnosis of gout by ultrasound. Rheumatology (Oxford) 2007;46(7):1116–21.
27. Thiele RG. Role of ultrasound and other advanced imaging in the diagnosis and management of gout. Curr Rheumatol Rep 2011;13(2):146–53.
28. D'Agostino MA, Aegerter P, Jousse-Joulin S, et al. How to evaluate and improve the reliability of power Doppler ultrasonography for assessing enthesitis in spondyloarthritis. Arthritis Rheum 2009;61(1):61–9.
29. D'Agostino MA, Said-Nahal R, Hacquard-Bouder C, et al. Assessment of peripheral enthesitis in the spondyloarthropathies by ultrasonography combined with power Doppler: a cross-sectional study. Arthritis Rheum 2003;48(2):523–33.
30. McGonagle D, Benjamin M, Marzo-Ortega H, et al. Advances in the understanding of entheseal inflammation. Curr Rheumatol Rep 2002;4(6):500–6.
31. McGonagle D, Lories RJ, Tan AL, et al. The concept of a "synovio-entheseal complex" and its implications for understanding joint inflammation and damage in psoriatic arthritis and beyond. Arthritis Rheum 2007;56(8):2482–91.
32. Gutierrez M, Filippucci E, Salaffi F, et al. Differential diagnosis between rheumatoid arthritis and psoriatic arthritis: the value of ultrasound findings at metacarpophalangeal joints level. Ann Rheum Dis 2011;70(6):1111–4.
33. Thiele RG, Paxton LA, Marston BA, et al. Erosive osteoarthritis is not associated with invading synovial tissue: an ultrasound study. Arthritis Rheum 2010;62(10):S674.
34. McCarthy GM. Crystal-related tissue damage. In: Smyth CJ, Holers VM, editors. Gout, hyperuricemia and other crystal-associated arthropathies. New York: Marcel Dekker; 1999. p. 39–57.
35. Thiele RG, Tabechian D, Anandarajah AP. Ultrasonographic features of rheumatoid synovium after treatment with TNF-alpha inhibitors suggest remission. Ann Rheum Dis 2008;67(Suppl II):646.
36. Scheel AK, Hermann KG, Ohrndorf S, et al. Prospective 7 year follow up imaging study comparing radiography, ultrasonography, and magnetic resonance imaging in rheumatoid arthritis finger joints. Ann Rheum Dis 2006; 65(5):595–600.
37. Naredo E, Moller I, Moragues C, et al. Interobserver reliability in musculoskeletal ultrasonography: results from a "Teach the Teachers" rheumatologist course. Ann Rheum Dis 2006;65(1):14–9.
38. Scheel AK, Schmidt WA, Hermann KG, et al. Interobserver reliability of rheumatologists performing musculoskeletal ultrasonography: results from a EULAR "Train the trainers" course. Ann Rheum Dis 2005;64(7):1043–9.
39. Hammer HB, Bolton-King P, Bakkeheim V, et al. Examination of intra and interrater reliability with a new ultrasonographic reference atlas for scoring of synovitis in patients with rheumatoid arthritis. Ann Rheum Dis 2011;70(11):1995–8.

40. Ohrndorf S, Naumann L, Grundey J, et al. Is musculoskeletal ultrasonography an operator-dependent method or a fast and reliably teachable diagnostic tool? Interreader agreements of 3 ultrasonographers with different training levels. Int J Rheumatol 2010;2010:164518.
41. Cheung PP, Dougados M, Gossec L. Reliability of ultrasonography to detect synovitis in rheumatoid arthritis: a systematic literature review of 35 studies (1,415 patients). Arthritis Care Res (Hoboken) 2010;62(3):323–34.
42. Koski JM, Saarakkala S, Helle M, et al. Assessing the intra- and inter-reader reliability of dynamic ultrasound images in power Doppler ultrasonography. Ann Rheum Dis 2006;65(12):1658–60.
43. Fukae J, Isobe M, Kitano A, et al. Radiographic prognosis of finger joint damage predicted by early alteration in synovial vascularity in patients with rheumatoid arthritis: potential utility of power Doppler sonography in clinical practice. Arthritis Care Res (Hoboken) 2011;63(9):1247–53.

Magnetic Resonance Imaging Applications in Early Rheumatoid Arthritis Diagnosis and Management

Orrin M. Troum, MD[a],*, Olga Pimienta, MD[b], Ewa Olech, MD[c]

KEYWORDS

• Early rheumatoid arthritis • Magnetic resonance imaging
• Diagnosis • Prognosis • Management

Key Points

- More sensitive imaging techniques were incorporated in the assessment of early aggressive rheumatoid arthritis (RA) because of the availability of effective biological therapies.

- Distinguishing between active treatments in modern trials is difficult using conventional radiography and is especially limited in early disease detection.

- Magnetic resonance imaging has the advantage of detecting both joint inflammation and damage and thus provides additional and unique data.

- This information is useful for early and accurate diagnosis, prediction of poor prognosis, and monitoring response to therapy in RA clinical trials.

According to its definition based on clinical studies, early rheumatoid arthritis (RA) ranges from 6 weeks to less than 5 years from the onset of symptoms. Microscopic changes, including osteoclastogenesis, occur early in the course of the disease. Radiographic damage is seen in 50% to 70% of patients within the first 2 years of disease onset,[1,2] indicating that early detection and prevention are of paramount importance. Lindqvist and colleagues[3] reported that 75% of the median radiographic

---

The authors have nothing to disclose.
[a] Keck School of Medicine, University of Southern California, 2336 Santa Monica Boulevard, Suite 207, Santa Monica, CA 90404, USA; [b] Orrin M. Troum, MD & Medical Associates, 2336 Santa Monica Boulevard, Suite 207, Santa Monica, CA 90404, USA; [c] Division of Rheumatology, Department of Internal Medicine, University of Nevada School of Medicine, 1707 West Charleston Boulevard, Suite 220, Las Vegas, NV 89102, USA
* Corresponding author.
E-mail address: otroum@troummd.org

Rheum Dis Clin N Am 38 (2012) 277–297
doi:10.1016/j.rdc.2012.04.001
0889-857X/12/$ – see front matter © 2012 Elsevier Inc. All rights reserved.

progression in RA occurs within the first 5 years. Lard and colleagues[4] suggested that structural damage progresses more quickly and that even a brief delay of therapy can affect the extent of damage that occurs.

More recently, attention has been focused on how early the active treatment of RA should be initiated. Finckh and colleagues[5] demonstrated that a shorter disease duration is the strongest predictor of improvement in disease activity over 5 years, and delayed treatment led to further radiographic progression. Bathon and colleagues[6] administered etanercept to patients within 1 year of onset of RA and reported that the bone erosion score showed a significantly slower rate of change in the etanercept group than in the methotrexate (MTX) group. Nell and colleagues[7] prospectively investigated the changes of disease activity (Disease Activity Score [DAS] 28) in patients with early RA (<3 months). The group reported that DAS28 improved significantly after 3 months of disease-modifying antirheumatic drug (DMARD) therapy; this trend continued over the following 3 years. Others have placed increasing emphasis on assessing and diagnosing RA within the first 6 weeks of patient symptoms, initiating treatment using DMARD therapy in a similar time frame. This is reflected in both the European League Against Rheumatism (EULAR) and the American College of Rheumatology (ACR) guidelines for patient care.[8,9]

The availability of DMARDs, including biological therapy for early aggressive RA, generated the need for more sensitive imaging techniques. These give further insight into the underlying pathophysiology of RA and assist the clinician in predicting prognosis and monitoring long-term treatment. Thus, an accurate early diagnosis of RA assisted by detailed joint imaging may be especially beneficial in preventing disability.

LIMITATIONS OF RADIOGRAPHY IN RA

The first study comparing magnetic resonance imaging (MRI) and radiography of the wrist joint in patients with RA was published in 1988.[10] There have been numerous subsequent publications using MRI in RA that have demonstrated the technique's utility in detecting early arthritic changes.[11] Many studies have compared the sensitivity of detecting bone erosions between MRI and conventional radiography. In addition, longitudinal studies have confirmed that many bone marrow lesions (osteitis) seen with MRI progress to radiographic erosions. Thus, in addition to lacking the capacity for multidimensional imaging (2-dimensional representation of 3-dimensional pathologic condition), radiographs do not detect early bone lesions because they are incapable of assessing osteitis (**Figs. 1–3**).

There is ongoing demand for better early predictors of progression and more sensitive erosion detection. Thus, the shift in approach from diagnosing bone erosions to identifying pre-erosive features is important but not possible with radiography. Technical limitations of radiography include lack of sensitivity for bone erosions because radiograph lucency primarily reflects cortical bone loss and projection superimposition obscures nontangential erosions. Radiography cannot accurately assess cartilage loss because joint space narrowing (JSN) only indirectly measures the magnitude of existing cartilage. In addition, radiography has a low sensitivity to change over time and, importantly, the cartilage, synovium, bone marrow, and tendons cannot be accurately visualized. Multiple studies have shown that MRI is at least twice as sensitive as radiography for detecting erosions.[12–16]

ADVANTAGES AND DISADVANTAGES OF MRI IN RA

The main advantages of MRI are no exposure to x-ray radiation, tomographic/3-dimentional viewing, high resolution, good soft tissue contrast, and reproducibility.

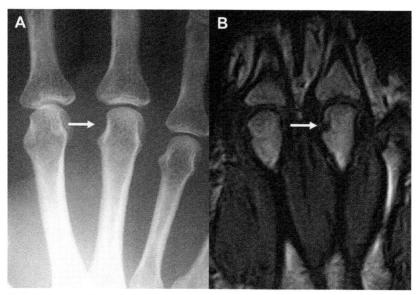

Fig. 1. Imaging in a 56-year-old man with recent-onset RA. (*A*) Radiograph of the right hand shows no erosions. (*B*) Coronal T1-weighted image (0.2-T extremity MRI) shows moderate-size erosion in the third metacarpal head (*arrow*).

This technique enables detailed visualization of bone marrow, synovium, cartilage, and tendons. Potential disadvantages of MRI are high cost and limited accessibility. In contrast-enhanced imaging protocols, there is a small risk of gadolinium toxicity, such as nephrogenic systemic fibrosis, especially in patients with renal impairment. Also, interpretation of magnetic resonance images is more complex and time consuming than radiographs, and they should be evaluated by an experienced musculoskeletal reader. High-quality images are assured only if patients remain immobile while the images are being obtained. In patients who are anxious, confused, or in severe pain, it is more challenging to obtain high-quality images. Claustrophobia also makes it difficult for some patients to cooperate with the study.

Contraindications to MRI also remain a problem in some patients. In addition, morbidly obese patients may not fit into a conventional MRI machine and patients with pacemakers, certain ferromagnetic appliances, and certain surgical clips and those with recent cardiac stent placement cannot be included in the study. Although there is no current evidence that MRI harms the fetus, pregnant women are usually advised not to undergo MRI examination unless medically necessary, but ultrasonography may be performed.

Ultrasonography is another viable imaging option for rheumatologists. Surface erosions can be detected with high-resolution ultrasonography because it is more sensitive than radiography, but less sensitive than MRI. Compared with MRI, ultrasonography is inexpensive, portable, and real time; it is also efficient than radiography for measuring soft tissue changes, including synovitis. The use of color Doppler and power Doppler aids in detecting the increased vascularity of synovitis, differentiating it from effusion. These are also useful for joint aspiration and injection techniques because they accurately identify the joint and periarticular structures. However, bone shadowing can obscure the medial and lateral aspects of the metacarpal and carpal bones. Standardization is difficult, limiting its use in clinical trials, because

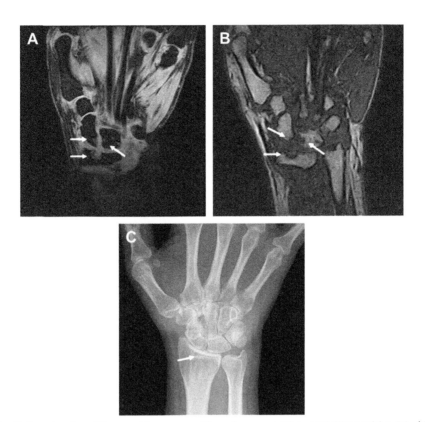

Fig. 2. Imaging in a 39-year-old woman with early seropositive, anti-CCP–positive RA. (*A*) Coronal T1-weighted fat-suppressed image of the right wrist performed on 1.5-T whole-body MRI system. Small erosions are seen in the right scaphoid, lunate, and distal radius (*arrows*). (*B*) Coronal T1-weighted image on 0.2-T extremity MRI (C-Scan). The same erosions are found (*arrows*). (*C*) Radiograph of the right wrist. Joint space narrowing of the radioulnar joint and subchondral sclerosis of the distal ulna are present (*arrow*) but no evidence of erosions.

the findings vary depending on the operator and there has been no validated scoring system to date.

Compared with ultrasonography, MRI has a relatively low resolution, and, because contrast administration is required to reliably distinguish synovium from effusion, the imaging of multiple joints can be difficult. In addition to increased availability and fewer financial constraints relative to MRI, ultrasonography allows the clinician to assess the patient at the time of imaging and to examine the contralateral side or additional joints if necessary.

TYPES OF MRI MACHINES

There are several types of MRI machines available. In general, they are divided into conventional (whole body) and extremity MRI (eMRI) systems, in which only the extremity of interest is positioned into the magnet bore while the rest of the body remains outside. Both conventional and eMRI systems come in various field strengths,

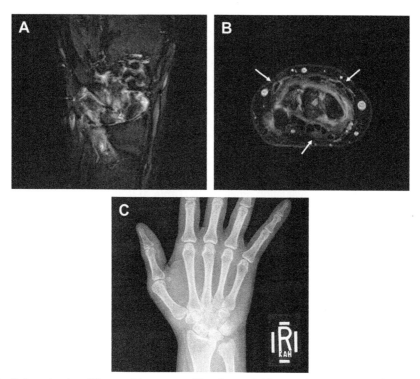

Fig. 3. Imaging in a 22-year-old woman with a 6-month history of severe seropositive, anti-CCP–positive RA. (*A*) Coronal short tau inversion recovery image of the right wrist shows synovitis (high-signal tissue in the synovial space) and bone marrow edema (increased signal within the bone marrow) in the carpal bones. (*B*) Postcontrast axial T1-weighted fat-saturated image confirming the previous findings. Tenosynovitis of extensor and flexor tendons is also seen (*arrows*). (*C*) Radiograph is incapable of visualizing synovitis, bone edema, or tendinitis.

ranging from a low 0.2 T to a high 1.5 T and more recently available 3.0-T magnets. Currently available eMRI systems include the 0.2-T C-Scan and E-Scan XQ (Opera), 0.25-T S-Scan, and 0.31-T O-Scan (Esaote SpA, Genoa, Italy), the portable 0.2-T MV-R by MagneVu (Carlsbad, CA, USA), and the high-field 1.0- and 1.5-T OrthOne (ONI Medical Systems, Wilmington, MA, USA). There are differences between these extremity scanners, ranging from the field of view available for scanning (smallest field: the MV-R) to the joints being visualized and whether special shielding is needed for the examination room.

Low-Field MRI

Detecting osteitis, synovitis, or erosions does not require a higher-Tesla magnet or whole-body machine. Taouli and colleagues[17] found that a stronger magnet is not needed to detect early RA. Crues and colleagues[14] compared radiography with MRI using a portable MRI machine with a focused field of view examining 227 wrists and the second and third metacarpal joints of 132 patients with RA with a median disease duration of 8 years. Erosions, as read by 2 musculoskeletal radiologists, were detected in 95% of patients by MRI and in only 59% by radiography in these different locations.

In a prospective study of 405 patients, the majority with established RA and receiving tumor necrosis factor (TNF) α inhibitors were examined at baseline with eMRI. Of them, 156 patients had 246 follow-up examinations (average of 8 months) over a 2-year period. A change in erosions or erosion diameter was considered significant when there was at least a change of 20%.[16] MRI detected new erosions or change in erosion size in 50% of patients, whereas radiography was not sensitive enough to detect these changes.

Since the introduction of extremity-dedicated low-field units (<1.0 T), there has been interest in comparing the diagnostic performance of low-field scanners with that of existing high-field (≥1.0 T) scanners.

Published data demonstrate excellent correlation between extremity units and whole-body systems. There are 6 published studies comparing eMRI with high-field conventional MRI evaluating small joints (**Table 1**).[17–22] Overall, in diagnosing and scoring RA pathology, the agreement between the 2 field strengths was high (see **Fig. 2**).

With high-field MRI as the gold standard and using the Artoscan (0.2 T), Ejbjerg and colleagues[18] found 93% sensitivity and 94% specificity for erosions and 90% sensitivity and 96% specificity for synovitis. However, the low-field unit displayed high specificity but only moderate sensitivity (39%) for detection of bone marrow edema. Bird and colleagues[21] found high specificity but only moderate sensitivity on low- compared with high-field MRI in scoring synovitis and bone edema.

One study evaluated interreader reliability of the Outcome Measures in Rheumatoid Arthritis Clinical Trials (OMERACT) RA MRI score assessing change in disease activity and bone erosions using eMRI in comparison with high-field MRI. The intraclass correlation coefficients and smallest detectable difference results for the change in scores were good for erosions and synovitis but not acceptable for bone edema.[23]

Table 1
Agreements in scoring RA pathologies between high and low-field MRI systems in published studies

Study	Savnik et al,[19] 2001	Taouli et al,[17] 2004	Ejbjerg et al,[18] 2005	Schirmer et al,[20] 2007	Bird et al,[21] 2007	Suzuki et al,[22] 2009
Number of Subjects	103	18	65	17	15	3
Anatomy	Unilateral wrist, MCP, PIP joints	Bilateral wrist, MCP joints	Unilateral wrist and MCP joints	Unilateral wrist, MCP, PIP joints	Dominant wrist and MCP joints	Bilateral wrist, MCP joints
eMRI Unit	0.2-T Artoscan	0.2-T Artoscan	0.2-T Artoscan	0.2-T C-Scan	0.2-T Artoscan	0.3-T CompacTscan
Synovitis	+	+	+	+	±	+
Osteitis	+	NA	±	NA	±	+
Erosions	+	+	+	+	+	+
JSN	NA	+	NA	NA	NA	NA
Tenosynovitis	NA	NA	NA	+	NA	NA

Abbreviations: +, high agreement; ±, moderate or low agreement; JSN, joint space narrowing; MCP, metacarpophalangeal; NA, not assessed; PIP, proximal interphalangeal.

Given these results, the optimal method for assessing bone edema may be high-field MRI. However, MRI systems, imaging protocols, and scoring methods differed amongst these studies.

Duer-Jensen and colleagues,[24] using computed tomography (CT) as the reference, compared the ability of 2 different eMRI units (Artoscan and MagneVu) and conventional radiography to identify bone erosions in patients with RA of the metacarpophalangeal and wrist joints. The Artoscan showed higher sensitivity than the MagneVu and conventional radiography.

When assessing the practicality of obtaining an eMRI for the rheumatologist's office or clinical setting, several issues must be addressed. It is now mandatory in the United States to get accreditation to perform MRI outside a radiology facility. Accreditation can be obtained through the American College of Radiology (ACR) or the Intersocietal Accreditation Commission.

In 2005, the International Society of Extremity MRI in Rheumatology (ISEMIR) was established with the purpose of bringing together rheumatologists, radiologists, and other specialties dedicated to MRI technology as applied to rheumatologic diseases.[25] ISEMIR, renamed in 2011 as the International Society of Musculoskeletal Imaging in Rheumatology, now incorporates ultrasonography.

MRI SCORING

The RA MRI score (RAMRIS) was developed at OMERACT 6 in April 2002. The aim was to provide a well-defined reproducible measurement system appropriate for multicenter use. The consensus by the OMERACT 6 MRI committee was that cortical erosion, bone marrow edema, and synovial volume were the most reproducible measurements.[26]

The RAMRIS system has limitations with significant variation in interreader correlation despite low intrareader variation.[27,28] However, this validated scoring system has been applied for diagnosis, assessment of disease activity, prognosis, and monitoring response to treatment. Hirose and colleagues[29] showed that RAMRIS is useful for assessing early response to TNF inhibitors.

RAMRIS is specific to the wrist and metacarpophalangeal joints but has been successfully modified to include the feet.[30] Baan and colleagues[31] demonstrated good to excellent interreader and intrareader reliability for MRI of the rheumatic foot using RAMRIS.

Other scoring methods have been developed. Crowley and colleagues[32] investigated the reliability, feasibility, and validity of a computer-assisted manual segmentation (outlining) technique for measuring MRI bone erosion and edema at the wrist in RA. Segmentation measures the volume of MRI bone edema and erosion. When compared with RAMRIS, outlining was less reliable for bone edema but had similar reliability for quantifying erosions. Ostergaard and colleagues[33] pioneered the segmentation technique in quantifying rheumatoid synovial membrane volume. Bird and colleagues[34] subsequently applied it to measuring bone erosion volume. Chand and colleagues[35] demonstrated excellent intraobserver and very good interobserver reliability, content validity (represented by strong correlation with RAMRIS synovitis), and moderate feasibility by measuring MRI synovitis using a computer-assisted manual segmentation method.

Cyteval and colleagues[36] assessed a simplified scoring method (Simplified Rheumatoid Arthritis Magnetic Resonance Imaging Score [SAMIS]) developed to shorten interpretation time while retaining both correlation with RAMRIS and same or better intrareader and interreader reliability. The results from SAMIS closely correlated with those of RAMRIS; however, the scoring time was dramatically reduced: 5 to 20 minutes for RAMRIS versus 2 to 7 minutes SAMIS.

Dynamic Contrast-Enhanced MRI

Rapid acquisition of sequential contrast-enhanced images following administration of contrast allows mapping of the time course of synovial enhancement.[37] Resultant measures depend on both synovial perfusion and capillary permeability. A rapid bolus injection, followed by sequential imaging from 2.6 to 69.0 seconds, allows measurement of multiple time-dependent variables.[38]

In several studies, dynamic contrast-enhanced MRI (DCE-MRI) findings correlated well with C-reactive protein (CRP) levels and erythrocyte sedimentation rate (ESR) as well as DAS, Health Assessment Questionnaire scores,[39] and erosions.[40] In follow-up studies, findings correlated with clinical and histologic changes and relapse, with erosions seen at 1 year.[41,42] DCE-MRI has also been successfully used to compare therapy effectiveness between DMARDs.[43]

RA JOINT PATHOLOGY

MRI allows assessment of all the structures involved in RA: synovial membrane, synovial fluid, tendons, tendon sheaths, ligaments, cartilage, and bone. Miniarthroscopy of the metacarpophalangeal joints in patients with RA confirmed the presence of bone pathology in all joints with MRI bone erosions and histologic synovitis in all joints with synovitis. The extent of synovitis in these joints correlated well not only between MRI and macroscopic findings on miniarthroscopy but also with clinical disease activity.[44] Recently, increased synovial vascularity assessed by magnetic resonance angiography has been shown to correlate well with both MRI and ultrasonography-detected synovitis in a pilot study involving 30 patients with early inflammatory arthritis.[45]

Several studies have confirmed that MRI bone edema represents a cellular infiltrate, indicating the presence of osteitis within the subchondral bone.[46–48] In contrast to radiographic erosions, which reflect fully developed bone damage with a break in the cortical bone, bone marrow edema comprises a link between joint inflammation and bone destruction.

Some remain skeptical as to whether erosions seen by MRI are true erosions. Many studies have confirmed that MRI erosions do reflect actual bone damage. MRI findings correlate closely with histopathologic signs of synovial inflammation.[33,49] Using high-resolution CT as the gold standard, nonradiographically visible MRI erosions have been proved to be true erosions. At follow-up, these erosions demonstrated a small degree of reversibility by MRI after patients initiated either anti-TNF or rituximab treatment.[50] In wrists and metacarpophalangeal joints, MRI and CT have a concordance of between 77% and 89%,[51–53] given that CT is often considered the gold standard for detection of bone destruction.

Cartilage assessment was initially excluded in RAMRIS because of poor interreader reliability, but an MRI JSN scoring system proposed by McQueen and colleagues[54] demonstrated excellent interreader and intrareader reliability. However, it was not capable of distinguishing JSN between those with early RA and healthy subjects. Subsequently, the OMERACT MRI group commenced the development of a JSN MRI score as a potential RAMRIS addendum for cartilage assessment. Preliminary use of this scoring method had good intrareader/interreader agreements.[55,56] A novel MRI technique, delayed gadolinium-enhanced MRI of cartilage, has emerged as most promising to assess cartilage quality.[57]

RA DIAGNOSIS
Synovitis

There are several ways in which MRI can assist the clinician in the diagnosis of RA. MRI is more sensitive than clinical examination, and confirming subclinical synovitis can allow differentiation of the patient with nonspecific joint pain from a patient with true inflammatory synovitis. Synovitis is the primary abnormality in RA, and MRI, unlike radiography, can be used to image the synovium. MRI can assess synovial volume and the level of synovial inflammation. Although clinical examination remains a cornerstone in diagnosing and monitoring disease progression in patients with RA, MRI is more sensitive than clinical examination for identifying synovitis. Sugimoto and colleagues[58] diagnosed 25 of 26 patients at RA disease onset using MRI criteria (presence of contrast enhancement), 23% more patients than were identified using ACR criteria. Another study compared the diagnostic utility of testing for anti–cyclic citrullinated protein (anti-CCP) antibodies with MRI to confirm the diagnosis of RA. This cohort of patients with recent-onset arthritis met at least 3 of the 4 ACR clinical criteria in the absence of serum rheumatoid factor (RF), nodules, or erosions.[59] The presence of MRI synovitis with bone erosions or bone edema of the hand had a specificity of 78% and a sensitivity of 100% for making the diagnosis of RA.

Erosions

MRI can assist in diagnosing RA by revealing erosive disease in the typical RA joint distribution. In 42 patients with early RA (<6 months), McQueen and colleagues[60] found 45% of patients with erosions at baseline by MRI, whereas only 15% showed erosions at baseline on radiography. A 5-year longitudinal study demonstrated that at baseline only 20% of MRI lesions were detected by radiography, in contrast to the 5-year follow-up where 60% of the initial lesions were detected radiographically.[61] In another study comparing MRI with radiography in detecting erosions, only approximately 10% of bone erosions by radiography were classified as small in size.[61,62] Erosions are visible by MRI at a median of 2 years before being detected by radiography and may become consistently noticeable by radiography of the metacarpophalangeal joints only after 20% to 30% of the bone is eroded on MRI.[63]

Tenosynovitis

MRI is a sensitive tool for detecting inflammation of periarticular tendons (tenosynovitis) (see **Fig. 3**).[64] Flexor tenosynovitis of the hand diagnosed by MRI is a strong predictor of early RA. Combining flexor tenosynovitis by MRI with positive serology test results (anti-CCP or RF) more strongly predicts early RA.[65]

Bone Marrow Edema (Osteitis)

MRI permits the visualization of subchondral bone abnormality in the form of marrow edema. This is clinically important because marrow edema identified by MRI is often present in patients with early RA.[66,67]

In a cross-sectional study of 40 healthy controls and 40 randomly chosen patients with RA, bilateral hand and wrist magnetic resonance images were assessed by 2 readers blinded to the diagnosis.[68] The presence of bone edema was found to be the best test for RA diagnosis, with a specificity of 82.5% and a sensitivity of 60%, and osteitis of the metacarpophalangeal joints was 100% specific for RA.

Using MRI in the diagnosis of early RA may be most useful when evaluating patients with undifferentiated arthritis (UA) with the ultimate goal to identify those who would benefit from earlier treatment. Tamai and colleagues[69] followed up 129 patients with UA for 1 year, with 75 ultimately developing RA. Baseline MRI together with RF and CCP level determination predicted the progression from UA to RA. MRI osteitis was better at predicting RA then synovitis or bone erosions. Duer-Jensen and colleagues[70] followed up 116 patients with UA for 1 year. Similar to the previous study, MRI bone edema independently predicted the development of RA. A prediction model, including clinical hand arthritis, morning stiffness, and positive RF and MRI bone edema score in MTP and wrist joints correctly identified the development of RA versus non-RA in 82% of patients.

Enthesitis

Clinical manifestations of the spondyloarthropathies that involve peripheral joints, especially in psoriatic patients presenting with polyarthritis, may be difficult to distinguish from those of RA. Identification of enthesitis (inflammation at the insertions of ligaments and tendons) using MRI may be helpful in making the correct diagnosis[71] when assessing peripheral involvement in patients with spondyloarthritis.

A recent study assessed the value of MRI to diagnose early RA, in which MRI detected nonradiographic lesions.[72] Of 20 patients with early RA (<2 years' duration), 75% with no radiographic erosions had abnormal results on hand MRI. This review found 36 erosions (50% in the carpal bones) and 55 joints with synovitis (mainly mid-carpal and metacarpophalangeal joints). Bone edema was found in the carpal bones, and tenosynovitis most frequently affected the flexor tendons. Ostendorf and colleagues[30] showed similar results in a cohort of 25 patients with early RA (<1 year). Radiographic results were negative in 60%; however, MRI erosions were detected in 36%, and 24% showed pre-erosive features, synovitis, and osteitis. In another study, bone edema, erosions, and synovitis were present in 26 patients with very early (<3 months) RA, with the prevalence being 100%, 96%, and 92%, respectively.[73]

A recent systematic review performed by Suter and colleagues[74] specifically addressed the question of diagnostic utility of MRI in RA. Eleven studies (606 subjects) were analyzed to determine the sensitivity and specificity of the diagnostic utility of MRI. The reported sensitivity and specificity ranged widely between 20% and 100% and 0% and 100%, respectively. The main difficulty in interpreting results across studies was related to nonuniformity in the use of MRI RA criteria, MRI definitions and scoring systems, and magnetic resonance systems. These findings suggest that well-designed studies are still needed in this area.

According to the new ACR/EULAR 2010 classification criteria, definite RA is based on the presence of definite synovitis (tenderness and swelling on clinical examination) in 1 or more joints, absence of an alternative diagnosis that explains the synovitis, and achievement of a total score of 6 or more (range, 0–10) from the individual scores in 4 domains: number/site of involved joints (range, 0–5), serologic abnormalities (range, 0–3), elevated acute phase reactants (range, 0–1), and duration of symptoms (range, 0–1).[75] Despite the fact that imaging is not part of the new RA classification criteria, there is consensus that MRI and ultrasonography may be used to detect synovitis and to count joints in the joint involvement domain.[76]

RA PROGNOSIS

There are multiple studies demonstrating that MRI is a useful biomarker for prognosis of early RA. MRI predicts erosive phenotype, worse clinical disease activity, inflammatory activity (higher ESR and CRP level), and functional disability.

Accurately predicting the rate of disease progression is important in the management of early RA. This crucial information allows early aggressive therapeutic intervention. Several studies have reported that MRI of the small joints in early RA predicts progression of erosive disease (**Table 2**). Some investigators have looked at the short-term predictive value of MRI after 1 year, whereas other studies had up to 10 years of follow-up. Structural progression was assessed by either conventional radiography or MRI. All these studies demonstrated MRI to be a highly significant predictor of structural joint damage.

Data from an uncontrolled prospective cohort of 42 patients demonstrated that baseline MRI bone edema score of the dominant wrist predicted radiographic erosions at 6 years.[78] The levels of CRP was the only clinical measure found to have predictive value, whereas tender and swollen joint scores did not. Boyesen and colleagues[83] showed that both baseline and 1-year cumulative measures of MRI synovitis and bone marrow edema independently predicted 3-year radiographic progression, suggesting these pathologic changes precede radiographic progression in early RA. However, in some studies, MRI synovitis did not reliably predict erosions, as opposed to bone edema, which was found to be the best predictor of structural damage. The largest data set in early RA using MRI is derived from the CIMESTRA (Cyclosporine, Methotrexate, Steroid in RA) trial in which hand and wrist bone edema was the strongest independent predictor of radiographic progression at 2 years.[84] It was superior to conventional radiography, immunologic serology tests (anti-CCP, IgM RF, and IgA RF), environmental factors (smoking, educational level), genetics (shared epitope), and disease activity markers. MRI bone edema and anti-CCP levels predicted radiographic progression in the 5-year extension of this study.[81]

Only one study on established RA (mean disease duration, 7 years), reported by Brown and colleagues,[85] demonstrated that MRI bone edema was less predictive of radiographic erosions in comparison with MRI synovitis. However, the investigators did not use T2-weighted or short tau inversion recovery sequences in their MRI protocol to detect bone edema, as recommended by OMERACT, which may have influenced the results.

MONITORING OF RA

The early course of RA is well depicted by MRI because both subchondral edema and synovitis are clearly characterized using this technique (**Fig. 4**). Recent studies have

Table 2
Studies evaluating the utility of MRI in predicting structural deterioration in early RA

Study	Number of Subjects	Study Duration (y)	Technique Assessing Structural Deterioration
Savnik et al,[77] 2002	22 early, 22 late RA	1	MRI
McQueen et al,[78] 2003	42 early RA	6	Radiography
Tanaka et al,[79] 2005	114 early RA	10	Radiography
Palosaari et al,[67] 2006	27 early RA	2	MRI
Lindegaard et al,[15] 2006	25 early RA	1	Radiography
Haavardsholm et al,[66] 2008	84 early RA	1	Radiography and MRI
Mundwiler et al,[80] 2009	50 early RA (<5 y)	1	Radiography
Hetland et al,[81] 2010	139 early RA	5	Radiography
Boyesen et al,[82] 2011	84 early RA	1	MRI
Boyesen et al,[83] 2011	55 early RA	5	Radiography

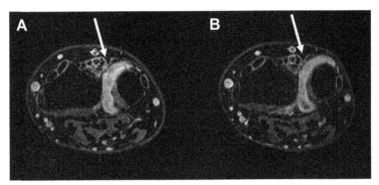

Fig. 4. The same patient as in **Fig. 2** treated with MTX. Postcontrast axial T1-weighted magnetic resonance images of the radioulnar joint at baseline (*A*) and 5 months later (*B*). Mild improvement in the synovitis and joint effusion is noticed (*arrow*).

shown the important role of early bone injury in determining both progression and long-term functionality in RA. Subchondral edema cannot be assessed on clinical examination, and reproducibility of the clinical examination to determine synovial inflammation is relatively low in comparison with ultrasonography and MRI.[86]

Ejbjerg and colleagues[87] compared MRI with radiographic scores, which were applied to different joint combinations. Independent of the number of joints imaged, MRI was superior in detecting progressive joint destruction. Similar results were seen in another study by Olech and colleagues in patients with early RA,[88] adding validity for using MRI as a tool to monitor RA.

In other clinical studies, MRI has been utilized longitudinally in assessing response to therapy. In a 2-year prospective study by Chen and colleagues,[16] 405 patients being aggressively treated for RA were followed up at 8-months intervals with MRI. Lindergaard and colleagues[15] also used MRI in a 1-year follow-up study of patients with early RA who were aggressively treated for RA. Troum and colleagues[89] reported that tocilizumab reduced synovitis within 2 weeks and pre-erosive osteitis within 12 weeks in patients with RA using low-field eMRI.

Subclinical Disease

Structural damage may be ongoing despite alleviation of pain, signs, and symptoms. MRI is a useful technique in assessing subclinical progression of RA, when synovial inflammation, subchondral edema, and nonradiographically identifiable erosions cannot be detected clinically. In a previously referenced study by Brown and colleagues,[90] MRI detected synovitis in 96% and bone marrow edema in 46% of patients with RA in clinical remission. In this group of patients, progression of radiographic joint damage continued in 19% over 1 year despite remaining in remission.[85] Gandjbakhch and colleagues[91] published pooled data from 6 patient cohorts, including 5 international centers (n = 81), confirming this important observation. These patients with RA were classified as being in clinical remission (DAS28-CRP <2.6) or having low disease activity (DAS28-CRP between 2.6 and 3.2). Wrist and/or hand synovitis and marrow edema on MRI were present in 95% and 35% of the patients, respectively.

The definition of remission in RA varies according to the composite measure utilized. With the advent of new more effective therapies for the treatment of RA, the concept of remission currently invokes more stringent criteria. This change is reflected in new provisional definitions of remission developed jointly by the American College of Rheumatology (ACR) and the EULAR.[92] A significant limitation in this new definition of remission is that imaging is not included and residual synovitis may exist in many patients whose disease appears inactive based on clinical examination. The accuracy of more stringent remission criteria for assessing the absence of inflammation was described by Saleem and colleagues[93] using ultrasonography as the gold standard. Despite reduced signs and symptoms of inflammation using these more stringent remission criteria, power Doppler activity persisted in joints with no signs or symptoms; these data suggest that clinical criteria are sufficiently insensitive to accurately detect low but clinically relevant levels of inflammation.

MRI AS AN OUTCOME MEASURE IN EARLY RA CLINICAL TRIALS

Although conventional radiography is still the only approved and most widely used imaging tool for monitoring RA progression, MRI offers clear advantages and is increasingly used in clinical trials on RA.[94] This imagining technique assesses structural joint damage (phase III/IV RA trials), evaluates a new compound's anti-inflammatory efficacy and its impact on pre-erosive lesions (proof-of-concept phase I/II studies), and aids in the diagnosis/prognosis of study subjects. As opposed to radiographic outcomes, multiple randomized clinical trials, including studies on early RA, have used MRI to demonstrate efficacy of various RA therapies in a shorter time frame using fewer subjects (**Table 3**).

Conaghan and colleagues[95] published the first randomized therapeutic trial using MRI as an outcome measure in early RA. MRI was used to monitor synovitis and erosions in patients randomized to MTX versus MTX plus intra-articular corticosteroids. Reduced MRI synovitis scores and significantly fewer joints with new erosions were found in the combination arm in comparison with MTX monotherapy. Quinn and colleagues[96] assessed efficacy of very early treatment of RA with infliximab added to MTX; synovitis and erosions detected on MRI were reduced significantly by this combination at 1 year in comparison with MTX monotherapy. Durez and colleagues[97] compared MTX, infliximab, and methylprednisolone in early RA (<1 year) using MRI and found significant differences between arms in synovitis, bone edema, and

Table 3
Published randomized clinical trials using MRI as an outcome measure in early RA

Study	Number of Patients	Therapy	MRI Outcome
Conaghan et al,[95] 2003	40	MTX/intra-articular corticosteroids vs MTX alone	Synovitis & number of joints with new erosions in 3 mo
Quinn et al,[96] 2005	20	Infliximab/MTX vs placebo/MTX	Synovitis & bone edema at 14 wk, new erosions at 24 wk
Durez et al,[97] 2007	44	MTX/methylprednisolone vs MTX/infliximab vs MTX alone	Synovitis & bone edema at wk 18
Emery et al,[98] 2010	56	Placebo vs abatacept	Synovitis, osteitis, erosions at 6 & 12 mo
Østergaard et al,[99] 2011	318	MTX/golimumab vs MTX alone	Synovitis, osteitis, erosions at 12 & 24 wk

erosions. Abatacept has been studied in 56 anti-CCP–positive patients with undifferentiated or very early RA. Active treatment per protocol was discontinued at 6 months. Beneficial effects demonstrated by hand/wrist RAMRIS synovitis, erosion, and osteitis scores persisted for 1 year in the abatacept group, providing evidence that early T-cell modulation may favorably alter the course of RA.[98] An MRI substudy of the GO-BEFORE trial evaluated MTX-naive patients with RA randomized to MTX monotherapy or a combination of MTX with golimumab. Serial measurements of synovitis, bone edema/osteitis, and bone erosion were obtained using the RAMRIS system. MRI revealed reductions in synovitis, osteitis, and bone erosion at week 12 and onward in patients receiving golimumab plus MTX in comparison with those receiving MTX monotherapy. MRI confirmed clinical and radiographic findings reported for the overall study population with less than half the follow-up time and half the number of patients.[99] There are also several early RA MRI studies currently ongoing, and an interest in incorporating this imaging technique into RA clinical trials has been rapidly increasing.

SUMMARY

Early diagnosis and treatment have been recognized as essential for improving clinical outcomes in patients with early RA. MRI is a sensitive modality that can assess both inflammatory and structural lesions. It is increasingly being utilized in assessing early RA due to its capacity to help identify the key pathologic features of this disease. MRI has demonstrated greater sensitivity for detecting synovitis and erosions than both clinical examination and conventional radiography and can help establish an early diagnosis of RA. In addition, it may assist in differentiating RA from subsets of peripheral spondyloarthropathies by detecting enthesitis. Unique to MRI is the ability to demonstrate bone marrow edema, a marker of active inflammation and the best predictor for developing erosions in early RA.

MRI can assist in following the disease course in patients treated with traditional DMARDs and biological therapies both in the clinic and in research trials. Therefore, it is expected that MRI becomes the diagnostic imaging modality of choice in RA clinical trials while remaining a useful tool for clinicians evaluating patients with RA.

REFERENCES

1. van der Heijde DM. Joint erosions and patients with early rheumatoid arthritis. Br J Rheumatol 1995;34(Suppl 2):74–8.
2. Sundy JS, Clair EW. Early DMARD therapy for RA: primary care physicians play a major role in diagnosis and follow-up. J Musculoskel Med 2002;19:395–403.
3. Lindqvist E, Jonsson K, Saxne T, et al. Course of radiographic damage over 10 years in a cohort with early rheumatoid arthritis. Ann Rheum Dis 2003;62:611–6.
4. Lard LR, Visser H, Speyer I, et al. Early versus delayed treatment in patients with recent-onset rheumatoid arthritis: comparison of two cohorts who received different treatment strategies. Am J Med 2001;111(6):446–51.
5. Finckh A, Choi H, Wolfe F. Progression of radiographic joint damage in different eras: trends towards milder disease in rheumatoid arthritis are attributable to improved treatment. Ann Rheum Dis 2006;65(9):1192–7.
6. Bathon JM, Martin RW, Fleischmann RM, et al. A comparison of etanercept and methotrexate in patients with early rheumatoid arthritis. N Engl J Med 2000; 343:1586–93.

7. Nell VP, Machold KP, Eberl G, et al. Benefit of very early referral and very early therapy with disease modifying antirheumatic drugs in patients with early rheumatoid arthritis. Rheumatology 2004;43:906–14.
8. Combe B, Landewe R, Lukas C, et al. EULAR recommendation for the management of early arthritis: report of a task force of the European Standing Committee for International Clinical Studies Including Therapeutics (ESCISIT). Ann Rheum Dis 2007;66(1):34–45.
9. American College of Rheumatology Subcommittee on Rheumatoid Arthritis Guidelines. Guidelines for the management of rheumatoid arthritis: 2002 update. Arthritis Rheum 2002;46(2):328–46.
10. Gilkeson G, Polisson R, Sinclair H, et al. Early detections of carpal erosions in patients with rheumatoid arthritis: a pilot study of magnetic resonance imaging. J Rheumatol 1988;15:1361–6.
11. Boesen M, Ostergaard M, Cimmino MA, et al. MRI quantification of rheumatoid arthritis: current knowledge and future perspectives. Eur J Radiol 2009;71:189–96.
12. Foley-Nolan D, Stack JP, Ryan M, et al. Magnetic resonance imaging in the assessment of rheumatoid arthritis—a comparison with plain film radiographs. Br J Rheumatol 1991;30:101–6.
13. Jorgensen C, Cyteval C, Anaya JM, et al. Sensitivity of magnetic resonance imaging of the wrist in very early rheumatoid arthritis. Clin Exp Rheumatol 1993;11:163–8.
14. Crues JV, Shellock FG, Dardashti S, et al. Identification of wrist and metacarpophalangeal joint erosions using a portable magnetic resonance imaging system compared to conventional radiographs. J Rheumatol 2004;31:676–85.
15. Lindergaard HM, Vallo J, Horslev-Petersen K, et al. Low-cost, low-field dedicated extremity magnetic resonance imaging in early rheumatoid arthritis: a 1-year follow up study. Ann Rheum Dis 2006;65:1208–12.
16. Chen TS, Crues JV, Ali M, et al. Magnetic resonance imaging is more sensitive than radiographs in detecting change in size of erosions in rheumatoid arthritis. J Rheumatol 2006;33:1957–67.
17. Taouli B, Zaim S, Peterfy CG, et al. Rheumatoid arthritis of the hand and wrist: comparison of three imaging techniques. Am J Roentgenol 2004;182:937–43.
18. Ejbjerg BJ, Narvestad E, Jacobsen S, et al. Optimised, low cost, low field dedicated extremity MRI is highly specific and sensitive for synovitis and bone erosions in rheumatoid arthritis wrist and finger joints: comparison with conventional high field MRI and radiography. Ann Rheum Dis 2005;64(9):1280–7.
19. Savnik A, Malmskov H, Thomsen HS, et al. MRI of the arthritic small joints: comparison of extremity MRI (0.2 T) vs high-field MRI (1.5 T). Eur Radiol 2001; 11(6):1030–8.
20. Schirmer C, Scheel AK, Althoff C, et al. Diagnostic quality and scoring of synovitis, tenosynovitis and erosions in low-field MRI of patients with rheumatoid arthritis: a comparison with conventional MRI. Ann Rheum Dis 2007;66(4):522–9.
21. Bird P, Ejbjerg B, Lassere M, et al. A multireader reliability study comparing conventional high-field magnetic resonance imaging with extremity low-field MRI in rheumatoid arthritis. J Rheumatol 2007;34(4):854–6.
22. Suzuki T, Ito S, Handa S, et al. A new low-field extremity magnetic resonance imaging and proposed compact MRI score: evaluation of anti-tumor necrosis factor biologics on rheumatoid arthritis. Mod Rheumatol 2009;19(4):358–65.
23. Conaghan PG, Ejbjerg B, Lassere M, et al. A multicenter reliability study of extremity-magnetic resonance imaging in the longitudinal evaluation of rheumatoid arthritis. J Rheumatol 2007;34(4):857–8.

24. Duer-Jensen A, Ejbjerg B, Albrecht-Beste E, et al. Does low field dedicated extremity MRI (E-MRI) reliably detect bone erosions in rheumatoid arthritis? A comparison of two different E-MRI units and conventional radiography with high-resolution CT scanning. Ann Rheum Dis 2009;68:1296–302.
25. International Society of Extremity MRI in Rheumatology (ISEMIR) web site. Available at: http://www.isemir.org. Accessed February 14, 2012.
26. Ostergaard M, Peterfy CG, Conaghan P, et al. OMERACT rheumatoid arthritis magnetic resonance imaging studies: Core set of MRI acquisitions, joint pathology definitions, and the OMERACT RA-MRI scoring system. J Rheumatol 2003;30:1385–6.
27. Haavardsholm EA, Ostergaard M, Ejbjerg BJ, et al. Reliability and sensitivity to the change of the OMERACT rheumatoid arthritis magnetic resonance imaging score in a multireader, longitudinal setting. Arthritis Rheum 2005;52(12):3860–7.
28. Ostergaard M, Klarlund M, Lassere M, et al. Interreader agreement in the assessment of magnetic resonance images of rheumatoid arthritis wrist and finger joints – An international multicenter study. J Rheumatol 2001;28:1143–50.
29. Hirose W, Nishikawa K, Hirose M, et al. Response of early active rheumatoid arthritis to tumor necrosis factor inhibitors: evaluation by magnetic resonance imaging. Mod Rheumatol 2009;19:20–6.
30. Ostendorf B, Scherer A, Modder U, et al. Diagnostic value of magnetic resonance imaging of the forefeet in early rheumatoid arthritis when findings on imaging of the metacarpophalangeal joints of the hands remain normal. Arthritis Rheum 2004;50:2094–102.
31. Baan H, Bezooijen R, Avenarius JK, et al. Magnetic resonance imaging of the rheumatic foot according to the RAMRIS system is reliable. J Rheumatol 2011;38:1003–8.
32. Crowley A, Dong J, McHaffie A, et al. Measuring bone erosion and edema in rheumatoid arthritis: a comparison of manual segmentation and RAMRIS methods. J Magn Reson Imaging 2011;33:364–71.
33. Ostergaard M, Stoltenberg M, Lovgreen-Nielsen P, et al. Magnetic resonance imaging-determined synovial membrane and joint effusion volumes in rheumatoid arthritis and osteoarthritis: comparison with the macroscopic and microscopic appearance of the synovium. Arthritis Rheum 1997;40:1856–67.
34. Bird P, Ejbjerg B, McQueen F, et al. OMERACT rheumatoid arthritis magnetic resonance imaging studies. Exercise 5: an international multicenter reliability study using computerized MRI erosion volume measurements. J Rheumatol 2003;30:1380–4.
35. Chand AS, McHaffie A, Clarke AW, et al. Quantifying synovitis in rheumatic arthritis using computer-assisted manual segmentation with 3 Tesla MRI scanning. J Magn Reson Imaging 2011;33:1106–11.
36. Cyteval C, Miquel A, Hoa D, et al. Rheumatoid Arthrtis of the hand: Monitoring with a simplied imaging scoring method- preliminary assessment. Radiology 2010;256(3):863–9.
37. Bliddal H, Boesen M, Christensen R, et al. Imaging as a follow-up tool in clinical trials and clinical practice. Best Pract Res Clin Rheumatol 2008;22(6):1109–26.
38. Chang J, Crues JV, Troum O. MRI in rheumatoid arthritis: Why start using it now? A review of imaging modalities, MR scoring, and pathophysiology in RA. Contemporary Topics in Rheumatoid Arthritis 2009;3(4):2–9.
39. Cimmino MA, Innocenti S, Livrone F, et al. Dynamic gadolinium-enhanced magnetic resonance imaging of the wrist in patients with rheumatoid arthritis can discriminate active from inactive disease. Arthritis Rheum 2003;48(5):1207–13.

40. Hermann KG, Backhaus M, Schneider U, et al. Rheumatoid arthritis of the shoulder joint: comparison of conventional radiography, ultrasound, and dynamic contrast-enhanced magnetic resonance imaging. Arthritis Rheum 2003;48(12): 3338–49.

41. Huang J, Stewart N, Crabbe J, et al. A 1-year follow up study of dynamic magnetic resonance imaging in early rheumatoid arthritis reveals synovitis to be increased in shared-epitope patients and predictive of erosions at 1-year. Rheumatology 2000;39:407–16.

42. Veale DJ, Reece RJ, Parsons W, et al. Intra-articular primatised anti-CD4: efficacy in resistant rheumatoid knee. A study of combined arthroscopy, magnetic resonance imaging, and histology. Ann Rheum Dis 1999;58(6):342–9.

43. Reece RJ, Kraan MC, Radjenovic A, et al. Comparative assessment of leflunomide and methotrexate for the treatment of rheumatoid arthritis, by dynamic enhanced magnetic resonance imaging. Arthritis Rheum 2002;46(2): 366–72.

44. Ostendorf B, Peters R, Dann P, et al. Magnetic Resonance Imaging and Miniarthroscopy of metacarpophalangeal joints: sensitive detection of morphologic changes in rheumatoid arthritis. Arthritis Rheum 2001;44(11):2492–502.

45. Vasanth LC, Foo LF, Potter HG, et al. Using magnetic resonance angiography to measure abnormal synovial blood vessels in early inflammatory arthritis: a new imaging biomarker? J Rheumatol 2010;37(6):1129–35.

46. Jimenez-Boj E, Nobauer-Huhmann I, Hanslik-Schnabel B, et al. Bone erosions and bone marrow edema as defined by magnetic resonance imaging reflect true bone marrow inflammation in rheumatoid arthritis. Arthritis Rheum 2007;56(4): 1118–24.

47. McQueen F, Gao A, Ostergaard M, et al. High-grade MRI bone edema is common within the surgical field in rheumatoid arthritis patients undergoing joint replacement and is associated with osteitis in subchondral bone. Ann Rheum Dis 2007;66(12):1581–7.

48. Dalbeth N, Smith T, Gray S, et al. Cellular characterization of magnetic resonance imaging bone edema in rheumatoid arthritis; implications for pathogenesis of erosive disease. Ann Rheum Dis 2009;68:279–82.

49. Konig H, Sieper J, Wolf KJ. Rheumatoid arthritis: evaluation by hypervascular and fibrous pannus with dynamic MR imaging enhanced with Gd-DTPA. Radiology 1990;176:473–7.

50. Dohn UM, Ostergaard M, Bird P, et al. Tendency towards erosive regression on magnetic resonance imaging at 12 months in rheumatoid arthritis patients treated with rituximab. Ann Rheum Dis 2009;68:1072–3.

51. Perry D, Stewart N, Benton N, et al. Detection of erosions in the rheumatoid hand; a comparative study of multidetector computerized tomography versus magnetic resonance scanning. J Rheumatol 2005;32:256–67.

52. Dohn UM, Ejbjerg BJ, Hasselquist M, et al. Detection of bone erosions in rheumatoid arthritis wrist joints with magnetic resonance imaging, computed tomography and radiography. Arthritis Res Ther 2008;10(1):R25.

53. Dohn UM, Ejbjerg B, Court-Payen M, et al. Are bone erosions detected by magnetic resonance imaging and ultrasound true erosions? A comparison with computed tomography in rheumatoid arthritis metacarpophalangeal joints. Arthritis Res Ther 2006;8:R110.

54. McQueen F, Clarke A, McHaffie A, et al. Assessment of cartilage loss at the wrist in rheumatoid arthritis using a new MRI scoring system. Ann Rheum Dis 2010; 69(11):1971–5.

55. Conaghan PG, McQueen FM, Bird P, et al. Update on research and future directions of the OMERACT MRI inflammatory arthritis group. J Rheumatol 2011;38(9): 2031–3.

56. Ostergaard M, Bøyesen P, Eshed I, et al. Development and preliminary validation of a magnetic resonance imaging joint space narrowing score for use in rheumatoid arthritis: potential adjunct to the OMERACT RA MRI scoring system. J Rheumatol 2011;38(9):2045–50.

57. Buchbender C, Scherer A, Kröpil P, et al. Cartilage quality in rheumatoid arthritis: comparison of T2* mapping, native T1 mapping, dGEMRIC, ΔR1 and value of pre-contrast imaging. Skeletal Radiol 2012;41(6):685–92.

58. Sugimoto H, Takeda A, Kyodoh K. Early-stage rheumatoid arthritis: prospective study of the effectiveness of MR imaging for diagnosis. Radiology 2000;216: 569–75.

59. Narváez J, Sirvent E, Narváez JA, et al. Usefulness of magnetic resonance imaging of the hand versus anticyclic citrullinated peptide antibody testing to confirm the diagnosis of clinically suspected early rheumatoid arthritis in the absence of rheumatoid factor and radiographic erosions. Semin Arthritis Rheum 2008;38(2):101–9.

60. McQueen FM, Stewart N, Crabbe J, et al. Magnetic resonance imaging of the wrist in early rheumatoid arthritis reveals a high prevalence of erosions at four months after symptom onset. Ann Rheum Dis 1998;57:350–6.

61. Albers JM, Paimela L, Kurki P, et al. Treatment strategy, disease activity, and outcome in four cohorts of patients with early rheumatoid arthritis. Ann Rheum Dis 2001;60:453–8.

62. Wakefield RJ, Gibbon WW, Conaghan PG, et al. The value of sonography in the detection of bone erosions in patients with rheumatoid arthritis: a comparison with conventional radiography. Arthritis Rheum 2000;43:2762–70.

63. Ejbjerg BJ, Vertergaard A, Jacobsen S, et al. Conventional radiography requires a MRI-estimated bone volume loss of 20% to 30% to allow certain detection of bone erosions in rheumatoid arthritis metacarpophalangeal joints. Arthritis Res Ther 2006;8:R59.

64. Kainberger F, Trattnig S, Czerny C, et al. MRI in assessment of the systemic manifestations of rheumatological disease. Br J Rheumatol 1996;35(Suppl 3): 40–4.

65. Eshed I, Feist E, Althoff CE, et al. Tenosynovitis of the flexor tendons of the hand detected by MRI: an early indicator of rheumatoid arthritis. Rheumatology 2009; 48:887–91.

66. Haavardsholm E, Boyesen P, Ostergaard M, et al. Magnetic resonance imaging findings in 84 patients with early rheumatoid arthritis: bone marrow edema predicts erosive progression. Ann Rheum Dis 2008;67:794–800.

67. Palosaari K, Vuotila J, Takalo R, et al. Bone edema predicts erosive progression on wrist MRI in early RA - A 2-year observational MRi and NC scintigraphy study. Rheumatology 2006;45(12):1542–8.

68. Olech E, Crues JV 3rd, Yocum DE, et al. Bone marrow edema is the most specific finding for rheumatoid arthritis (RA) on noncontrast magnetic resonance imaging of the hands and wrists: a comparison of patients with RA and healthy controls. J Rheumatol 2010;37(2):265–74.

69. Tamai M, Kawakami A, Uetani M, et al. A prediction rule for disease outcome in patients with undifferentiated arthritis using magnetic resonance imaging of the wrists and finger joints and serologic autoantibodies. Arthritis Rheum 2009; 61(6):772–8.

70. Duer-Jensen A, Hørslev-Petersen K, Hetland ML, et al. Bone edema on magnetic resonance imaging is an independent predictor of rheumatoid arthritis development in patients with early undifferentiated arthritis. Arthritis Rheum 2011;63(8): 2192–202.

71. Schoellnast H, Deutschmann HA, Hermann J, et al. Psoriatic arthritis and rheumatoid arthritis: findings in contrast-enhanced MRI. AJR Am J Roentgenol 2006; 187(2):351–7.

72. Mrabet D, Mizouni H, Charfi O, et al. Usefulness of magnetic resonance imaging in the diagnosis of early rheumatoid arthritis: a prospective study about 20 cases. Tunis Med 2012;90(2):154–60.

73. Kosta PE, Voulgari PV, Zikou AK, et al. The usefulness of magnetic resonance imaging of the hand and wrist in very early rheumatoid arthritis. Arthritis Res Ther 2011;13(3):R84.

74. Suter LG, Fraenkel L, Braithwaite RS. Role of magnetic resonance imaging in the diagnosis and prognosis of rheumatoid arthritis. Arthritis Care Res (Hoboken) 2011;63(5):675–88.

75. Aletaha D, Neogi T, Silman AJ, et al. 2010 Rheumatoid arthritis classification criteria: an American College of Rheumatology/European League Against Rheumatism collaborative initiative. Ann Rheum Dis 2010;69:1580–8.

76. Aletaha D, Hawker G, Neogi T, et al. Re: Clarification of the role of ultrasonography, magnetic resonance imaging and conventional radiography in the ACR/EULAR 2010 rheumatoidarthritis classification criteria—comment to the article by Aletaha, et al. Ann Rheum Dis 2011 [E-letter published online January 11].

77. Savnik A, Malmskov H, Thomsen HS, et al. MRI of the wrist and finger joints in inflammatory joint diseases at 1-year interval: MRI features to predict bone erosions. Eur Radiol 2002;12(5):1203–10.

78. McQueen FM, Benton N, Perry D, et al. Bone edema scored on magnetic resonance imaging scans of the dominant carpus at presentation predicts radiographic joint damage of the hands and feet six years later in patients with rheumatoid arthritis. Arthritis Rheum 2003;48(7):1814–27.

79. Tanaka N, Sakahashi H, Ishii S, et al. Synovial membrane enhancement and bone erosion by magnetic resonance imaging for prediction of radiologic progression in patients with early rheumatoid arthritis. Rheumatol Int 2005;25(2): 103–7.

80. Mundwiler M, Maranian P, Brown DH, et al. The utility of MRI in predicting radiographic erosions in the metatarsophalangeal joints of the rheumatoid foot: a prospective longitudinal cohort study. Arthritis Res Ther 2009;11:R94.

81. Hetland ML, Stengaard-Pedersen K, Junker P, et al. Radiographic progression and remission rates in early rheumatoid arthritis – MRI bone edema and anti-CCP predicted radiographic progression in the 5-year extension of the double blind randomized CIMESTRA trial. Ann Rheum Dis 2010;69:1789–95.

82. Bøyesen P, Haavardsholm EA, van der Heijde D, et al. Prediction of MRI erosive progression: a comparison of modern imaging modalities in early rheumatoid arthritis patients. Ann Rheum Dis 2011;70(1):176–9.

83. Boyesen P, Haavardsholm EA, Ostergaard M, et al. MRI in early rheumatoid arthritis: synovitis and bone marrow edema are independent predictors of subsequent radiographic progression. Ann Rheum Dis 2011;70:428–33.

84. Hetland ML, Ejbjergb B, Horslev-Petersen K, et al. MRI bone edema is the strongest predictor of subsequent radiographic progression in early rheumatoid arthritis: results from a 2-year randomized controlled trial (CIMESTRA). Ann Rheum Dis 2009;68:384–90.

85. Brown AK, Conaghan PG, Karim Z, et al. An explanation for the apparent disso-ciation between clinical remission and continued structural deterioration in rheu-matoid arthritis. Arthritis Rheum 2008;58(10):2958–67.
86. Naredo E, Moller I, Moragues C, et al. Interobserver reliability in musculoskeletal ultrasonography: results from a "Tech the teachers" rheumatologist course. Ann Rheum Dis 2006;65(1):14–9.
87. Ejbjerg BJ, Vestergaard A, Jacobsen S, et al. The smallest detectable difference and sensitivity to change of magnetic resonance imaging and radiographic scoring of structural joint damage in rheumatoid arthritis finger, wrist, and toe joints: a comparison of the OMERACT rheumatoid arthritis magnetic resonance imaging score applied to different joint combinations and the Sharp/van der Heijde radiographic score. Arthritis Rheum 2005;52(8):2300–6.
88. Olech E, Freeston JE, Conaghan PG, et al. Using extremity magnetic resonance imaging to assess and monitor early rheumatoid arthritis: the optimal joint combi-nation to be scanned in clinical practice. J Rheumatol 2008;35(4):580–3.
89. Troum O, Peterfy C, Kaine J, et al. Tocilizumab reduces synovitis within 2 weeks and pre-erosive osteitis within 12 weeks in patients with RA: results from a multi-site low-field MRI study. Ann Rheum Dis 2010;69(Suppl 3):98.
90. Brown AK, Quinn MA, Karim Z, et al. Presence of significant synovitis in rheuma-toid arthritis patients with disease modifying antirheumatic drug-induced clinical remission. Arthritis Rheum 2006;54:3761–73.
91. Gandjbakhch F, Conaghan PG, Ejbjerg B, et al. Synovitis and osteitis are very frequent in rheumatoid arthritis clinical remission: results from an MRI study of 294 patients in clinical remission or low disease activity state. J Rheumatol 2011;38(9):2039–44.
92. Felson DT, Smolen JS, Wells G, et al. American College of Rheumatology/Euro-pean League against Rheumatism provisional definition of remission in rheuma-toid arthritis for clinical trials. Ann Rheum Dis 2011;70(3):404–13.
93. Saleem B, Brown AK, Keen H, et al. Should imaging be a component of rheuma-toid arthritis remission criteria? A comparison between traditional and modified composite remission scores and imaging assessments. Ann Rheum Dis 2011; 70(5):792–8.
94. Olech E. MRI in rheumatoid arthritis clinical trials: expensive imaging techniques may ultimately save money. Expert Rev Clin Pharmacol 2009;2(5):443–7.
95. Conaghan PG, O'Connor P, McGonagle D, et al. Elucidation of the relationship between synovitis and bone damage: a randomized magnetic resonance imaging study of individual joints in patients with early rheumatoid arthritis. Arthritis Rheum 2003;48:64–71.
96. Quinn MA, Conaghan PG, O'Connor PJ, et al. Very early treatment with inflix-imab in addition to methotrexate in early, poor-prognosis rheumatoid arthritis reduces magnetic resonance imaging evidence of synovitis and damage, with sustained benefit after infliximab withdrawal: results from a twelve-month randomized, double-blind, placebo-controlled trial. Arthritis Rheum 2005;52: 27–35.
97. Durez P, Malghem J, Nzeusseu Toukap A, et al. Treatment of early rheumatoid arthritis: a randomized magnetic resonance imaging study comparing the effects of methotrexate alone, methotrexate in combination with infliximab, and metho-trexate in combination with intravenous pulse methylprednisolone. Arthritis Rheum 2007;56:3919–27.
98. Emery P, Durez P, Dougados M, et al. Impact of T-cell costimulation modulation in patients with undifferentiated inflammatory arthritis or very early rheumatoid

arthritis: a clinical and imaging study of abatacept (the ADJUST trial). Ann Rheum Dis 2010;69(3):510–6.
99. Østergaard M, Emery P, Conaghan PG, et al. Significant improvement in synovitis, osteitis, and bone erosion following golimumab and methotrexate combination therapy as compared with methotrexate alone: a magnetic resonance imaging study of 318 methotrexate-naive rheumatoid arthritis patients. Arthritis Rheum 2011;63(12):3712–22.

Disease Activity Assessment and Patient-Reported Outcomes in Patients with Early Rheumatoid Arthritis

Tuulikki Sokka, MD, PhD[a], Tuomas Rannio, MD[a],
Nasim A. Khan, MD[b],*

KEYWORDS

- Arthritis • Rheumatoid • Disease activity • Clinical evaluation
- Outcomes

Key Points

- Objective rheumatoid arthritis (RA) disease activity assessment and target to treatment strategy are crucial to improve outcomes for patients with RA, with benefits particularly pronounced for patients with early RA.
- The purpose of RA assessment is to achieve a rapid and continuous remission in all patients with RA and to improve quality of life and long-term outcomes of these patients.
- Hurdles for the implementation of routine clinical assessment are many, and they must be recognized and overcome.
- Inexpensive, easy-to-use electronic devices have been developed to monitor RA disease activity as part of routine clinical care.
- Extensive clinical assessment including laboratory, doctor-performed, and patient self-reported measures should be the right of every patient with RA anywhere in the world.

Statement acknowledging funding support: Academy of Finland.
Financial disclosure: The authors have nothing to disclose.
[a] Department of Rheumatology, Jyväskylä Central Hospital, Keskussairaalantie 19, 40620 Jyväskylä, Finland; [b] Division of Rheumatology, Department of Internal Medicine, University of Arkansas for Medical Sciences and Central Arkansas Veterans Healthcare System, Little Rock, AR, USA
* Corresponding author. University of Arkansas for Medical Sciences, 4301 West Markham Street, # 509, Little Rock, AR 72205.
E-mail address: nakhan@uams.edu

Rheum Dis Clin N Am 38 (2012) 299–310
doi:10.1016/j.rdc.2012.04.005
0889-857X/12/$ – see front matter Published by Elsevier Inc.

INTRODUCTION

Objective assessment of disease activity is recommended in the current clinical practice guidelines and treatment recommendations for rheumatoid arthritis (RA).[1,2] This is in contrast to common practice 30 years ago, which was described by Dr Wright as "clinicians may all too easily spend years writing 'doing well' in the notes of a patient who has become progressively crippled before their eyes ...."[3]

Last 30 years have provided new insights to RA management. It was recognized that most patients with early RA had a progressive disease with joint damage, disability, and early death.[4] Evidence from variety of clinical studies have shown that disease-modifying antirheumatic drugs (DMARDs) have to be used more early, aggressively, continuously, and often in combinations to improve outcomes.[5,6] New potent biologic treatments came to market. A treatment target and routine clinical monitoring to reach that target were found to be crucial for better outcomes.[7]

The evidence for the benefits of objective disease activity assessment and target to treatment strategy to improve functional and structural outcomes is particularly pronounced for patients with early RA.[8] Moreover, good treatment response early in the disease predicts improved long-term outcomes. Disease activity at the baseline, and especially after 3 months, is significantly related to disease activity at 1 year.[9] Achieving remission early in the disease provides sustained reduction in radiographic progression.[10] Failure to achieve low disease activity 3 months after the diagnosis of early RA, as assessed by Disease Activity Score based on 28 joint assessment (DAS28), was found to be associated with high direct and indirect costs over the following 4 years.[11]

Ingredients to reach good clinical outcomes of RA exist. However, data from real life settings indicate that most patients with RA have an active disease, especially in countries with low gross domestic product,[12] and many still become work disabled during the first year of the disease.[13] Traditions rather than data influence treatment decisions.[14] Most of the usual clinical rheumatology care is based on the physicians' impressions rather than quantitative measures.[15]

CHALLENGES OF CLINICAL MEASURES OF RA DISEASE ACTIVITY AND PATIENT-REPORTED OUTCOMES
No Single Gold Standard

Quantitative clinical monitoring of musculoskeletal conditions and inflammatory joint diseases is challenging compared with the quantitative monitoring of conditions, such as hypertension or hyperlipidemia, for which single measures can be used as an indicator of disease status and change. A single gold standard for patient assessment, which can be used to assess all individual patients in clinical trials, clinical research, and clinical care is not available for any rheumatic disease, and hence, different types of measures are used in assessment of patients with rheumatic diseases. Because no individual measure reflects RA activity in a valid and reliable fashion, composite indices, derived from multiple individual variables, have been developed for RA activity assessment. The commonly used indices for RA activity assessment are summarized in **Table 1**, with each index described in greater details elsewhere.[16–21] Traditional measures to assess RA, such as joint assessment, laboratory tests, imaging, and patient-reported outcomes (PROs) have limitations and provide only a reflection of the underlying inflammatory process.

CHALLENGES IN PHYSICIAN MEASURES: JOINT ASSESSMENT

A careful joint examination is required to establish a diagnosis of RA, and a count of swollen and tender joints is the most specific quantitative clinical measures for RA

Table 1
Commonly used composite indices for rheumatoid arthritis (RA) disease activity assessment

Index	Formula	Range	RA Activity State			
			Remission	Low	Moderate	High
DAS28[a]	$0.56 \times \sqrt{(TJC28)} + 0.28 \times \sqrt{(SJC28)} + 0.70 \times \ln(ESR) + 0.014 \times GH$	0–9.4	<2.6	2.6 to ≤3.2	>3.2 to ≤5.1	>5.1
SDAI[b,c]	TJC28 + SJC28 + CRP + MDGL + PTGL	0.1–86	≤3.3	>3.3 to <11	>11 to ≤26	>26
CDAI[c]	TJC28 + SJC28 + MDGL + PTGL	0–76	≤2.8	>2.8 to ≤10	>10 to ≤22	>22
RAPID3[c]	MDHAQ × 3.3 + Pain + PTGL	0–30	<3	3 to <6	>6 to ≤12	>12
PASII[c]	(HAQII × 3.3 + Pain + PTGL)/10	0–10	≤1	>1 to 1.9	>1.9 and ≤5.3	>5.3
RADAI[d]	components and calculation[e]	0–10	–	<2.2	≥2.2 to ≤4.9	>4.9

Abbreviations: CRP, C-reactive protein; CDAI, clinical disease activity index; ESR, erythrocyte sedimentation rate; GH, patient's assessment of general health; HAQII, health assessment questionnaire II; MDGL, physician's global assessment of disease activity; MDHAQ, multidimensional health assessment questionnaire; PTGL, patient's global assessment of disease activity; PASII, patient activity score II; RAPID3, routine assessment of patient index data 3; RADAI, rheumatoid arthritis disease activity index; SJC28, swollen joint count on 28 joint evaluation; SDAI, simplified disease activity index; TJC28, tender joint count on 28 joint evaluation.

[a] GH rating is scored on a 0 to 100 scale.

[b] CRP in mg/dl.

[c] PTGL rating is scored on a 0 to 10 scale.

[d] No values of remission reported for RADAI.

[e] RADAI has 5 components: current disease activity with respect to joint tenderness and swelling; arthritis pain; global disease activity in the last 6 months; morning stiffness (scored as 0 = none, 1 = <30 minutes, 2 = 30 minutes to 1 hour, 3 = 1–2 hours, 4 = 2–4 hours, 5 = >4 hours, and 6 = all day); and joint list score (16 joint or joint groups scored from 0 indicating no pain to 3 indicating severe pain). All 5 components are calculated or transformed to a 0 to 10 scale, and sum of all component scores is divided by 5 to get the RADAI score.

patient assessment.[22] Several limitations of the joint count have been described as summarized below and described in greater detail elsewhere.[23]

Joint counts are poorly reproducible in formal studies.[24,25] Variations in the results of joint count can be reduced by training rheumatologists or other assessors to standardize scores.[26] Nonetheless, all protocols for clinical trials and other clinical research studies in RA require that a joint count must be performed by the same observer at each assessment. The need for the same person to perform each joint count of a given patient presents a considerable limitation to the use of joint counts as rigorous indicators of a need for changes in therapy, responses to therapy, or to document quality of care. Possible collaborative care between rheumatologists and family practitioners or other health professionals to manage patients is limited by a requirement for the same observer because joint counts by different observers cannot be compared reliably.

In clinical trials, patients who receive placebo or control treatments almost always show improvement in swollen and tender joint counts as great as or greater than in other disease activity measures.[27] Furthermore, several studies indicate that formal swollen and tender joint counts are not as sensitive as ultrasonography or magnetic resonance imaging to detect synovitis.[28]

CHALLENGES IN THE USE OF LABORATORY TESTS

The discovery of rheumatoid factor in 1940s[29] led to hopes that laboratory tests could serve as gold standard measures in rheumatic diseases. In many diseases, laboratory tests provide the most definitive information in diagnosis, management, prognosis, and documentation of course of the disease. According to a biomedical model, laboratory test results are often seen as the most important information from a rheumatology visit.

Erythrocyte Sedimentation Rate and C-Reactive Protein Are Not Specific for RA

Many patients with RA have an elevated erythrocyte sedimentation rate (ESR) and C-reactive protein (CRP) although ESR and CRP are normal in about 40% of patients with RA.[30] Moreover, many patients with active RA have normal ESR/CRP, whereas many with inactive disease have abnormal values.[31] Mean ESR levels in RA cohorts with baseline have declined from 50 mm/h in 1954 to 1980 to 41 mm/h in 1981 to 1984 to 35 mm/h after 1985.[32] Comorbidities are common in patients with RA, including comorbidities with elevated laboratory markers for inflammation.[33] Furthermore, higher ESR levels are considered normal in women than men, especially in older age groups.[34]

Different Methods to Measure ESR and CRP Challenge Comparison of Patient Status Across Clinics

ESR is traditionally measured according to the Westergren method, which has been replaced in some laboratories with more modern methods. In some clinics, CRP has replaced ESR for RA assessment. Despite attempts at standardization, there remains heterogeneity in measurement methods, normal range at local laboratories and reporting methods for CRP. This introduces challenges in the calculation of disease activity indices. In the Quantitative Standard Monitoring of Patients with RA (QUEST-RA) study, which has recruited more than 9000 patients from 34 countries, 45 different ways of CRP reporting (normal range or measurement units) were noted, making any comparative assessment difficult (Nasim A. Khan, MD, unpublished observation, 2011).

Laboratory research is essential to provide new insights into pathogenesis and new treatments for rheumatic diseases. However, in usual clinical care, laboratory tests often have limited specificity and sensitivity, with high levels of false-positive and -negative results. Physicians and patients may attribute disproportionate importance to laboratory tests in rheumatic diseases.

CHALLENGES OF PATIENT SELF-REPORTED MEASURES

Patient self-report has become prominent in rheumatology assessment because the patient himself or herself is the only source for information concerning functional capacity, pain, patient's global assessment of disease activity (PTGL), patient's assessment of general health (GH), fatigue, psychological distress, and so forth. The health assessment questionnaire (HAQ) is the most commonly used tool for assessing physical function.[35] Several modifications have been developed, such as a multidimensional HAQ, which also includes 4 psychological items.[36] Pain, PTGL, GH, and fatigue are generally assessed on a 10-cm visual analog scale. Patient questionnaires concerning functional status provide the most significant prognostic clinical measure for all important long-term outcomes of RA, including functional status,[4,37] work disability,[13,38] costs,[39] joint replacement surgery,[40] and premature death.[4,41]

In RA, inflammation of joints and other systems affects patient functional status and causes pain, fatigue, and other symptoms, which improve or resolve as inflammation responds to treatments. Therefore, PROs perform well as measures of disease activity. However, several aspects need to be taken into account in the interpretation of PROs as RA disease activity measures.

Patient Questionnaires Are Not Specific to the Degree of Inflammatory Activity

A patient's pain score might improve or decline considerably because of developments other than direct changes in inflammatory status, for example, a score might improve based on good news, but could be higher (more pain) as a result of negative life events. Non-RA–related characteristics such as self-efficacy and learned helplessness also affect patient's perception of disease.[42] Furthermore, polymorphisms in genes involved in symptom modulation, such as pain, strongly affect its perception.[43]

There Are No Universal Normative Values for PROs

Patient questionnaires can be subject to cultural and linguistic differences. Older people generally have more symptoms than younger people. Furthermore, throughout the history of the HAQ, women have been found to report poorer scores than men,[44,45] which is understandable because women have lesser strength than men,[46] which has a major effect on the functional status of patients with RA and in a healthy population.[47]

CHALLENGES TO IMPLEMENT RA DISEASE ACTIVITY ASSESSMENT AND PROs IN CLINICAL CARE

Many clinicians have suggested that it is not possible to acquire outcomes data in usual rheumatology clinical care. Over the decades, many programs have been established, to collect outcomes data in collaborative clinics, but these efforts have faded away because data collection was unpaid extra work and responsibility was laid on treating rheumatologists. Therefore, solutions to acquire outcomes data on patients with RA include direct communication between a research center and patients, as exemplified by the National Data Bank for Rheumatic Disease by Wolfe and Michaud.[48]

A program called QUEST-RA was established in 2005 to promote quantitative assessment in usual rheumatology care and to develop a cross-sectional database of consecutive patients with RA seen outside of clinical trials in regular care in many countries. Three or more rheumatologists were asked to enroll 100 consecutive unselected patients in each country.[49] This program represents an important accomplishment with numerous interesting observations published but is limited thus far to a cross-sectional database. It seemed that data were collected primarily for the purpose of a collaborative database. There are doubts whether QUEST-RA reached its goal to introduce routine data collection as part of usual clinical practice to clinics in which routine data collection was not a standard already.

CHALLENGES OF MOTIVATION

Research can serve as motivation for data collection for some time. Internal assessment of quality of care or treatment outcomes may motivate in some circumstances. However, the only universal motivation comes from health care payers or other official agencies, which may set requirements for collection of quality measures and outcomes.

The Institute of Medicine defines quality as the "degree to which health services for individuals and populations increase the likelihood of desired health outcomes and are consistent with current professional knowledge."[50] In some countries, attention has been paid to quality indicators and ways of compensating physicians accordingly. In 2006, the US Congress established G codes—quality indicators that physicians must meet to receive increased Medicare payments. In most countries, regulations for quality indicators have not been implemented and compensation for health services is not related to quality of care or achieved health outcomes.

CHALLENGES OF RESOURCES

Some of the complexities of performing a rigorous formal quantitative joint count in each patient are noted previously. Moreover, careful joint count assessment takes time,[51] which may be considered as a limitation in busy clinical practices. Careful joint count assessment may also require partial undressing of patients that may also consume time in the examination room especially in regions with colder climate.

CHALLENGES OF DEVICES

A simple tool for quantitative measure for patient's functional status, pain, fatigue, PTGL, and so forth is a short patient questionnaire that each patient completes at each visit in the waiting room with a pencil and paper. Attention to certain issues, as listed below, may enhance feasibility and acceptance of such questionnaires in the routine clinical practice.

The questionnaire has to be short, preferably only 1 sheet (2 sides a page).
Use "one-size" questionnaire that is same for all patients irrespective of diagnosis.
The questionnaire is to be completed by every patient at every visit.
The patient completes the questionnaire, not a health professional.
The clinician must review results of the questionnaire. This should preferably be done with the patient so as to reinforce the importance of questionnaire to the patient.

Historically, a pencil and paper method was the only way to collect quantitative data in clinical care. However, this method has its own challenges. Patients may have difficulties in questionnaire completion arising from use of small font, visual impairment, and problems with pen/pencil gripping with painful/deformed hands. Clinicians may also have issues with difficulty in longitudinal time-oriented follow-up for changes in patient status because data are present on separate pieces of paper; data for groups of patients is time-consuming and costly because of the work of data entry; the need for separate documentation of joint counts and laboratory tests and a calculator for disease activity assessment; and the inability to save paper questionnaires (unless scanned) in electronic medical records (EMRs).

Electronic solutions have been built, to collect real-time data from each patient, including PROs, disease-activity measures, and history of RA, comorbidities, joint surgeries, and all medications received.[49] The patient is asked to arrive in clinic 15 minutes before the scheduled visit to complete an expanded self-report health questionnaire on a touch screen. Data are stored in a central server. Patient self-report of clinical status is available for the health professional as calculated scores and as raw data, to scan ("eye-ball") before the patient enters the room and to facilitate a focused discussion. Physicians record a tender and swollen joint count on a homunculus pointing each of the joints with positive findings on the screen, which provides immediate scores for disease activity on DAS28 and other composite measures. Disease activity, PROs, and the use of DMARDs over time are also shown in time-oriented graphics.

CHALLENGES OF ATTITUDE OF PERSONNEL

Attitude of personnel is the most important hurdle to RA assessment. One would consider medical care inadequate if physicians caring for people with hypertension said that they did not have time to measure the blood pressure, or physicians managing a patient with diabetes said that the staff will not cooperate to draw blood for hemoglobin A1C? Yet, disease activity assessment and PROs are not included in care by most rheumatologists. The 3 most common reasons for not performing quantitative disease assessment by rheumatologists in routine clinical practice were: takes too much time (29%); staff will not cooperate (21%); and patients will not cooperate (13%).[15]

EXAMPLES ON HOW TO MEASURE DISEASE ACTIVITY AND PROs IN PATIENTS WITH EARLY RA

One author (NAK) uses paper questionnaire for the collection of PROs. The summary scores from the questionnaire and 28 joint-count are sequentially noted in the clinical note in an EMR for the patients visit. The questionnaires are scanned, and become part of the patient's medical records.

At a county hospital rheumatology unit in Jyväskylä Central Hospital, Finland, which serves a population of 275,000 people, the authors (TS and TR) use an electronic data-capturing system, which is in use in several clinics in Finland, Norway, and other countries. Each year, roughly 100 patients are diagnosed with early RA. DMARD therapy is started on the day of the diagnosis, tailored according to the disease activity level, with a treatment target of remission at 3 months and continuously thereafter. Routine clinic visits are scheduled at 3 and 6 months and at years 1, 2, 5, and 10 in all patients. Patients with continuously active disease and those who are treated with biologics are seen as often as clinically needed. At every visit, patient completes a self-report health questionnaire on a touch screen in the waiting area before the visit. The physician records the tender and swollen joint counts on an electronic homunculus and an estimate of overall disease activity. Disease activity on DAS28 and Clinical Disease Activity Index are automatically calculated as data are being entered. Disease activity,

Date	25.01.2012
ID	
Name	
Age, Gender	65, Male
Work status	Pensioner
Diagnosis	Rheumatoid Arthritis
Diagnosis criteria	- Symptoms (ACR RA): Polyarticular 3.2011
	- Clinical diagnosis (ACR RA): 6.2011
Highest RF (IgM)	Positive (390) 4.2011
Highest (aCCP)	Positive (147) 6.2011
Erosions	Positive 6.2011
Drug (now)	Sulfasalazine 6.2011
	- 2 000,00 mg Peroral Every day
	Methotrexate 6.2011
	- 25,00 mg Subcutaneous Once a week
	Hydroxychloroquine 6.2011
	- 300,00 mg Peroral Every day
	Prednisolone 5.2011
	- 5,00 mg Peroral Every day
Surgery	Left MTP Joint resection 1.2010
	Right MTP Joint resection 1.2010
Data confirmed	05.12.2011, miina_I

Latest score

Date			06.06.2011	16.09.2011	05.12.2011
HEALTH STATUS					
Pain			50	0	0
Fatigue			42	0	0
Morning stiffness			2,50	0,25	0,00
Rheumatic activity			53	0	0
Physical exercise				>=3/week	>=3/week
M-HAQ (0-3)			1,13	0	0
MDHAQ (FN) (0-3)			1,9	0	0
MDHAQ (PS) (0-3)			0,5	0	0
HAQ (0-3)			1,63	0	0
Raw HAQ (0-24)			12	0	0
DISEASE ACT.					
Inv. global			40	9	6
ESR			44	17	23
CRP			24	4	5
TJC 28/32			10/10	0/0	0/0
SJC 28/32			9/9	1/1	0/0
TJC 46			10	0	0
SJC 46			9	1	0
Patient global			21	0	0
DAS28 (4)			5,6	2,3	2,2
DAS28 (3)			5,8	2,6	2,5
DAS28-CRP(4)			5	1,8	1,6
DAS28-CRP(3)			5,3	2,1	1,9
CDAI			25,1		0,6
ANTHR.DATA					
Weight			85	86	86
BMI			27,1	27,5	27,5

Fig. 1. Data for rheumatoid arthritis assessment are available to the health professionals as raw data and as automated calculated scores.

PROs, and the use of DMARDs over time are shown on a flow sheet (**Fig. 1**). The electronic software is also configured to display time-oriented graphics, as well as comorbidities, extra-articular RA manifestations, and surgeries. Radiographs of hands and feet are scheduled at 1-, 2-, 5-, and 10-year visits. Each patient receives education individually from a rheumatology nurse specialist and is invited for group education sessions.

Consultation of a physical therapist is an essential part of patient education. Patients with early RA are tested for muscle strength and aerobic capacity. An individualized exercise program is planned, to include with a minimum of 2.5 hours of aerobic exercises a week and twice a week muscle strength exercises. Patient is scheduled follow-up visits with a physical therapist at 1 and 2 years.

This early RA program has been developed since 1997 with a prospective follow-up of patients. In a clinical evaluation of all patients with RA in 2010 (one-third diagnosed before 1997), 54% were in DAS28 remission (Tuulikki Sokka, MD, PhD, unpublished observation, 2010). Although these remission rates are among the best in usual clinical practice, space for improvement remains.

SUMMARY

Interest in the measurement of disease activity and PROs is increasing at this time. The value of assessment of RA is emphasized in treatment guidelines, editorials, and reports from clinical studies. Hurdles of the implementation of clinical assessment can be recognized and overcome. Relatively inexpensive, easy-to-use electronic devices are available for solo practices and large university practices. Therefore, clinical assessment of disease activity and PROs should be easier than ever. The purpose of RA assessment is to achieve a rapid and continuous remission in all patients with RA and to improve quality of life and long-term outcomes of these patients.

REFERENCES

1. Saag KG, Teng GG, Patkar NM, et al. American College of Rheumatology 2008 recommendations for the use of nonbiologic and biologic disease-modifying anti-rheumatic drugs in rheumatoid arthritis. Arthritis Rheum 2008;59:762–84.
2. Schoels M, Knevel R, Aletaha D, et al. Evidence for treating rheumatoid arthritis to target: results of a systematic literature search. Ann Rheum Dis 2010;69:638–43.
3. Smith T. Questions on clinical trials. Br Med J (Clin Res Ed) 1983;287:569.
4. Pincus T, Callahan LF, Sale WG, et al. Severe functional declines, work disability, and increased mortality in seventy-five rheumatoid arthritis patients studied over nine years. Arthritis Rheum 1984;27:864–72.
5. Luukkainen R, Kajander A, Isomaki H. Effect of gold on progression of erosions in rheumatoid arthritis. Better results with early treatment. Scand J Rheumatol 1977; 6:189–92.
6. Fries JF. Reevaluating the therapeutic approach to rheumatoid arthritis: the "sawtooth" strategy. J Rheumatol Suppl 1990;22:12–5.
7. O'Dell JR, Mikuls TR. To improve outcomes we must define and measure them: toward defining remission in rheumatoid arthritis. Arthritis Rheum 2011;63:587–9.
8. Schoels M, Aletaha D, Smolen JS, et al. Follow-up standards and treatment targets in rheumatoid arthritis: results of a questionnaire at the EULAR 2008. Ann Rheum Dis 2010;69:575–8.
9. Aletaha D, Funovits J, Keystone EC, et al. Disease activity early in the course of treatment predicts response to therapy after one year in rheumatoid arthritis patients. Arthritis Rheum 2007;56:3226–35.
10. Rantalaiho V, Korpela M, Laasonen L, et al. Early combination disease-modifying antirheumatic drug therapy and tight disease control improve long-term radiologic outcome in patients with early rheumatoid arthritis: the 11-year results of the Finnish Rheumatoid Arthritis Combination Therapy trial. Arthritis Res Ther 2010;12:R122.
11. Hallert E, Husberg M, Skogh T. 28-Joint count disease activity score at 3 months after diagnosis of early rheumatoid arthritis is strongly associated with direct and indirect costs over the following 4 years: the Swedish TIRA project. Rheumatology (Oxford) 2011;50:1259–67.

12. Sokka T, Kautiainen H, Pincus T, et al. Disparities in rheumatoid arthritis disease activity according to gross domestic product in 25 countries in the QUEST-RA database. Ann Rheum Dis 2009;68:1666–72.

13. Sokka T, Kautiainen H, Pincus T, et al. Work disability remains a major problem in rheumatoid arthritis in the 2000s: data from 32 countries in the QUEST-RA study. Arthritis Res Ther 2010;12:R42.

14. Sokka T, Envalds M, Pincus T. Treatment of rheumatoid arthritis: a global perspective on the use of antirheumatic drugs. Mod Rheumatol 2008;18:228–39.

15. Pincus T, Sokka T. Complexities in the quantitative assessment of patients with rheumatic diseases in clinical trials and clinical care. Clin Exp Rheumatol 2005; 23:S1–9.

16. Prevoo ML, van 't Hof MA, Kuper HH, et al. Modified disease activity scores that include twenty-eight-joint counts. Development and validation in a prospective longitudinal study of patients with rheumatoid arthritis. Arthritis Rheum 1995;38: 44–8.

17. Smolen JS, Breedveld FC, Schiff MH, et al. A simplified disease activity index for rheumatoid arthritis for use in clinical practice. Rheumatology (Oxford) 2003;42: 244–57.

18. Aletaha D, Nell VP, Stamm T, et al. Acute phase reactants add little to composite disease activity indices for rheumatoid arthritis: validation of a clinical activity score. Arthritis Res Ther 2005;7:R796–806.

19. Pincus T, Yazici Y, Bergman M. A practical guide to scoring a Multi-Dimensional Health Assessment Questionnaire (MDHAQ) and Routine Assessment of Patient Index Data (RAPID) scores in 10-20 seconds for use in standard clinical care, without rulers, calculators, websites or computers. Best Pract Res Clin Rheumatol 2007;21:755–87.

20. Wolfe F, Michaud K, Pincus T. A composite disease activity scale for clinical practice, observational studies, and clinical trials: the patient activity scale (PAS/PAS-II). J Rheumatol 2005;32:2410–5.

21. Fransen J, Hauselmann H, Michel BA, et al. Responsiveness of the self-assessed rheumatoid arthritis disease activity index to a flare of disease activity. Arthritis Rheum 2001;44:53–60.

22. Scott DL, Houssien DA. Joint assessment in rheumatoid arthritis. Br J Rheumatol 1996;35(Suppl 2):14–8.

23. Sokka T, Pincus T. Joint counts to assess rheumatoid arthritis for clinical research and usual clinical care: advantages and limitations. Rheum Dis Clin North Am 2009;35:713–22, v–vi.

24. Eberl DR, Fasching V, Rahlfs V, et al. Repeatability and objectivity of various measurements in rheumatoid arthritis. A comparative study. Arthritis Rheum 1976;19:1278–86.

25. Lassere MN, van der Heijde D, Johnson KR, et al. Reliability of measures of disease activity and disease damage in rheumatoid arthritis: implications for smallest detectable difference, minimal clinically important difference, and analysis of treatment effects in randomized controlled trials. J Rheumatol 2001;28:892–903.

26. Scott DL, Choy EH, Greeves A, et al. Standardising joint assessment in rheumatoid arthritis. Clin Rheumatol 1996;15:579–82.

27. Strand V, Cohen S, Crawford B, et al. Patient-reported outcomes better discriminate active treatment from placebo in randomized controlled trials in rheumatoid arthritis. Rheumatology (Oxford) 2004;43:640–7.

28. Ostergaard M, Pedersen SJ, Dohn UM. Imaging in rheumatoid arthritis–status and recent advances for magnetic resonance imaging, ultrasonography, computed

tomography and conventional radiography. Best Pract Res Clin Rheumatol 2008; 22:1019–44.

29. Rose HM, Ragan C. Differential agglutination of normal and sensitized sheep erythrocytes by sera of patients with rheumatoid arthritis. Proc Soc Exp Biol Med 1948;68:1–6.

30. Sokka T, Pincus T. Erythrocyte sedimentation rate, C-reactive protein, or rheumatoid factor are normal at presentation in 35%-45% of patients with rheumatoid arthritis seen between 1980 and 2004: analyses from Finland and the United States. J Rheumatol 2009;36:1387–90.

31. Wolfe F. The many myths of erythrocyte sedimentation rate and C-reactive protein. J Rheumatol 2009;36:1568–9.

32. Abelson B, Sokka T, Pincus T. Declines in erythrocyte sedimentation rates in patients with rheumatoid arthritis over the second half of the 20th century. J Rheumatol 2009;36:1596–9.

33. Isomaki HA, Hakulinen T, Joutsenlahti U. Excess risk of lymphomas, leukemia and myeloma in patients with rheumatoid arthritis. J Chronic Dis 1978;31:691–6.

34. Miller A, Green M, Robinson D. Simple rule for calculating normal erythrocyte sedimentation rate. Br Med J (Clin Res Ed) 1983;286:266.

35. Fries JF, Spitz P, Kraines RG, et al. Measurement of patient outcome in arthritis. Arthritis Rheum 1980;23:137–45.

36. Pincus T, Swearingen C, Wolfe F. Toward a multidimensional Health Assessment Questionnaire (MDHAQ): assessment of advanced activities of daily living and psychological status in the patient-friendly health assessment questionnaire format. Arthritis Rheum 1999;42:2220–30.

37. Wolfe F, Cathey MA. The assessment and prediction of functional disability in rheumatoid arthritis. J Rheumatol 1991;18:1298–306.

38. Wolfe F, Hawley DJ. The longterm outcomes of rheumatoid arthritis: work disability: a prospective 18 year study of 823 patients. J Rheumatol 1998;25:2108–17.

39. Kobelt G, Eberhardt K, Jonsson L, et al. Economic consequences of the progression of rheumatoid arthritis in Sweden. Arthritis Rheum 1999;42:347–56.

40. Wolfe F, Zwillich SH. The long-term outcomes of rheumatoid arthritis: a 23-year prospective, longitudinal study of total joint replacement and its predictors in 1,600 patients with rheumatoid arthritis. Arthritis Rheum 1998;41:1072–82.

41. Sokka T, Hakkinen A, Krishnan E, et al. Similar prediction of mortality by the health assessment questionnaire in patients with rheumatoid arthritis and the general population. Ann Rheum Dis 2004;63:494–7.

42. Ward MM. Rheumatology care, patient expectations, and the limits of time. Arthritis Rheum 2004;51:307–8.

43. Diatchenko L, Slade GD, Nackley AG, et al. Genetic basis for individual variations in pain perception and the development of a chronic pain condition. Hum Mol Genet 2005;14:135–43.

44. Thompson PW, Pegley FS. A comparison of disability measured by the Stanford Health Assessment Questionnaire disability scales (HAQ) in male and female rheumatoid outpatients. Br J Rheumatol 1991;30:298–300.

45. Sokka T, Toloza S, Cutolo M, et al. Women, men, and rheumatoid arthritis: analyses of disease activity, disease characteristics, and treatments in the QUEST-RA study. Arthritis Res Ther 2009;11:R7.

46. Hakkinen A, Kautiainen H, Hannonen P, et al. Muscle strength, pain, and disease activity explain individual subdimensions of the Health Assessment Questionnaire disability index, especially in women with rheumatoid arthritis. Ann Rheum Dis 2006;65:30–4.

47. Krishnan E, Sokka T, Hakkinen A, et al. Normative values for the Health Assessment Questionnaire disability index: benchmarking disability in the general population. Arthritis Rheum 2004;50:953–60.
48. Wolfe F, Michaud K. A brief introduction to the National Data Bank for Rheumatic Diseases. Clin Exp Rheumatol 2005;23:S168–71.
49. Sokka T, Haugeberg G, Pincus T. Assessment of quality of rheumatoid arthritis care requires joint count and/or patient questionnaire data not found in a usual medical record: examples from studies of premature mortality, changes in clinical status between 1985 and 2000, and a QUEST-RA global perspective. Clin Exp Rheumatol 2007;25:86–97.
50. Agnew-Blais JC, Coblyn JS, Katz JN, et al. Measuring quality of care for rheumatic diseases using an electronic medical record. Ann Rheum Dis 2009;68: 680–4.
51. Fransen J, Stucki G, van Riel P. Rheumatoid arthritis measures: Disease Activity Score (DAS), Disease Activity Score-28 (DAS28), Rapid Assessment of Disease Activity in Rheumatology (RADAR), and Rheumatoid Arthritis Disease Activity Index (RADAI). Arthritis Care Res 2003;49:S214–24.

Initial Management of Rheumatoid Arthritis

Anna Gramling, MD[a,b,*], James R. O'Dell, MD[a,b]

KEYWORDS

- Rheumatoid arthritis • Disease-modifying antirheumatic drug
- DMARD

Key Points

- Half of patients who have rheumatoid arthritis (RA) which is diagnosed and treated early by a rheumatologist with the goal of remission or low disease activity can expect to achieve remission while taking their disease-modifying antirheumatic drugs.
- Recently, the recognized benefits of very early therapy of RA highlighted the need to make the diagnosis of RA as early as possible.
- Therapeutic goals and the ability to measure them are critically important in treating any disease.

The prognosis for the patient with newly diagnosed rheumatoid arthritis (RA) has dramatically changed over the last two decades. If a patient is diagnosed and treated early by a rheumatologist with the goal of remission or low disease activity, half of patients can expect to achieve remission while taking their disease-modifying antirheumatic drugs (DMARDs). Strong evidence exists that early diagnosis and aggressive treatment alter the natural history of RA. Clearly, prevention of permanent structural damage to joints, including both erosions and joint-space narrowing as measured on radiographs, but also the prevention of deformities that can occur without erosions, is a strong rationale for early RA treatment.[1,2] Structural damage, when it reaches a critical level, is associated with functional impairment. Although there is evidence in some cases that erosions may heal (at least radiographically), joint-space narrowing and subluxations are permanent.[3-6] A meta-analysis of 12 studies demonstrated significant reduction of radiographic progression in subjects treated early when compared with the subjects treated later. An average delay of 9 months in starting DMARDs significantly

[a] Division of Rheumatology and Immunology, University of Nebraska Medical Center, 983025 Nebraska Medical Center, Omaha, NE 68198-3025, USA; [b] Department of Veterans Affairs Nebraska-Western Iowa Health Care System, 4101 Woolworth Avenue, Omaha, NE 68105, USA
* Division of Rheumatology and Immunology, University of Nebraska Medical Center, 983025 Nebraska Medical Center, Omaha, NE 68198-3025.
E-mail address: anna.gramling@unmc.edu

Rheum Dis Clin N Am 38 (2012) 311–325
doi:10.1016/j.rdc.2012.05.003
0889-857X/12/$ – see front matter © 2012 Elsevier Inc. All rights reserved.

rheumatic.theclinics.com

increased radiographic progression. Subjects with more aggressive erosive disease benefited the most from early therapy.[7] However, it is important to note that most patients who have RA fall into the category of poor prognosis by virtue of erosions at baseline, or rheumatoid factor (RF) or cyclic citrullinated peptide (CCP) positivity, and clearly need early intervention.

Some investigators have suggested that there is a window of opportunity in early disease during which therapy is somehow particularly effective. Much data, some referenced above, clearly show that the earlier physicians treat, the better patients do. Most large trials in early disease show a strong correlation of disease duration to outcomes.[8–10] No one can argue that earlier is better, but the window of opportunity concept can be, and sometimes is, carried too far. It should not be assumed that this window somehow closes and then patients do not benefit from therapy. Excellent data demonstrate that in the face of active disease, patients benefit from appropriate DMARD treatment regardless of disease duration.[11–17] It remains debatable whether early therapy can reset the radiographic progression rate of patients for years to come. The Finnish Rheumatoid Arthritis Combination Therapy (FIN-RACo) and the Combination Therapy in Patients with Early Rheumatoid Arthritis (COBRA) trials (see later discussion), among others, suggest this may be true. It is important to keep in mind the many limitations of the open long-term observational nature of these results and how aggressively subjects from these trials were treated to target.

Long-term results (5-year and 11-year) of the FIN-RACo trial suggest that effect of early aggressive intervention on radiologic progression is longlasting.[18–20] In this study, subjects were randomized into two groups. From the start, one group received a combination of DMARDs, including methotrexate (MTX), sulfasalazine (SSZ) and hydroxychloroquine (HCQ), and the other group received SSZ as monotherapy. The first group had prednisolone as part of their regimen; in the second group it was used as needed. After the initial 2 years, the drug regimen became unrestricted and, therefore, similar. At 5 and 11 years, radiologic progression in the SSZ-alone group was significantly higher than in the group treated with the combination of DMARDs. Similar results were demonstrated in the COBRA trial.[21–23] In this trial, 155 subjects were randomized to COBRA therapy (SSZ 2 g/day, MTX 7.5 mg/week, prednisolone starting at 60 mg/day and tapered to 7.5 mg by the seventh week) or SSZ (2 g/day) monotherapy. At 28 weeks, prednisolone was tapered and withdrawn and, after 40 weeks, MTX was stopped. After this, treatment in both groups became unrestricted. Analysis at 5 and 11 years showed a significantly higher rate of radiologic progression in the SSZ group. Both the COBRA and FIN-RACo studies support the hypothesis that aggressive therapy in the early phase of RA results in long-term radiologic benefit that may translate into better functional outcome.

How soon is soon enough? There really is no answer to this question. Treatment within the first 3 months of onset is a goal. A study of a cohort of subjects with early RA with disease duration less than 12 months, treated with tight-control protocol, showed that a major predictor of an American College of Rheumatology (ACR) clinical remission at 12 months is the duration of disease at the time of initiation of treatment. Very early RA was defined as disease with symptoms of less than 12 weeks. Multivariate analysis demonstrated that the only independent predictor of erosives at 12 months was an increase in duration of disease at the time of initiation of treatment (odds ratio [OR] 2.4; CI 1.1–5.6).[24]

EARLY DIAGNOSIS (CLASSIFICATION) OF RA

Recently, the recognized benefits of very early therapy of RA highlighted the need to make the diagnosis of RA as early as possible. With this goal in mind, the ACR and

European League Against Rheumatism (EULAR) collaborated on a new set of criteria that were meant to distinguish inflammatory arthritis (arthritis that needed MTX treatment) from noninflammatory arthritis. The results were the ACR-EULAR 2010 Classification Criteria (**Table 1**).[25] The 1987 ACR classification criteria for RA remain very useful for discriminating inflammatory from noninflammatory arthritis. However, because 6 weeks of symptoms are required and they do not include anti-CCP positivity, the 1987 criteria are not as useful in early disease.[26,27] The goal of the new criteria was to provide a uniform approach to identify individuals with undifferentiated synovitis who have the highest probability of developing persistent RA and structural damage and, therefore, individuals who would benefit from early DMARD intervention. The new classification criteria will also allow more uniform disease definition and subject recruitment into clinical and epidemiologic studies in early RA.

Importantly, compared with the 1987 criteria, 6 weeks of symptoms is not required and anti-CCP antibody positivity is included. In the new criteria, 6 weeks or more of symptoms are not required, but they do give an extra point and increase the specificity for ongoing disease. Analysis of 2010 RA criteria performance by Cader and colleagues[28] demonstrated, not surprisingly, that 2010 criteria identify more subjects with RA earlier than 1987 criteria (42% vs 23%, respectively; $P<.0001$). However, more subjects whose arthritis resolved spontaneously were classified initially as definite RA

Table 1 The 2010 ACR-EULAR classification for RA	
A. Joint involvement	0–5
1 large joint[a]	0
2–10 large joints	1
1–3 small joints[b] (with or without involvement of large joints)	2
4–10 small joints (with or without involvement of large joints)	3
>10 joints (at least 1 small joint)	5
B. Serology (at least 1 test result is needed for classification)	0–3
Negative[c] RF and negative ACPA	0
Low-positive[d] RF or low-positive ACPA	2
High-positive[e] RF or high-positive ACPA	3
C. Acute-phase reactants (at least 1 test result is needed for classification)	0–1
Normal CRP and normal ESR	0
Abnormal CRP or abnormal ESR	1
D. Duration of symptoms	0–1
<6 wk	0
≥6 wk	1

When RF information is available only as positive or negative, a positive result should be scored as low-positive.

Abbreviations: ACPA, anticitrullinated protein antibody; CRP, C-reactive protein; ESR, erythrocyte sedimentation rate.

[a] Shoulders, elbows, hips, knees, ankles.

[b] Metacarpophalangeal joints, proximal interphalangeal joints, second to fifth metatarsophalangeal joints, thumb interphalangeal joints, and wrists.

[c] Values less than or equal to the upper limit of normal for the laboratory and assay.

[d] Values higher than the upper limit of normal but three or less times the upper limit of normal.

[e] Values more than three times the upper limit of normal for the laboratory and assay.

Adapted from Aletaha D, Neogi T, Silman AJ, et al. 2010 Rheumatoid arthritis classification criteria: an American College of Rheumatology/European League Against Rheumatism collaborative initiative. Arthritis Rheum 2010;62(9):2569–81.

by 2010 criteria than 1987 criteria (8% vs 2%, respectively; $P = .01$). After 18 months, both criteria performed the same in identifying subjects with RA. A retrospective study by Kaneko and colleagues[29] showed that 2010 criteria have better sensitivity in identifying RA than 1987 criteria (73.5% vs 47.1%, respectively), but less specificity (71.4% vs 92.9%, respectively). Conversely, in the subgroup of subjects who are negative for RF and anti-CCP antibody, the 2010 criteria have a sensitivity of only 15.8%. Although useful to identify disease early, clinicians have to be mindful of potential limitations of 2010 criteria: lower specificity than the old criteria and potentially low sensitivity in seronegative RA.

ANTI-CCP IN EARLY DIAGNOSIS OF RA

Many studies have shown that autoantibodies are seen in people who have no symptoms or physical findings of arthritis but who will develop RA years later.[30-37] Anti-CCP antibodies seem to be the most important of these. Anti-CCP has been shown to be reasonably sensitive (65%–80%) and highly specific for RA (98%).[38-43] Importantly, a study by van Gaalen and colleagues[44] demonstrated that presence of anti-CCP antibodies predicts progression of undifferentiated arthritis to RA independently of other factors. For 3 years, 318 subjects with undifferentiated arthritis (**Table 2**) were followed. After 3 years, 93% of the subjects who were CCP-positive developed RA by the 1987 criteria (99% by 2010 criteria) compared with only 25% of the subjects who were CCP-negative. This demonstrates the usefulness of this test in patients with undifferentiated inflammatory arthritis. Because of the inclusion of CCP positivity in the 2010 criteria, many of the subjects in the above study would have been classified as RA at baseline.

THE NEXT STEP? THE CONCEPT OF PRECLINICAL RA

As mentioned above, people who later develop RA frequently have CCP and RF antibodies present in their serum for years before they develop clinical RA. This takes the discussion of early treatment to a whole new level and leads to speculation about the possibility of treating or modifying risk factors in these people to prevent the onset of clinical disease.[45-49] Obviously, this raises several questions, not the least of which are how to identify these people in the first place and what risks of therapy are acceptable in people who do not yet have clinical disease? RA has a prevalence of less than 1%. Therefore, CCP used in the general population is not a good screening test, even with sensitivity between 96% and 98%. Far more false positives would be identified than true positives if used in the general population. Despite all these issues,

Table 2
Anti-CCP antibodies and prediction of RA in patients with undifferentiated arthritis

	Patients Fulfilling ACR RA Criteria, Number (%)		
	After 1 y	After 2 y	After 3 y
Anti-CCP–positive (n = 69)	57 (83)	62 (90)	64 (93)
Anti-CCP–negative (n = 249)	46 (18)	60 (24)	63 (25)

Multivariate analysis showed that anti-CCP positivity in undifferentiated arthritis is the most important predictor of future diagnosis of RA (OR = 38.6, CI 9.9–151.0).

Adapted from van Gaalen FA, Linn-Rasker SP, van Venrooij WJ, et al. Autoantibodies to cyclic citrullinated peptides predict progression to rheumatoid arthritis in patients with undifferentiated arthritis: a prospective cohort study. Arthritis Rheum 2004;50(3):709–15.

preventive trials are in the planning stages for people at high risk for the future development of RA.

Goals for Early RA Treatment

Therapeutic goals and the ability to measure them are critically important in treating any disease. This is certainly true in RA treatment and, until recently, clear goals have been elusive. Rheumatologists have long envied the endocrinologists with their hemoglobin (Hgb) A1C or the cardiologists with their blood pressure measurements and low-density lipoprotein levels. Recently, the rheumatologic world has embraced the concept of having a goal or target for therapy in RA as important, and the ACR has endorsed several different measures of disease activity in RA. These include the Disease Activity Score (DAS) 28, the Clinical Disease Activity Index (CDAI), the Simplified Disease Activity Index (SDAI), the Routine Assessment of Patient Index Data, and the Patient Activity Scale.[50–57] Although it may seem intuitively obvious that having a target and treating to this would be beneficial, the Tight Control for Rheumatoid Arthritis (TICORA) study showed this for the first time. In TICORA, subjects were randomly assigned to intensive management or routine care. Escalation of therapy in the intensive group was based on monthly measured DAS. If the DAS was greater than 2.4, therapy was escalated. Escalation of therapy in the routine group was done at the discretion of the rheumatologist without particular disease activity index recordings. At 18 months, subjects in intensive therapy were doing better in all respects—clinically and radiographically.[58]

Rheumatoid arthritis treatment guidelines from the ACR and EULAR recommend monitoring disease activity and treating it to a target of at least low disease activity.[59–61] Remission is the ultimate goal of treatment, but it is unclear whether this should be the target for all patients. If a patient is on MTX alone (or any other therapy), is very close to remission, is happy, and has no problems with activities of daily living, does it make sense to add a biologic to their program? This is when the art of medicine still plays an important role. As these decisions are made, efficacy, toxicity, and the cost of adding and not adding additional therapy must be carefully weighed. The endocrinologists have taught that lower is not always better; aggressive HgbA1C lowering trials pushed too far result in unacceptable toxicities.[62]

Recognition of remission in RA has been difficult because of the many different definitions used.[63–69] Fortunately, there is now one uniform definition, at least for clinical trials: the new ACR-EULAR remission guidelines. It was proposed that, in the setting of clinical trials, a subject is in remission when scores of swollen-joint count, tender-joint count, patient global assessment, and CRP are all less than or equal to 1 or when the score on the (SDAI) is less than or equal to 3.3. Importantly, analysis by Felson and colleagues[70] showed that DAS 28 at cutpoint less than 2.6 or less than 2.0 did not ensure good radiologic outcomes. The new ACR-EULAR proposed definition is still waiting for further validation.[71] What the remission definition for clinical practice should be remains an important question. One set of criteria might not be suitable for heterogeneous groups of patients who are not in a trial setting. CDAI less than or equal to 2.8 and a cumulative score of less than or equal to 1 for swollen-joint count, tender-joint count, and patient global assessment seem to have good predictive validity for remission in the clinical setting.[72–74]

An international task force developed treat-to-target recommendations to achieve optimal therapeutic outcomes in RA.[75] This task force had the following suggestions or recommendations:

- Sustained clinical remission is the primary target in treating RA.

- In some circumstances, when a state of complete remission is not possible (eg, significant joint damage, failure of multiple treatment regiments, toxicities, or cost issues), low disease activity could be an acceptable alternative target.
- A patient's disease activity should be followed every 1 to 3 months until the target is reached, with subsequent assessments every 3 to 6 months.
- Validated composite disease activity indices should be used in routine clinical practice.

The Dutch Rheumatoid Arthritis Monitoring (DREAM) remission induction cohort study demonstrated that adapting treat-to-target strategy aiming at remission in the setting of clinical practice is realistic.[76] Because this trial was done before the new remission definition was available, several definitions were evaluated. Full ACR, modified-ACR criteria, DAS 28 with different cutoffs, SDAI less than 3.3, and CDAI less than 2.8 were used to define remission in this trial.

INITIAL THERAPY IN EARLY RA: MONOTHERAPY OR COMBINATION, BIOLOGIC OR NONBIOLOGIC

Despite tremendous advances in RA treatment, many questions remain about initial therapy, and the art of medicine is again important. Many studies have shown that combination of DMARDs is more effective than monotherapy.[19,22,77–88] Four potential approaches in combining DMARDs are (1) parallel administration of DMARDs (eg, MTX, SSZ, and HCQ combinations; triple therapy) from the start, (2) the step-up approach (addition of second and, potentially, third DMARD in patients with initial inadequate response, (3) the step-down approach (initial administration of combination therapy with subsequent withdrawal of drugs if good control of disease is achieved), and (4) initial combination of nonbiologic and biologic DMARDs. Goekoop-Ruiterman and colleagues[77,78] examined four different initial treatment approaches in RA. In the Behandel-Strategieën (BeSt) study, subjects were randomly assigned to (1) methotrexate monotherapy, (2) step-up combination to three DMARDs (triple therapy), (3) combination of MTX, SSZ, and high dose prednisone, or (4) combination of MTX with infliximab. Therapy in all groups was adjusted every 3 months if the DAS was greater than or equal to 2.4. If the DAS was less than 2.4 for more than 6 months, medications were withdrawn until one drug remained for maintenance. Groups 3 and 4 (the initial combination groups) had more rapid clinical improvement during the first year and less progression of radiographic joint damage. However, after 2 years, similar clinical and functional improvement was noted across all four groups even though, by that time, subjects in all groups were on many different therapies. This study highlights two very important points:

1. Therapy should be individualized for each patient.
2. Treating to a target as per the TICORA trial is the critical factor to achieve outcomes regardless of the therapy used.

With the results of the BeSt trial, some rheumatologists have advocated combinations up front for all patients, based on the radiographic benefit; others have advocated the step-up approach because clinical outcomes of all groups in the BeSt trail were indistinguishable at 2 years. The Treatment of Early Aggressive Rheumatoid Arthritis (TEAR) trial addressed this question in early (mean duration 3.6 months), poor prognosis (all subjects who were RF-positive, CCP-positive, or had at least two erosions) RA.[89] This trial was the largest (755 subjects) investigator-initiated, double-blind, randomized trial ever in early RA. Half of the subjects were randomized to receive combinations up front (either MTX and etanercept or MTX, SSZ, and HCQ [triple]) while the other half received MTX alone (20 mg/week). At 6 months, subjects who took the MTX alone stepped up to combinations if the DAS28 score was greater than 3.2 (step-up occurred for 72% of subjects). The primary outcome was the mean DAS28 for subjects between weeks 48 and 102. No difference was seen between step-up and initial-combination subjects (mean DAS28 3.2 vs 3.2, respectively; $P = .75$). There was also no difference for radiographic progression. In this trial, 28% of subjects started on MTX had a great response (DAS28 <3.2) and did not need additional therapy. This number is very similar to that found in the BeSt trial and Swedish Farmacotherapy trial (SWEFOT). Thirty percent of subjects with early RA did well on MTX monotherapy.[90,91] Importantly, TEAR teaches that those patients who do need a step-up do well and have clinical and radiographic outcomes identical to those of the patients who received combinations up front. Therefore, it seems prudent to initiate therapy with MTX and then, at 3 to 6 months, step up to combinations only with patients that still have DAS28 greater than 3.2. With regard to which combination to step up to, in the TEAR trial there was no advantage of etanercept over SSZ- HCQ; therefore, it would seem prudent to use the far less expensive SSA-HCQ first.[92,93]

HEALTH CARE MAINTENANCE IN EARLY RA

When faced with a patient with recent onset RA, rheumatologists have rightly focused on getting the disease under control as rapidly as possible. However, with the excellent outcomes of most patients, attention should also be directed to important health-care maintenance issues. In particular, concern should be on cardiovascular risk factors, immunization status, and bone health. With the well-known excess morbidity and mortality in this patient population attributable to cardiovascular disease, risk factors such as obesity, hypertension, sedentary lifestyle, and lipids should be addressed by the rheumatologist or addressed in a close partnership with the primary care physician.[94–96] If statins are necessary, they have the added benefit of decreasing the DAS of the RA.[97–99] All patients with RA should be up-to-date on all immunizations. It is prudent to think about this early in the course of disease because many of the DMARDs, including MTX, will blunt the response to immunization.[100–103] Therefore, if at all possible, all appropriate patients should receive their pneumococcal vaccination before MTX therapy. Further, all indicated live vaccines (usually zoster vaccine) should be given at least 2 weeks before biologicals. Therefore, it is better to do it in the very beginning than to have to delay biologic therapy later.[104] Finally, especially in postmenopausal women, bone density status should be known and appropriate treatment, usually bisphosphonate, prescribed.[105] Unless contraindicated, all patients with RA should be on adequate calcium and vitamin D. Although lung cancers and lymphomas are overrepresented in patients with RA, other health-care maintenance should be appropriate for the patient's age.

UNANSWERED QUESTIONS: THE WAY FORWARD

Currently there are at least three major questions that, when answered, will allow major steps forward:

1. How can we predictably select the best therapy for each individual patient?
2. Would patients benefit from induction approaches in RA and, if so, which patients?
3. What should the goal or target be in RA, and is the current definition of remission adequate for this?

The next major advance in treatment in early RA will occur when differential selection can identify which patients will benefit most from which therapies and, perhaps, which patients are at risk for toxicities from the therapies. Who are those 30% of patients that need only MTX initially? Which patients need triple therapy up front? Which patients need a biologic from the onset and which biologic? Which patients might have great responses to HCQ or SSZ monotherapy? To address these questions, clinical trials are needed designed to answer these questions and, importantly, biomarkers are needed that are linked to well-defined clinical outcomes, preferably from randomized clinical trials.

Recently, the ACR published the results of a workshop on RA clinical trial issues.[106] This group of experts highlighted these priorities and highlighted the need for biomarkers to be included in all trials. The trials needed to address these questions will, for the most part, not come from the pharmaceutical industry because most of the questions will require comparison of different medications and approaches, and not necessarily new products. It is unclear where funding for these needed trials and biomarker collection will come from, but partnerships between all interested parties are a must. Recently, health care systems, such as the Department of Veterans Affairs, have stepped up and funded important trials that will ultimately make treatment of RA, not only better, but more economical. Although new medications are always welcome, if current medications were used to the best advantage, it would be a huge leap forward for patients with RA.

REFERENCES

1. Smolen JS, van der Heijde DM, Aletaha D, et al. Progression of radiographic joint damage in rheumatoid arthritis: independence of erosions and joint space narrowing. Ann Rheum Dis 2009;68(10):1535–40.
2. Sokka T, Kautiainen H, Mottonen T, et al. Erosions develop rarely in joints without clinically detectable inflammation in patients with early rheumatoid arthritis. J Rheumatol 2003;30(12):2580–4.
3. Aletaha D, Funovits J, Smolen JS. Physical disability in rheumatoid arthritis is associated with cartilage damage rather than bone destruction. Ann Rheum Dis 2011; 70(5):733–9.
4. Smolen JS, Aletaha D, Grisar JC, et al. Estimation of a numerical value for joint damage-related physical disability in rheumatoid arthritis clinical trials. Ann Rheum Dis 2010;69(6):1058–64.
5. van der Heijde D, Landewe R, van Vollenhoven R, et al. Level of radiographic damage and radiographic progression are determinants of physical function: a longitudinal analysis of the TEMPO trial. Ann Rheum Dis 2008;67(9):1267–70.
6. Drossaers-Bakker KW, de Buck M, van Zeben D, et al. Long-term course and outcome of functional capacity in rheumatoid arthritis: the effect of disease activity and radiologic damage over time. Arthritis Rheum 1999;42(9):1854–60.
7. Finckh A, Liang MH, van Herckenrode CM, et al. Long-term impact of early treatment on radiographic progression in rheumatoid arthritis: a meta-analysis. Arthritis Rheum 2006;55(6):864–72.
8. Kyburz D, Gabay C, Michel BA, et al. The long-term impact of early treatment of rheumatoid arthritis on radiographic progression: a population-based cohort study. Rheumatology (Oxford) 2011;50(6):1106–10.
9. Anderson JJ, Wells G, Verhoeven AC, et al. Factors predicting response to treatment in rheumatoid arthritis: the importance of disease duration. Arthritis Rheum 2000;43(1):22–9.

10. Nell VP, Machold KP, Eberl G, et al. Benefit of very early referral and very early therapy with disease-modifying anti-rheumatic drugs in patients with early rheumatoid arthritis. Rheumatology (Oxford) 2004;43(7):906–14.
11. Garnero P, Thompson E, Woodworth T, et al. Rapid and sustained improvement in bone and cartilage turnover markers with the anti-interleukin-6 receptor inhibitor tocilizumab plus methotrexate in rheumatoid arthritis patients with an inadequate response to methotrexate: results from a substudy of the multicenter double-blind, placebo-controlled trial of tocilizumab in inadequate responders to methotrexate alone. Arthritis Rheum 2010;62(1):33–43.
12. Heiberg MS, Rodevand E, Mikkelsen K, et al. Adalimumab and methotrexate is more effective than adalimumab alone in patients with established rheumatoid arthritis: results from a 6-month longitudinal, observational, multicentre study. Ann Rheum Dis 2006;65(10):1379–83.
13. Maini RN, Breedveld FC, Kalden JR, et al. Therapeutic efficacy of multiple intravenous infusions of anti-tumor necrosis factor alpha monoclonal antibody combined with low-dose weekly methotrexate in rheumatoid arthritis. Arthritis Rheum 1998;41(9):1552–63.
14. Smolen JS. Efficacy and safety of the new DMARD leflunomide: comparison to placebo and sulfasalazine in active rheumatoid arthritis. Scand J Rheumatol Suppl 1999;112:15–21.
15. Takeuchi T, Tanaka Y, Amano K, et al. Clinical, radiographic and functional effectiveness of tocilizumab for rheumatoid arthritis patients–REACTION 52-week study. Rheumatology (Oxford) 2011;50(10):1908–15.
16. Tanaka Y, Harigai M, Takeuchi T, et al. Golimumab in combination with methotrexate in Japanese patients with active rheumatoid arthritis: results of the GO-FORTH study. Ann Rheum Dis 2012;71(6):817–24.
17. O'Dell JR, Haire CE, Erikson N, et al. Treatment of rheumatoid arthritis with methotrexate alone, sulfasalazine and hydroxychloroquine, or a combination of all three medications. N Engl J Med 1996;334(20):1287–91.
18. Mottonen T, Hannonen P, Leirisalo-Repo M, et al. Comparison of combination therapy with single-drug therapy in early rheumatoid arthritis: a randomised trial. FIN-RACo trial group. Lancet 1999;353(9164):1568–73.
19. Korpela M, Laasonen L, Hannonen P, et al. Retardation of joint damage in patients with early rheumatoid arthritis by initial aggressive treatment with disease-modifying antirheumatic drugs: five-year experience from the FIN-RACo study. Arthritis Rheum 2004;50(7):2072–81.
20. Rantalaiho V, Korpela M, Laasonen L, et al. Early combination disease-modifying antirheumatic drug therapy and tight disease control improve long-term radiologic outcome in patients with early rheumatoid arthritis: the 11-year results of the Finnish Rheumatoid Arthritis Combination Therapy trial. Arthritis Res Ther 2010;12(3):R122.
21. Boers M, Verhoeven AC, Markusse HM, et al. Randomised comparison of combined step-down prednisolone, methotrexate and sulphasalazine with sulphasalazine alone in early rheumatoid arthritis. Lancet 1997;350(9074): 309–18.
22. Landewe RB, Boers M, Verhoeven AC, et al. COBRA combination therapy in patients with early rheumatoid arthritis: long-term structural benefits of a brief intervention. Arthritis Rheum 2002;46(2):347–56.
23. van Tuyl LH, Boers M, Lems WF, et al. Survival, comorbidities and joint damage 11 years after the COBRA combination therapy trial in early rheumatoid arthritis. Ann Rheum Dis 2010;69(5):807–12.

24. Bosello S, Fedele AL, Peluso G, et al. Very early rheumatoid arthritis is the major predictor of major outcomes: clinical ACR remission and radiographic non-progression. Ann Rheum Dis 2011;70(7):1292–5.
25. Aletaha D, Neogi T, Silman AJ, et al. 2010 Rheumatoid arthritis classification criteria: an American College of Rheumatology/European League Against Rheumatism collaborative initiative. Arthritis Rheum 2010;62(9):2569–81.
26. Arnett FC, Edworthy SM, Bloch DA, et al. The American Rheumatism Association 1987 revised criteria for the classification of rheumatoid arthritis. Arthritis Rheum 1988;31(3):315–24.
27. Harrison BJ, Symmons DP, Barrett EM, et al. The performance of the 1987 ARA classification criteria for rheumatoid arthritis in a population based cohort of patients with early inflammatory polyarthritis. American Rheumatism Association. J Rheumatol 1998;25(12):2324–30.
28. Cader MZ, Filer A, Hazlehurst J, et al. Performance of the 2010 ACR/EULAR criteria for rheumatoid arthritis: comparison with 1987 ACR criteria in a very early synovitis cohort. Ann Rheum Dis 2011;70(6):949–55.
29. Kaneko Y, Kuwana M, Kameda H, et al. Sensitivity and specificity of 2010 rheumatoid arthritis classification criteria. Rheumatology (Oxford) 2011;50(7):1268–74.
30. Nielen MM, van Schaardenburg D, Reesink HW, et al. Specific autoantibodies precede the symptoms of rheumatoid arthritis: a study of serial measurements in blood donors. Arthritis Rheum 2004;50(2):380–6.
31. van der Woude D, Rantapaa-Dahlqvist S, Ioan-Facsinay A, et al. Epitope spreading of the anti-citrullinated protein antibody response occurs before disease onset and is associated with the disease course of early arthritis. Ann Rheum Dis 2010;69(8):1554–61.
32. van de Stadt LA, de Koning MH, van de Stadt RJ, et al. Development of the anti-citrullinated protein antibody repertoire prior to the onset of rheumatoid arthritis. Arthritis Rheum 2011;63(11):3226–33.
33. Koivula MK, Heliovaara M, Ramberg J, et al. Autoantibodies binding to citrullinated telopeptide of type II collagen and to cyclic citrullinated peptides predict synergistically the development of seropositive rheumatoid arthritis. Ann Rheum Dis 2007;66(11):1450–5.
34. Bos WH, Wolbink GJ, Boers M, et al. Arthritis development in patients with arthralgia is strongly associated with anti-citrullinated protein antibody status: a prospective cohort study. Ann Rheum Dis 2010;69(3):490–4.
35. Rantapaa-Dahlqvist S, de Jong BA, Berglin E, et al. Antibodies against cyclic citrullinated peptide and IgA rheumatoid factor predict the development of rheumatoid arthritis. Arthritis Rheum 2003;48(10):2741–9.
36. Chibnik LB, Mandl LA, Costenbader KH, et al. Comparison of threshold cut-points and continuous measures of anti-cyclic citrullinated peptide antibodies in predicting future rheumatoid arthritis. J Rheumatol 2009;36(4):706–11.
37. Shadick NA, Cook NR, Karlson EW, et al. C-reactive protein in the prediction of rheumatoid arthritis in women. Arch Intern Med 2006;166(22):2490–4.
38. Nishimura K, Sugiyama D, Kogata Y, et al. Meta-analysis: diagnostic accuracy of anti-cyclic citrullinated peptide antibody and rheumatoid factor for rheumatoid arthritis. Ann Intern Med 2007;146(11):797–808.
39. Schellekens GA, Visser H, de Jong BA, et al. The diagnostic properties of rheumatoid arthritis antibodies recognizing a cyclic citrullinated peptide. Arthritis Rheum 2000;43(1):155–63.

40. van Gaalen FA, van Aken J, Huizinga TW, et al. Association between HLA class II genes and autoantibodies to cyclic citrullinated peptides (CCPs) influences the severity of rheumatoid arthritis. Arthritis Rheum 2004;50(7):2113–21.
41. Bas S, Perneger TV, Seitz M, et al. Diagnostic tests for rheumatoid arthritis: comparison of anti-cyclic citrullinated peptide antibodies, anti-keratin antibodies and IgM rheumatoid factors. Rheumatology (Oxford) 2002;41(7):809–14.
42. Goldbach-Mansky R, Lee J, McCoy A, et al. Rheumatoid arthritis associated autoantibodies in patients with synovitis of recent onset. Arthritis Res 2000; 2(3):236–43.
43. Kroot EJ, de Jong BA, van Leeuwen MA, et al. The prognostic value of anti-cyclic citrullinated peptide antibody in patients with recent-onset rheumatoid arthritis. Arthritis Rheum 2000;43(8):1831–5.
44. van Gaalen FA, Linn-Rasker SP, van Venrooij WJ, et al. Autoantibodies to cyclic citrullinated peptides predict progression to rheumatoid arthritis in patients with undifferentiated arthritis: a prospective cohort study. Arthritis Rheum 2004;50(3): 709–15.
45. Bykerk VP. Strategies to prevent rheumatoid arthritis in high-risk patients. Curr Opin Rheumatol 2011;23(2):179–84.
46. Deane KD, Norris JM, Holers VM. Preclinical rheumatoid arthritis: identification, evaluation, and future directions for investigation. Rheum Dis Clin North Am 2010;36(2):213–41.
47. Gerlag DM, Raza K, van Baarsen LG, et al. EULAR recommendations for terminology and research in individuals at risk of rheumatoid arthritis: report from the Study Group for Risk factors for Rheumatoid Arthritis. Ann Rheum Dis 2012; 71(5):638–41.
48. Kolfenbach JR, Deane KD, Derber LA, et al. A prospective approach to investigating the natural history of preclinical rheumatoid arthritis (RA) using first-degree relatives of probands with RA. Arthritis Rheum 2009;61(12):1735–42.
49. van de Sande MG, de Hair MJ, van der Leij C, et al. Different stages of rheumatoid arthritis: features of the synovium in the preclinical phase. Ann Rheum Dis 2011;70(5):772–7.
50. van der Heijde DM, van 't Hof M, van Riel PL, et al. Validity of single variables and indices to measure disease activity in rheumatoid arthritis. J Rheumatol 1993;20(3):538–41.
51. Prevoo ML, van 't Hof MA, Kuper HH, et al. Modified disease activity scores that include twenty-eight-joint counts. Development and validation in a prospective longitudinal study of patients with rheumatoid arthritis. Arthritis Rheum 1995; 38(1):44–8.
52. McInnes IB, O'Dell JR. State-of-the-art: rheumatoid arthritis. Ann Rheum Dis 2010;69(11):1898–906.
53. Smolen JS, Breedveld FC, Schiff MH, et al. A simplified disease activity index for rheumatoid arthritis for use in clinical practice. Rheumatology (Oxford) 2003; 42(2):244–57.
54. Aletaha D, Nell VP, Stamm T, et al. Acute phase reactants add little to composite disease activity indices for rheumatoid arthritis: validation of a clinical activity score. Arthritis Res Ther 2005;7(4):R796–806.
55. Wolfe F, Michaud K, Pincus T. A composite disease activity scale for clinical practice, observational studies, and clinical trials: the patient activity scale (PAS/PAS-II). J Rheumatol 2005;32(12):2410–5.
56. Yazici Y, Bergman M, Pincus T. Time to score quantitative rheumatoid arthritis measures: 28-Joint Count, Disease Activity Score, Health Assessment

Questionnaire (HAQ), Multidimensional HAQ (MDHAQ), and Routine Assessment of Patient Index Data (RAPID) scores. J Rheumatol 2008;35(4):603–9.

57. Soubrier M, Lukas C, Sibilia J, et al. Disease activity score-driven therapy versus routine care in patients with recent-onset active rheumatoid arthritis: data from the GUEPARD trial and ESPOIR cohort. Ann Rheum Dis 2011;70(4):611–5.

58. Grigor C, Capell H, Stirling A, et al. Effect of a treatment strategy of tight control for rheumatoid arthritis (the TICORA study): a single-blind randomised controlled trial. Lancet 2004;364(9430):263–9.

59. Saag KG, Teng GG, Patkar NM, et al. American College of Rheumatology 2008 recommendations for the use of nonbiologic and biologic disease-modifying antirheumatic drugs in rheumatoid arthritis. Arthritis Rheum 2008;59(6):762–84.

60. Smolen JS, Landewe R, Breedveld FC, et al. EULAR recommendations for the management of rheumatoid arthritis with synthetic and biological disease-modifying antirheumatic drugs. Ann Rheum Dis 2010;69(6):964–75.

61. Singh JA, Furst DE, Bharat A, et al. 2012 update of the 2008 American College of Rheumatology recommendations for the use of disease-modifying antirheumatic drugs and biologic agents in the treatment of rheumatoid arthritis. Arthritis Care Res (Hoboken) 2012;64(5):625–39.

62. ACCORD Study Group, Gerstein HC, Miller ME, et al. Long-term effects of intensive glucose lowering on cardiovascular outcomes. N Engl J Med 2011;364(9): 818–28.

63. Aletaha D, Ward MM, Machold KP, et al. Remission and active disease in rheumatoid arthritis: defining criteria for disease activity states. Arthritis Rheum 2005; 52(9):2625–36.

64. Fransen J, Creemers MC, Van Riel PL. Remission in rheumatoid arthritis: agreement of the disease activity score (DAS28) with the ARA preliminary remission criteria. Rheumatology (Oxford) 2004;43(10):1252–5.

65. Fransen J, van Riel PL. DAS remission cut points. Clin Exp Rheumatol 2006; 24(6 Suppl 43):S29–32.

66. Smolen JS, Aletaha D. What should be our treatment goal in rheumatoid arthritis today? Clin Exp Rheumatol 2006;24(6 Suppl 43):S7–13.

67. van der Heijde D, Klareskog L, Boers M, et al. Comparison of different definitions to classify remission and sustained remission: 1 year TEMPO results. Ann Rheum Dis 2005;64(11):1582–7.

68. van Tuyl LH, Vlad SC, Felson DT, et al. Defining remission in rheumatoid arthritis: results of an initial American College of Rheumatology/European League Against Rheumatism consensus conference. Arthritis Rheum 2009;61(5): 704–10.

69. Wells GA, Boers M, Shea B, et al. Minimal disease activity for rheumatoid arthritis: a preliminary definition. J Rheumatol 2005;32(10):2016–24.

70. Felson DT, Smolen JS, Wells G, et al. American College of Rheumatology/European League against rheumatism provisional definition of remission in rheumatoid arthritis for clinical trials. Arthritis Rheum 2011;63(3):573–86.

71. Vermeer M, Kuper HH, van der Bijl AE, et al. The provisional ACR/EULAR definition of remission in RA: a comment on the patient global assessment criterion. Oxford (UK): Rheumatology; 2012.

72. O'Dell JR, Mikuls TR. To improve outcomes we must define and measure them: toward defining remission in rheumatoid arthritis. Arthritis Rheum 2011;63(3): 587–9.

73. Shahouri SH, Michaud K, Mikuls TR, et al. Remission of rheumatoid arthritis in clinical practice: application of the American College of Rheumatology/European

League Against Rheumatism 2011 remission criteria. Arthritis Rheum 2011; 63(11):3204–15.

74. Block SR. Definition of rheumatoid arthritis remission in clinical practice: comment on the article by Felson et al. Arthritis Rheum 2011;63(11):3642 [author's reply: 3644].

75. Smolen JS, Aletaha D, Bijlsma JW, et al. Treating rheumatoid arthritis to target: recommendations of an international task force. Ann Rheum Dis 2010;69(4): 631–7.

76. Vermeer M, Kuper HH, Hoekstra M, et al. Implementation of a treat-to-target strategy in very early rheumatoid arthritis: results of the Dutch rheumatoid arthritis monitoring remission induction cohort study. Arthritis Rheum 2011; 63(10):2865–72.

77. Goekoop-Ruiterman YP, de Vries-Bouwstra JK, Allaart CF, et al. Clinical and radiographic outcomes of four different treatment strategies in patients with early rheumatoid arthritis (the BeSt study): a randomized, controlled trial. Arthritis Rheum 2005;52(11):3381–90.

78. Goekoop-Ruiterman YP, de Vries-Bouwstra JK, Allaart CF, et al. Comparison of treatment strategies in early rheumatoid arthritis: a randomized trial. Ann Intern Med 2007;146(6):406–15.

79. Kameda H, Ueki Y, Saito K, et al. Etanercept (ETN) with methotrexate (MTX) is better than ETN monotherapy in patients with active rheumatoid arthritis despite MTX therapy: a randomized trial. Mod Rheumatol 2010;20(6):531–8.

80. Breedveld FC, Weisman MH, Kavanaugh AF, et al. The PREMIER study: a multi-center, randomized, double-blind clinical trial of combination therapy with ada-limumab plus methotrexate versus methotrexate alone or adalimumab alone in patients with early, aggressive rheumatoid arthritis who had not had previous methotrexate treatment. Arthritis Rheum 2006;54(1):26–37.

81. Calguneri M, Pay S, Caliskaner Z, et al. Combination therapy versus monother-apy for the treatment of patients with rheumatoid arthritis. Clin Exp Rheumatol 1999;17(6):699–704.

82. Emery P, Breedveld FC, Hall S, et al. Comparison of methotrexate monotherapy with a combination of methotrexate and etanercept in active, early, moderate to severe rheumatoid arthritis (COMET): a randomised, double-blind, parallel treat-ment trial. Lancet 2008;372(9636):375–82.

83. Lipsky PE, van der Heijde DM, St Clair EW, et al. Infliximab and methotrexate in the treatment of rheumatoid arthritis. Anti-tumor necrosis factor trial in rheuma-toid arthritis with concomitant therapy Study Group. N Engl J Med 2000;343(22): 1594–602.

84. van der Heijde D, Klareskog L, Rodriguez-Valverde V, et al. Comparison of etanercept and methotrexate, alone and combined, in the treatment of rheumatoid arthritis: two-year clinical and radiographic results from the TEMPO study, a double-blind, randomized trial. Arthritis Rheum 2006; 54(4):1063–74.

85. Kremer JM, Russell AS, Emery P, et al. Long-term safety, efficacy and inhibition of radiographic progression with abatacept treatment in patients with rheuma-toid arthritis and an inadequate response to methotrexate: 3-year results from the AIM trial. Ann Rheum Dis 2011;70(10):1826–30.

86. Kuriya B, Arkema EV, Bykerk VP, et al. Efficacy of initial methotrexate monother-apy versus combination therapy with a biological agent in early rheumatoid arthritis: a meta-analysis of clinical and radiographic remission. Ann Rheum Dis 2010;69(7):1298–304.

87. O'Dell JR, Elliott JR, Mallek JA, et al. Treatment of early seropositive rheumatoid arthritis: doxycycline plus methotrexate versus methotrexate alone. Arthritis Rheum 2006;54(2):621–7.

88. Smolen JS, Van Der Heijde DM, St Clair EW, et al. Predictors of joint damage in patients with early rheumatoid arthritis treated with high-dose methotrexate with or without concomitant infliximab: results from the ASPIRE trial. Arthritis Rheum 2006;54(3):702–10.

89. Moreland LW, O'Dell JR, Paulus HE, et al. A randomized comparative effectiveness study of oral triple therapy versus etanercept plus methotrexate in early, aggressive rheumatoid arthritis. Arthritis Rheum 2012. [Epub ahead of print].

90. van Vollenhoven RF, Ernestam S, Geborek P, et al. Addition of infliximab compared with addition of sulfasalazine and hydroxychloroquine to methotrexate in patients with early rheumatoid arthritis (Swefot trial): 1-year results of a randomised trial. Lancet 2009;374(9688):459–66.

91. Saevarsdottir S, Wallin H, Seddighzadeh M, et al. Predictors of response to methotrexate in early DMARD naive rheumatoid arthritis: results from the initial open-label phase of the SWEFOT trial. Ann Rheum Dis 2011;70(3):469–75.

92. Michaud K, Messer J, Choi HK, et al. Direct medical costs and their predictors in patients with rheumatoid arthritis: a three-year study of 7,527 patients. Arthritis Rheum 2003;48(10):2750–62.

93. Wolfe F, Michaud K. The loss of health status in rheumatoid arthritis and the effect of biologic therapy: a longitudinal observational study. Arthritis Res Ther 2010;12(2):R35.

94. Friedewald VE, Ganz P, Kremer JM, et al. AJC editor's consensus: rheumatoid arthritis and atherosclerotic cardiovascular disease. Am J Cardiol 2010; 106(3):442–7.

95. De Vera MA, Choi H, Abrahamowicz M, et al. Statin discontinuation and risk of acute myocardial infarction in patients with rheumatoid arthritis: a population-based cohort study. Ann Rheum Dis 2011;70(6):1020–4.

96. Avina-Zubieta JA, Thomas J, Sadatsafavi M, et al. Risk of incident cardiovascular events in patients with rheumatoid arthritis: a meta-analysis of observational studies. Ann Rheum Dis 2012. [Epub ahead of print].

97. Jick SS, Choi H, Li L, et al. Hyperlipidaemia, statin use and the risk of developing rheumatoid arthritis. Ann Rheum Dis 2009;68(4):546–51.

98. Leung BP, Sattar N, Crilly A, et al. A novel anti-inflammatory role for simvastatin in inflammatory arthritis. J Immunol 2003;170(3):1524–30.

99. McCarey DW, McInnes IB, Madhok R, et al. Trial of Atorvastatin in Rheumatoid Arthritis (TARA): double-blind, randomised placebo-controlled trial. Lancet 2004;363(9426):2015–21.

100. Bingham CO 3rd, Looney RJ, Deodhar A, et al. Immunization responses in rheumatoid arthritis patients treated with rituximab: results from a controlled clinical trial. Arthritis Rheum 2010;62(1):64–74.

101. Fomin I, Caspi D, Levy V, et al. Vaccination against influenza in rheumatoid arthritis: the effect of disease modifying drugs, including TNF alpha blockers. Ann Rheum Dis 2006;65(2):191–4.

102. Kobie JJ, Zheng B, Bryk P, et al. Decreased influenza-specific B cell responses in rheumatoid arthritis patients treated with anti-tumor necrosis factor. Arthritis Res Ther 2011;13(6):R209.

103. van Assen S, Holvast A, Benne CA, et al. Humoral responses after influenza vaccination are severely reduced in patients with rheumatoid arthritis treated with rituximab. Arthritis Rheum 2010;62(1):75–81.

104. Heijstek MW, Ott de Bruin LM, Borrow R, et al. Vaccination in paediatric patients with auto-immune rheumatic diseases: a systemic literature review for the European league against rheumatism evidence-based recommendations. Autoimmun Rev 2011;11(2):112–22.

105. Grossman JM, Gordon R, Ranganath VK, et al. American College of Rheumatology 2010 recommendations for the prevention and treatment of glucocorticoid-induced osteoporosis. Arthritis Care Res (Hoboken) 2010; 62(11):1515–26.

106. O'Dell JR, Mikuls TR, Colbert RA, et al. American College of Rheumatology clinical trial priorities and design conference. Arthritis Rheum 2011;63:2151–6.

Tight Disease Control in Early RA

Deepali Sen, MD*, Richard Brasington, MD

KEYWORDS

• Early RA • Treatment • Tight control • Rheumatoid arthritis

Key Points

- Early diagnosis and early treatment of rheumatoid arthritis (RA) leads to improved long-term outcomes.
- Treatment in early RA should be targeted to achieve low levels of disease activity or remission.
- Indices that measure disease activity are helpful to guide changes in therapy.

WHY IS TREATMENT OF EARLY RHEUMATOID ARTHRITIS IMPORTANT?

The past decade has witnessed a dramatic change in the management of rheumatoid arthritis (RA). In contrast to the textbook description of patients with joint deformities, today patients who receive adequate treatment often bear no stigmata of the disease. The era of biologic disease-modifying antirheumatic drugs (DMARDs) has done more than just place new medications at our disposal; there has been a paradigm shift in the way we view disease management, especially in early disease. We now know that erosive joint disease can occur within months of symptom onset.[1,2] Loss of function can also occur early in the disease course and may be irreversible thereafter. Recent studies indicate that the high inflammatory burden of early RA may cause the progression of atherosclerotic disease earlier than previously anticipated.[3] The disease process may start earlier than the onset of symptoms suggested by the presence of autoantibodies before disease manifestation.[4]

Early RA is thought to offer a window of opportunity whereby the disease is more sensitive to treatment and during which therapeutic intervention has the potential to alter the disease course. Therefore, the emphasis is on early diagnosis and treatment.

Funding support: None for both authors.
Disclosure: None for both authors.
Division of Rheumatology, Department of Medicine, Washington University School of Medicine, 660 South Euclid Avenue, St Louis, MO 63110, USA
* Corresponding author.
E-mail address: dsen@dom.wustl.edu

Rheum Dis Clin N Am 38 (2012) 327–343
doi:10.1016/j.rdc.2012.04.004
0889-857X/12/$ – see front matter © 2012 Elsevier Inc. All rights reserved.
rheumatic.theclinics.com

Good response early in the disease course is thought to be predictive of better long-term outcomes.[5–7] Although there is no clear definition of early RA, most clinical trials use disease duration of 3 to 24 months from symptom onset. A survey of rheumatologists indicated that most physicians considered early RA as disease duration of less than 3 months.[8] In 2010, The American College of Rheumatology (ACR) and the European League Against Rheumatism (EULAR) developed new RA classification criteria to aid the recognition of and facilitate clinical studies in early disease.[9]

TREAT TO TARGET: BUT WHAT TARGET?

If we accept the concept of treating to a target, a critical question is: what is the target to which we should treat? Today remission is thought to be an achievable goal of treatment. Remission may be thought of as a state of total absence of articular or extraarticular inflammation, therefore, a complete arrest of disease progression. However, it is impossible to ascertain a complete lack of inflammation and, thus the concept of clinical remission was developed, which would be defined by the absence of activity on measurable parameters and could be widely applicable.[10] It is important to remember that clinical remission does not reflect a true absence of inflammation, and joint damage is known to progress in patients with clinical remission. Also, it may not be possible to attain clinical remission in all patients. If clinical remission cannot be attained in an individual, a state of low disease activity or minimal disease activity is an acceptable alternative. A variety of disease indices have been developed that measure disease activity and define clinical remission; most were developed for randomized control studies. These indices use composite scores reflecting joint counts, inflammatory markers, and physician and patient assessment of disease activity. The international task force on treating RA to target suggests: "The primary target for treatment of rheumatoid arthritis should be a state of clinical remission."[11] This statement underscores the need of a tool that clearly defines remission, detects minimal levels of disease activity, and is easily applicable to clinical practice.

Of the various indices, the disease activity score (DAS) and the DAS 28 are among the earliest and most widely used in clinical trials. The DAS is a composite score of a 53 tender or 44 swollen joint count, erythrocyte sedimentation rate (ESR), and a patient global assessment on a visual analog scale of 1 to 100. A computational device is required to calculate the score. Possible scores range from 0 to 9. Remission is defined as DAS less than 1.6.[12] The DAS 28 is similar to the DAS except it uses a 28 joint count for tender and swollen joints; the hips, ankles, and feet findings are excluded from the score. The scores can range from 0 to 9, with remission being defined as DAS 28 less than 2.6.[13] This score has been validated to be as effective as the DAS but allows for multiple tender or swollen joints in the lower extremities while achieving scores consistent with remission.

The ACR[14] and EULAR[15] response criterion were both developed to quantify the changes occurring with treatment with an active drug versus placebo. ACR 20, 50, and 70 is defined as a 20%, 50%, and 70% improvement, respectively, in the number of swollen and tender joint counts and a similar improvement in 3 of 5 variables: patient and physician global assessment, health assessment questionnaire (HAQ), ESR, or C-reactive protein (CRP). The EULAR response criterion define good, moderate, and no response based on the current level of disease activity and the decrease in disease activity from a prior time point by a DAS or DAS 28. For example, a reduction in a DAS 28 by more than 1.2 combined with a current DAS 28 less than 2.6 would be a good response. A reduction in a DAS 28 by more than 1.2 combined with a current DAS 28 of 4.0 would qualify as a moderate response. Because both the ACR and

EULAR response require the measurement of disease activity at 2 time points, they are difficult to implement in clinical practice. The EULAR criteria are thought to more accurately reflect disease activity as compared with the ACR criteria.

The simplified disease activity index (SDAI)[16] is the numeric value of a 28 swollen and tender joint count, CRP, and a patient and physician global assessment of disease activity on a visual analog scale of 1 to 10. SDAI scores can range from 0 to 86. Remission is defined as a score of less than 3.3. The clinical disease activity index (CDAI)[17] is similar to the SDAI except it does not need the measurement of CRP. Scores range from 0 to 76, and remission is defined as a score of less than 2.8. Both of these indices use a more stringent cutoff, allowing for less swollen and tender joint counts as compared with the DAS 28. The CDAI has the advantage of not requiring a laboratory parameter and can be completed at the time of the office visit, making it more suitable for office practice.

Pincus and colleagues[18] developed an index, the Routine Assessment of Patient Index Data 3 (RAPID 3), that is based purely on patient-reported measures. Patients rate 3 measures: a multidimensional HAQ questionnaire (10 questions), a pain visual analog scale from 1 to 10, and a global status visual analog scale from 1 to 10. The sum of these divided by 3 gives a number from 1 to 10, which constitutes the RAPID 3 score. This score has been validated to correlate significantly with the DAS 28 and the CDAI indices. This index, however, does not take into account any joint assessment for tender or swollen joints.

In 2011, the ACR and EULAR proposed that remission for clinical trials can be defined in one of two ways. A Boolean based definition where patients satisfy all three criteria of tender joint count less than or equal to 1, swollen joint count less than or equal to one and CRP less than or equal to 1. Alternatively an index based definition may be used where remission is defined as SDAI of less than or equal to 3.3. This definition can be modified for clinical practice by substituting CRP with a patient global assessment score.

If remission cannot be attained, minimal disease activity is an alternative goal. Outcome Measures in Rheumatoid Arthritis Clinical Trials (OMERACT) has proposed 2 definitions for minimal disease activity (MDA). Five out of 7 criterion had to be met: a patient pain visual analog scale less than or equal to 2 (1–10), swollen joint count less than or equal to 1 (1–28), tender joint count less than or equal to 1 (1–28), HAQ less than or equal to 0.5 (1–3), physician global assessment less than or equal to 1.5 (1–10), patient global assessment less than or equal to 2 (1–10), and an ESR less than or equal to 10. A DAS 28 less than 2.8 was also thought to reflect MDA.[19–21] The EULAR task force recommendations on treating RA to target emphasize the importance of using a validated composite measure that includes joint assessment in clinical practice.[11]

TREATMENT OF EARLY RA: EARLY INITIATION OF DMARD THERAPY

While treating RA, earlier and more intensive therapy has been shown to be superior to conventional care. If treated within a few months, the disease may be more responsive to DMARD therapy and it may eventually be possible to scale back therapy, signifying a window of opportunity. There is a long history of studies supporting the early administration of DMARDs. One of the first studies to demonstrate this was conducted by Egsmose and colleagues,[22] which showed that the immediate administration of auranoffin was clearly superior to waiting 8 months to begin this agent. There was both functional and radiographic advantage to the former approach that was maintained for an additional 3 years of follow-up. It is noteworthy that this difference was shown with an agent that is not generally considered one of the more effective DMARDs.

Similarly, an open-label study from the Mayo Clinic studied patients with early RA of less than 1-year for response to hydroxychloroquine, if patients did not have an ACR 50 response on hydroxychloroquine alone, methotrexate was added. At 24 months, 59 of 94 patients achieved an ACR 50 response on hydroxychloroquine alone. High pain scores, presence of rheumatoid factor, higher number of swollen joints were factors associated with inability to achieve an ACR 50 response on hydroxychloroquine alone.[23]

The Computer Assisted Management of Early Rheumatoid Arthritis (CAMERA) study looked at 299 patients with a disease duration of less than 1 year who were treated with methotrexate. One group received monthly follow-up with rapid up-titration of methotrexate dose and the addition of cyclosporine. Change of therapy was guided to meet predefined criteria by a computerized decision-making program. The other group had a follow-up every 3 months and received conventional therapy. Fifty percent of the patients in the intensive therapy arm achieved remission compared with 37% in conventional therapy at some point during the 2-year study. The 5-year follow-up results from the CAMERA study found that patients who had a good EULAR response at 6 months had favorable radiographic and disease activity outcomes at 5 years regardless of the therapy used.[24]

A study by Nell and colleagues[25] compared the treatment response of a very-early group (mean disease duration of 3 months) to a late-early group (mean duration of 12 months). Both groups were treated with oral DMARD therapy. At 36 months of follow-up, the very-early RA group had a mean improvement in the DAS 28 of 2.8 ± 1.5 compared with 1.7 ± 1.2 in the late-early RA group ($P<.05$). Radiographic progression as measured by the Larsen score increased by 3.6 ± 6.5 in the very-early group versus 14.7 ± 9.9 in the late-early group ($P<.05$). This finding suggests that very-early disease may be more responsive to DMARD therapy.[25]

The Finnish Rheumatoid Arthritis Combination Therapy (FIN RaCO) trial was one of the first studies to demonstrate long-term benefits of initial combination therapy.[26] The initial cohort of 195 patients with disease duration less than 2 years was recruited between 1993 and 1995 and followed up to 11 years. Ninety-seven of 195 patients received combination therapy with sulfasalazine, methotrexate, hydroxychloroquine, and prednisolone. Ninety-eight patients received single drug therapy with sulfasalazine or methotrexate with or without prednisolone. The aim of therapy was the induction of remission as measured by the ACR criteria. At the end of 2 years, 37% of the patients in combination therapy versus 18% of patients in single drug therapy were in remission. There was also a significantly higher ACR 50 response and less radiographic progression (measured by Larsen scores) in the combination therapy group. At the end of 2 years, more patients in the single drug therapy were on steroids.

After 2 years, therapy was unrestricted and all patients were treated at their rheumatologist's discretion, with treatment targeted to remission. After 11 years, follow-up was complete with 68 patients from the initial combination group and 70 patients from the single drug therapy group. The modified MDAs were met by 63% in the initial combination therapy group versus 43% in the initial single therapy group. DAS 28 remission was reached in 57% of the patients in the initial combination therapy versus 49% of the patients in the initial single drug therapy group. The ACR remission criteria were met more often at 2, 5, and 11 years in the combination therapy group. Early combination therapy improved the long-term radiographic outcome at 11 years.[27,28] This finding shows that intensive treatment of early active disease, perhaps with initial combination therapy, can result in improved long-term outcomes both in terms of functional outcomes and radiographic stability.

TREATMENT OF EARLY RA: EARLY INITIATION OF BIOLOGIC THERAPY

Since the advent of the biologic DMARDs, there has been much discussion and speculation about whether such agents should be used in the initial treatment regimen of RA. The argument for so doing relies on the consistent observation in numerous studies for Food and Drug Administration approval that radiographic change, in the aggregate, progresses less in the patients treated with biologics as compared with methotrexate in established RA. For example, the Anti TNF Therapy in RA with Concomitant Therapy (ATTRACT) study found that in 428 patients who were randomized to receive methotrexate plus infliximab versus methotrexate plus placebo, median change from baseline at week 102 in Sharp scores was 4.25 in patients who received methotrexate alone versus 0.5 in patients who received infliximab plus methotrexate (P<.001).[29] Furthermore, when patients with early disease are studied, the difference in radiographic progression between the two treatment groups is even more striking. A subgroup analysis of 82 patients with early disease (<3 years duration) from the ATTRACT study, the median change in Sharp scores at 102 weeks was 12.21 in the methotrexate alone group versus 0.49 in the methotrexate plus infliximab combination group (P<.001).[30]

Similar results have been observed with other tumor necrosis factor (TNF) inhibitors. The PREMIER study included 799 patients with RA with a mean disease duration of 1 year. Patients were randomized to methotrexate monotherapy, adalimumab monotherapy, or a combination of methotrexate and adalimumab. The primary end point at 2 years was an ACR 20 response and change from baseline in the Sharp score. At 1 year of therapy, 62% in the combination group, 41% in adalimumab group, and 46% in methotrexate group achieved an ACR 50 response. Superior response and significantly less radiographic progression were seen in the combination group at the end of 2 years. A change in Sharp scores at 1 and 2 years were 1.3 and 1.9 in the combination group, 3.0 and 5.5 in the adalimumab monotherapy group, and 5.7 and 10.4 in the methotrexate monotherapy groups, respectively. There was no difference in serious adverse events across groups.[31]

Etanercept versus methotrexate in early rheumatoid arthritis (ERA) trial, 632 patients with a mean disease duration of 1 year were treated with etanercept monotherapy versus methotrexate monotherapy. At 24 months, the patients treated with etanercept 25 mg twice every week had a significantly greater response than the methotrexate monotherapy group ACR 20 response 72% and 59% respectively (P<.005). A change in the Sharp score and erosion score in the etanercept group was 1.3 and 0.66 units, respectively, compared with 3.2 and 1.86 in the methotrexate group. The study also reported a significant improvement in the HAQ disability index.[32] A subset of 148 patients who received etanercept from this trial was compared with 464 patients with late disease (mean duration of 12 years) who also received etanercept. The mean HAQ score was similar at the onset of therapy in both groups; however, at the end of 3 years of treatment, 26% of the patients with early disease had an HAQ score of 0, whereas only 14% of patients in the late therapy achieved the same result (P<.0095). This finding signifies that early treatment can have significant benefits at limiting disability.[33]

The Active-Controlled Study of Patients Receiving Infliximab for the treatment of Rheumatoid Arthritis of Early Onset[34] study group studied the effects of elevated levels of ESR and CRP as well as swollen joint count on radiographic progression in patients on methotrexate monotherapy versus a combination of methotrexate and infliximab. They reported that ESR, CRP, and swollen joint counts were associated with joint damage in patients treated with methotrexate but not associated with joint damage in patients treated with a combination therapy of methotrexate and infliximab. The mean changes in the Sharp score among patients with a CRP of more than 3 and an ESR of more than 52 in the methotrexate-only group were 5.62 and 5.89, respectively, compared with 0.73 and 1.12 in the combination group ($P<.001$). This finding suggests that very active early disease may benefit from initial TNF therapy. The same group also studied radiographic progression in patients of different disease activity states by an SDAI[35] in methotrexate monotherapy versus a combination therapy of methotrexate and infliximab. A total of 1049 patients with early disease were randomized into 3 groups: methotrexate monotherapy, combination therapy with infliximab 3 mg/kg, or combination therapy with infliximab 6 mg/kg. They found that in patients on methotrexate monotherapy, radiographic progression was halted only in those who achieved SDAI remission. In both combination therapy groups radiographic progression was halted in patients who achieved remission. In patients who achieved low to moderate activity by SDAI radiographic progression was halted or retarded respectively. Results such as these have given rise to the thought that there may be uncoupling of inflammation and bone damage in the setting of anti-TNF therapy.

However, caution is warranted on several grounds. First, the Sharp score differences in the short-term trials are small, and it is unclear what the implications are for damage and function in the long-term. More importantly, probability analysis has consistently demonstrated that the aggregate difference in radiographic change results from only about 20% of the study cohort; in other words, for approximately 80% of patients in such studies, there is no difference between the two treatment groups in radiographic progression.[36] Regrettably, we currently have no way to reliable prospectively identify the patients most likely to enjoy the difference in radiograph progression.

TREATMENT OF EARLY RA: TIGHT CONTROL

Clearly, there is abundant data supporting the institution of DMARD therapy early in the course of RA. The concept of tight control of RA developed by analogy to tight control of diabetes, which has been shown to result in better long-term outcomes. In diabetes, this is achieved by treating to a target, the glycosylated hemoglobin level. Similarly, tight control of RA would entail modifying therapy toward the goal of achieving a quantitative clinical target rather than relying on the traditional subjective assessment of physician and patient as to whether the results of treatment were adequate. Several studies have since shown that tight control yields better results.

The Tight Control in Rheumatoid Arthritis (TICORA) was among the first to demonstrate long-term benefits of early aggressive therapy. This trial studied 110 European patients with RA of less than 5 years duration. All patients were treated with oral DMARDs. Patients were randomized to receive intensive treatment versus routine care, and the outcome was measured by DAS score. Intensive care involved monthly assessments by a rheumatologist; for DAS more than 2.4, DMARD treatment was escalated by protocol, all swollen joints were injected at each visit (unless injected within the past 3 months, maximum of 3 joints injected each visit). Patients in the routine care group were evaluated every 3 months, DAS was not used for clinical decision making, and change of therapy was at the discretion of the rheumatologist. After 18 months, patients in the intensive care group were more likely than the routine care group to have a good EULAR response (44% vs 82%), EULAR remission (16% vs 65%), ACR 50 response (40% vs 84%), and ACR 70 response (18% vs 71%). Thus, the differences in remission by both DAS and ACR criteria were striking. Patients in the intensive care arm also had greater improvement in their physical function and quality of life. There was no increase in adverse effects or cost of treatment; outpatient costs were higher in the intensive treatment group, whereas inpatient costs were higher in the routine treatment group, with no overall difference between the 2 groups. Interestingly, this study that tested the hypothesis that tight control of RA would lead to better outcomes was conducted before the availability of TNF antagonists.[37]

The Combinatietherapie Bij Rheumatoide Artritis protocol,[38] one of the first to demonstrate the superiority of a combination step-down regimen, was applied in a pilot study of 21 patients with very early active disease (mean DAS 5.3, mean disease duration of 3 months). The initial therapy consisted of methotrexate, sulfasalazine, and prednisolone starting at 60 mg. Treatment adjustments were made for a DAS 28 more than 3.2 or by the measurement of C terminal cross linking of type II collagen, a marker of cartilage degradation. Therapy could be stepped up by adding hydroxychloroquine or infliximab, and low-dose prednisone could be continued. The study had high remission rates (DAS 28 <2.6) of 90%, and the mean DAS at the end of the study was 1.6. However, some patients were maintained on low-dose prednisone at 7.5 mg.[39]

The head-to-head comparison between step-up versus initial combination therapy with conventional DMARD and TNF inhibitors have been studied by the 2007 Behandel Strategieen (BeST) trial.[40] The BeST study was a multicenter clinical trial that compared 4 different treatment strategies. Although designed to compare different treatment regimens, BeST also applied a treat-to-target strategy in its execution. A total of 508 patients with early active disease (mean disease duration of 24 weeks, mean DAS 4.4, HAQ 1.4) were randomized to one of 4 treatment groups: sequential monotherapy (group 1), step-up combination therapy (group 2), initial combination therapy with tapered high-dose prednisone (group 3), and initial combination with infliximab and DMARD (group 4). For each group, the target was to obtain a low disease activity level DAS of less than or equal to 2.4. Medications were adjusted every 3 months based on the DAS. For a DAS more than 2.4, therapy was escalated to the next step for the allocated group. If DAS remained at less than 2.4 for 6 months, medications were gradually withdrawn (steroids and infliximab were the first to be tapered) until monotherapy was achieved. The primary end point was functional ability measured by HAQ and radiographic damage as assessed by the change in Sharp scores. Secondary response was ACR 20 and ACR 70 response and disease remission by DAS. During the first year follow-up, patients in groups 3 and 4 (initial combination therapy) regained physical function earlier as measured by HAQ. Although the combination therapy groups did better over 1 year, at the end of 2 years, groups 1 and 2 achieved almost the same improvement in disease activity as groups 3 and 4. However, groups 1 and 2 needed more medication adjustments to reach a DAS less than 2.4. Also, more patients in groups 3 and 4 were maintained on monotherapy at 2 years.

At the 2-year follow-up, patients in groups 3 and 4 had less progression of radiographic joint damage than groups 1 and 2. The patients in group 4 had less, although not statistically significant, progression of radiographic scores compared with group 3. Infliximab therapy could be stepped down in 56% of the patients in group 4 who maintained a low disease activity state of a DAS less than 2.4. Infliximab therapy had to be withdrawn in certain cases because of new guidelines regarding contraindication of TNF inhibitors in the setting of congestive heart failure.[41] The BeST study showed rapid initial improvement of clinical symptoms with an initial combination therapy and favored an initial intensive regimen with subsequent step-down rather than a step-up therapy. Like the TICORA trial, BeST demonstrated that treatment to a target resulted in excellent results.

The question of whether the administration of an initial combination therapy would be superior to methotrexate monotherapy stepped up to combination therapy was tested in the Treatment of Early Aggressive Rheumatoid Arthritis (TEAR) trial.[42] This was a multispecialty, randomized, double-blind protocol that was investigator initiated. A treat-to-target strategy was applied with intensification of therapy for DAS 28 more than 3.2. A total of 755 patients were randomized to 4 groups. Two groups got step-up therapy, one group got methotrexate that was stepped up to triple oral DMARD therapy, the second group got methotrexate stepped up to the addition of etanercept. Two groups got initial combination therapy: one with initial triple oral DMARD therapy and another with initial methotrexate and etanercept combination therapy. At 6 months, there was a superior ACR 20, 50, and 70 response in both initial combination therapy groups ($P<.0001$ for all responses); however, at 2 years, there were no significant differences among the 4 groups in DAS scores. At 102 weeks, the same cohort showed a significant radiographic benefit in both etanercept groups over both triple-therapy groups.[43]

The Swedish Pharmacotherapy (SWEFOT) trial studied 258 patients with early RA (duration <1 year) who had not achieved low disease activity levels with methotrexate alone. One hundred thirty patients received combination therapy with methotrexate, sulfasalazine, and hydroxychloroquine; 128 patients received a combination of methotrexate and infliximab. The primary end point defined by a good EULAR response was met by 25% of the patients in the oral DMARD group versus 39% of the patients in the infliximab group ($P = .0160$).[44]

The Dutch Rheumatoid Arthritis Monitoring (DREAM) remission induction cohort studied a DAS 28–guided escalation protocol with treatment targeted to remission. This cohort had 534 patients with early RA of less than 1 year (mean duration of 24 weeks). They used an escalating regimen starting with methotrexate followed by the addition of sulfasalazine, followed by the substitution of sulfasalazine by a biologic agent that is reflective of current-day practice. Patients were monitored by the DAS 28, and treatment was aimed to remission defined as a DAS 28 of less than 2.6. With this regimen, 46% of the patients achieved remission.[45]

Together, these data emphasize the importance of aggressively treating early RA. Data support that the use of initial combination therapy in active disease may lead to early control. However, good results may be obtained with a step-up therapy as long as patients are closely monitored and treatment is modified to achieve rapid remission. The initial use of biologic therapy may have a benefit over conventional DMARD therapy in terms of radiographic progression, although the clinical significance of this is unclear.

IS THERE A RISK TO EARLY AGGRESSIVE TREATMENT?

Although aggressive treatment to remission seems to be beneficial in early active disease, this may not hold true in patients with mild early disease activity. The Strategies in Early Rheumatoid Arthritis Management (STREAM) trial randomized 82 patients with mild early RA of less than 2 years, with 2 to 4 swollen joints and a Sharp score of less than 5. Patients were randomized to an aggressive group aimed to maintain remission DAS less than 1.6 with methotrexate and the addition of adalimumab versus a traditional group treated without a DAS-based guideline with DMARD therapy at the treating physician's discretion. No biologics or oral steroids were used in the traditional group. The mean DAS at 0 and 2 years was 2.2 and 1.4, respectively, in the aggressive group and 2.4 and 1.7 in the traditional group. After 2 years of therapy, there was no significant difference in the remission rates, change in Sharp score, or decrease in the HAQ score between the two groups. The number of adverse events was 62 in the aggressive therapy group compared with 35 in the conventional group (P = .034). Five serious adverse events occurred in the aggressive therapy group versus 3 in the conventional group.[46]

A significant number of patients with early arthritis may also present with undifferentiated disease. Up to half of such patients may undergo spontaneous remission. The rest remain undifferentiated or progress to RA or other defined inflammatory disease. It is known that the treatment of undifferentiated arthritis with DMARD therapy can prevent the development of RA and subsequent joint damage.[47] It may, however, be difficult to determine an individual's chance of progression and, therefore, identify the right candidates for treatment. The 2010 ACR/EULAR guidelines provide a much-needed standard for the diagnosis of early RA. The new diagnostic criteria for RA have helped reclassify patients who had undifferentiated disease by the 1987 criteria with a high likelihood of progression to RA.[9] Therefore, fewer patients are now classified to have undifferentiated disease; such patients tend to have mild disease and are more likely to undergo spontaneous remission. It is thought that close to a quarter of patients with undifferentiated disease by the new criteria will still progress to RA.[48] It is important to note that most studies in early RA enrolled patients who satisfied the 1987 criteria, this may represent a substantially different cohort of patients than patients who are diagnosed now diagnosed with early RA by the new criteria. Because patients with milder disease are now diagnosed with RA, it is unclear if the same benefits of aggressive therapy would hold true in this population.

CLOSING THE GAP

The patient population in clinical practice is more heterogeneous than a study population. Indeed, a study by Sokka and Pincus[49] suggests that most patients in practice would not meet the criteria for enrollment in clinical trials. How can we apply this data in clinical practice? Here several questions remain unanswered. What disease activity measure would provide reliable information without being cumbersome or time consuming? The different indices, for example, may give variable results on remission in an individual patient[50]: Tender joints may reflect concomitant fibromyalgia, swollen joints may reflect chronic deformities, checking inflammatory markers may not be feasible at each visit, and abnormal values may reflect a multitude of causes. Similarly, patient-centered questionnaires may be dependent on an individual patient's perception of pain and functioning.

Furthermore, most practicing rheumatologists do not perform DAS, SDAI, or CDAI scores at each visit and not all document joint counts.[51] One study estimated the average time to perform a 28 joint count was 94 seconds. The mean time to score the DAS 28, CDAI, RAPID 3 (0–10 scale), and RAPID 3 (0–30 scale) was 114.0, 106.0, 9.6, and 4.6 seconds, respectively. Results on all indices seem to correlate significantly. The investigators suggest that RAPID 3 may provide equivalent information to a DAS 28 or CDAI in a fraction of time.[52] Thus, the outcome measures used in clinical trials remain largely inapplicable to clinical practice, and there is no clear consensus which measure is optimum. The EULAR task force recommendations on treating RA to target emphasize the importance of using a validated composite measure that includes joint assessment in clinical practice. However, it leaves the choice of which measure to apply up to the physician.

Today most patients are treated at their physician's discretion and most start with monotherapy. Data suggest that protocol-based treatment may be superior to decision making by the physician.[24,37] Initial combination therapy with subsequent step down may be beneficial at least in active disease to achieve rapid disease control.[40,42] Should treatment of RA be protocol driven like chemotherapy regimens? On the other hand, step-up therapy also yields good results over time, as long as there is intensive monitoring and rapid titration of therapy to achieve remission.[42,45] Intensive monitoring and rapid titration of therapy until remission is achieved is of paramount importance. It is also unclear what regimen is best for initial treatment; both oral DMARD and anti-TNF therapy seem to be effective at achieving clinical remission; however, biologics may be better at preventing radiographic progression even if an equivalent clinical response can be obtained by DMARD therapy.

Table 1
Oral DMARD therapy in early RA

Trial Year Number of Patients Disease Duration Follow-up	Study Design	Medications	Results
Egmose et al[22] 1995 No of patients 137 Disease duration <2y Follow-up 5 y	Double blind, placebo controlled Early group treated immediately at diagnosis Delayed group: initiation of treatment delayed 8 mo as compared with early group	Auranoffin Single oral DMARD of auranoffin D-penicillamine HCQS, SSZ, azathioprine, and so forth	At 5 y, change in Larsen scores and erosion scores were twice as much in the delayed treatment as compared with early treatment
Matteson et al[23] 2004 No of patients 111 Disease duration <1 y Follow-up 2 y	Open-label study All patients Failure to achieve ACR 50 response or requiring prednisone >10 mg	HCQS ± NSAID ± prednisone Addition of MTX 7.5–20 mg	At 24 mo, most patients achieved ACR 50 response on HCQS alone
CAMERA[24] 2007 No of patients 299 Disease duration <1 y Follow-up 2 y	2 arms Intensive group: monthly follow-up treatment adjustments based on computerized decision-making program Conventional care 3-mo follow-up	Rapid up titration of MTX followed by addition of cyclosporine Dose adjustment dependent on rheumatologist	Remission 50% with intensive care vs 37% in conventional care Good EULAR response at 6 mo predicted favorable radiographic and disease activity outcomes at 5 y regardless of the therapy used
FIN RaCo[26] 1999 No of patients 195 Disease duration <2 y Follow-up 2 y	Multicenter, randomized, open parallel group trial 2 arms Single-drug therapy Combination therapy	SSZ or MTX ± prednisolone SSZ + MTX + HCOS + prednisolone	At 2 y Combination vs single drug therapy Remission 37% vs 18% Median increase in Larsen scores 2 vs 10

Abbreviations: HCQS, hydroxychloroquine; MTX, methotrexate; SSZ, sulfasalazine.

Clinical remission, however, does not guarantee radiographic remission; new erosions may occur in patients who seem to be in remission.[53,54] This finding may reflect the presence of subclinical disease that remains undetected by routine measures causing progressive joint destruction. Both magnetic resonance imaging (MRI) and ultrasound have higher sensitivity to detect synovitis than clinical examination. Power Doppler activity on musculoskeletal ultrasound and bone edema on MRI are strong predictors of subsequent joint damage.[55,56]

Table 2
Biologic therapy in early RA

Trial Year Number of Patients Disease Duration Follow-up	Study Design	Clinical Results	Radiographic Results

ERA[32]
2002
No of patients 632
Disease duration <3 y
Follow-up 2 y
	Randomized
	  controlled study
	3 arms
	Etanercept 10 mg
	  twice weekly
	Etanercept 25 mg
	  twice weekly
	Oral MTX: mean
	  dosage 19 mg
	  weekly
		Response
		  etanercept 25 mg
		  vs MTX
		ACR 20
		72% vs 59%
		ACR 50
		49% vs 42%
		ACR 70
		29% vs 24%
			Mean change in
			  Sharp scores
			1.3 units in 25 mg
			  etanercept vs 3.2 in
			  MTX group
			Mean change in
			  erosion scores
			0.66 units in 25 mg
			  etanercept vs 1.86
			  in MTX group

ATTRACT[30]
2004
(subgroup analysis
  of patients with
  early RA)
No of patients 61
Disease duration <3 y
Follow-up 2 y
	Randomized
	  controlled study
	5 arms
	MTX only
	MTX + infliximab
	  3 mg/kg every
	  4 wk
	MTX + infliximab
	  3 mg/kg every 8
	  wk MTX +
	  infliximab 10 mg/
	  kg every 4 wk
	MTX + infliximab
	  10 mg/kg every
	  8 wk
			Progression of
			  erosion scores at
			  102 wk
			MTX only −12.21
			Total MTX +
			  infliximab -0.49
			Joint space
			  narrowing scores
			MTX only 12.82
			Total MTX +
			  infliximab 0.05
			(all infliximab
			  regimens gave
			  comparable
			  results)

PRIMIER[31]
2006
No of patients 799
Disease duration <3 y
Follow-up 2 y
	Multicenter, double
	  blind,
	  comparator
	  controlled
	3 arms
	adalimumab + MTX
	adalimumab
	  monotherapy
	MTX monotherapy
		Response at 2 y
		  combination
		  therapy,
		  adalimumab
		  monotherapy and
		  MTX monotherapy,
		  respectively
		ACR 20%–69%,
		  49%, 56%
		ACR 50
		59%, 37%, 43%
		ACR70
		47%, 28%, 28%
			Radiographic
			  progression at
			  1 and 2 y,
			  respectively
			Combination therapy
			  1.3 and 1.9 units
			adalimumab
			  monotherapy 3.0
			  and 5.5 units
			MTX 5.7 and
			  10.4 units

Abbreviations: HCQS, hydroxychloroquine; MTX, methotrexate; SSZ, sulfasalazine.

Table 3
Treat-to-target trials in early RA

Trial Year Number of Patients Target Disease Duration	Design	Medications	Results
TICORA[37] 2004 Number of patients 110 Target DAS <2.4 Disease duration <5 y	Single-blind randomized controlled trial 2 groups Intensive care group Followed every month therapy escalation for DAS >2.4 All swollen joints injected Routine care Follow-up every 3 mo Change in therapy was not guided by measurement of disease activity	Oral DMARD + intraarticular/injected steroids Oral DMARD	Good EULAR response 44% in routine care vs 82% intensive care EULAR remission 16% in routine care vs 65% in intensive care ACR 50 response 40% in routine care vs 84% in intensive care ACR 70 response 18% in routine care vs 71% in intensive care
BeST[40] 2007 Number of patients 508 Target DAS <2.4 Disease duration <2 y	Randomized controlled trial 4 treatment groups: group 1: sequential monotherapy group 2: step-up combination therapy group 3: initial oral DMARD combination therapy with tapered high-dose prednisone group 4: initial combination with infliximab	MTX to SSZ then per protocol MTX to MTX + SSZ then per protocol MTX + SSZ + prednisone MTX + infliximab	79% of patients in all groups attained DAS <2.4 67%, 69%, 42%, 28% of patients in groups 1, 2, 3, and 4, respectively, needed treatment adjustments to achieve the goal Mean increase in Sharp scores was 2.0, 2.0, 1.0, 1.0 in groups 1, 2, 3, and 4, respectively Improvement in HAQ scores occurred earlier in groups 3 and 4 as compared with groups 1 and 2

Swefot[44] 2009 No of Patients 258 Target DAS 28 <3.2 Disease duration <1 y	Patients with DAS 28 >3.2 on MTX randomized to Combination therapy MTX +oral DMARD Combination of MTX with infliximab	MTX + SSZ + HCQS MTX + infliximab	Good EULAR response 25% in MTX + SSZ + HCQS group v/s 37% in MTX + infliximab group
TEAR[42,43] 2009 No of patients 755 Target DAS 28 <3.2 Disease duration <3 y	Multicenter randomized study 4 groups: Immediate triple DMARD Immediate anti-TNF Step-up triple DMARD Step-up to anti-TNF	MTX + SSZ + HCQ MTX + etanercept MTX to MTX + SSZ + HCQ MTX to MTX + etanercept	Patients with initial combination therapy had significantly better ACR 20, 50, 70 responses at 6 mo All groups had similar responses at 2 y Treatment with MTX + etanercept had significantly better radiologic outcome than triple therapy
DREAM[45] 2011 No of patients 534 Target DAS 28 <2.6 Disease duration <1 y	Cohort study To study remission with a treat-to-target approach	MTX to MTX + SSZ to MTX + anti-TNF therapy	At 6 months 42% DAS 28 <2.6 57% good EULAR response 32% ACR remission At 12 mo 58% DAS 28 <2.6 67.9% good EULAR response 46.45 ACR remission

Abbreviations: HCQS, hydroxychloroquine; MTX, methotrexate; SSZ, sulfasalazine.

Brown and colleagues[57] studied 102 patients on conventional therapy who were judged to be in remission by their treating rheumatologist. Patients were evaluated with conventional radiographs, ultrasound, and MRI at baseline and 1 year. Nineteen percent of the patients in remission by ACR and DAS criterion still had radiographic progression. Scores on musculoskeletal ultrasound for synovial hypertrophy, power Doppler, and MRI synovitis at baseline were significantly associated with worsening radiographic changes. These changes occurred at sites detected to have active synovitis by ultrasound and MRI. They reported a 12 times higher odds of damage in joints with increased power Doppler signals.[57]

These modalities are clearly superior to clinical examination and conventional radiographs at detecting joint disease. There are currently no clear guidelines that indicate how these imaging techniques can help define response to therapy or remission and if treatment should be guided by these findings of subclinical disease.

To facilitate early treatment, early diagnosis is essential. This point needs increased awareness among primary care physicians to aid diagnostic workup in the early phase. Prompt referral systems need to be set up so that these patients do not wait for weeks before getting to a rheumatologist. Although complete clinical remission with no tender or swollen joints and normal inflammatory markers remains the ultimate aim, in clinical practice, it may not be feasible to escalate therapy to meet these goals in all patients. Treatment ultimately has to be individualized to the patient.

SUMMARY

Early diagnosis and early treatment of RA leads to better long-term outcomes. There is clear evidence that aggressive treatment and close monitoring is of paramount importance in treating early active disease. The treat-to-target approach leads to better outcomes. Under ideal circumstances, clinical remission is the goal of therapy. DMARD therapy should be initiated early; good results can be obtained with conventional oral DMARD therapy as long as clinical remission is obtained. However, anti-TNF therapy may improve radiologic outcomes as compared with oral DMARDs. Multiple indices have been designed to measure disease activity and define remission, and it is recommended that physicians use these indices to guide decision making in clinical practice. While translating the data from studies into clinical practice, physicians need to adapt therapy to each individual patient. Determining the role of newer imaging modalities in diagnosing and treating early disease remains a work in progress (**Tables 1–3**).

REFERENCES

1. van Der Heijde D. Joint erosions in patients with early rheumatoid arthritis. Br J Rheumatol 1995;34:74–8.
2. Machold K, Stamm T, Eberl G, et al. Very recent onset arthritis clinical, laboratory and radiologic findings during the first year of disease. J Rheumatol 2002;29: 2278–87.
3. Giles J, Post W, Blumenthal R, et al. Longitudinal predictors of progression of carotid atherosclerosis in rheumatoid arthritis. Arthritis Rheum 2011;63: 3216–25.
4. Nielen M, Van Schaardenberg D, Reesink H, et al. Specific auto antibodies precede the symptoms of rheumatoid arthritis –a study of serial measurements in blood donors. Arthritis Rheum 2004;50:350–6.

5. Lard L, Visser H, Speyer I, et al. Early versus delayed treatment in patients with recent onset rheumatoid arthritis: comparison of two cohorts who received different treatment strategies. Am J Med 2001;111:446–51.
6. Anderson J, Wells G, Verhoeven A, et al. Factors predicting response to rheumatoid arthritis: the importance of disease duration. Arthritis Rheum 2000;43: 22–9.
7. Quinn M, Emery P. Window of opportunity in early rheumatoid arthritis: possibility of altering the disease process with early intervention. Clin Exp Rheumatol 2003; 21:S154–7.
8. Aletaha G, Eberl G, Nell V, et al. Attitudes to early rheumatoid arthritis: changing patterns. Results of a survey. Ann Rheum Dis 2002;61:630–4.
9. Aletaha D, Neogi T, Silman A, et al. 2010 Rheumatoid arthritis classification criterion a ACR/EULAR collaborative initiative. Arthritis Rheum 2010;62:2569–81.
10. Pinals R, Masi A, Larsen R, et al. Preliminary criteria for clinical remission in rheumatoid arthritis. Arthritis Rheum 1981;24:1308–15.
11. Smolen J, Aletaha D, Bijlsma J, et al. Treating rheumatoid arthritis to target: recommendation of a international task force. Ann Rheum Dis 2010;69:631–7.
12. van der Heijde D, van't Hof M, van Riel P, et al. Judging disease activity in clinical practice in RA: first step to developing a disease activity score. Ann Rheum Dis 1990;49:916–20.
13. Prevoo M, van't Hof M, Kuper H, et al. Modified disease activity scores that include 28 joint counts. Arthritis Rheum 1998;38:44–8.
14. Felson D, Anderson J, Boers M, et al. American College of Rheumatology, preliminary definition of improvement in RA. Arthritis Rheum 1995;38:727–35.
15. van Gestel A, Prevoo M, van't Hof M, et al. Development and validation of EULAR response criterion for RA. Comparison with preliminary ACR and WHO/International League Against Rheumatism criterion. Arthritis Rheum 1996;39:34–40.
16. Smolen J, Breedveld F, Schiff M, et al. A simplified disease activity index in rheumatoid arthritis for use in clinical practice. Rheumatology 2003;42:244–57.
17. Aletaha D, Nell V, Stamm T, et al. Acute phase reactant adds little to composite disease activity indices for rheumatoid arthritis. Validation of a clinical activity score. Arthritis Res Ther 2005;7:R796–806.
18. Pincus T, Swearingen C, Bergmen M, et al. "Routine assessment of patient index data 3" RAPID 3 a rheumatoid arthritis index without formal joint count for routine care: proposed severity categories compared to disease activity scores and clinical disease activity index categories. J Rheumatol 2008;35:2136–47.
19. Wells G, Boers M, Shea B, et al. Minimal disease activity for rheumatoid arthritis: a preliminary definition. J Rheumatol 2005;32:2016–24.
20. Wells G, Boers M, Shea B, et al. Low disease activity state workshop: low disease activity in rheumatoid arthritis. J Rheumatol 2003;30:1110–1.
21. Khanna D, Oh M, Furst D, et al. Evaluation of minimal disease activity and remission in early seropositive rheumatoid arthritis. Arthritis Rheum 2007;57: 440–7.
22. Egsmose C, Lund B, Borg G, et al. Patients with rheumatoid arthritis benefit from early second line therapy. J Rheumatol 1995;22:2208–13.
23. Matteson E, Weyland C, Fulbright J, et al. How aggressive should initial therapy for rheumatoid arthritis be? Factors associated with non response to non aggressive DMARD treatment and perspective from a 2-yr open label trial. Rheumatology 2004;43:619–25.
24. Bakker M, Jacobs J, Welsing P, et al. Early clinical response to treatment predicts 5 year outcome in RA patients. Ann Rheum Dis 2011;70:1099–103.

25. Nell V, Machold K, Ebler G, et al. Benefit of very early referral and very early therapy with disease modifying anti rheumatic drugs in patients with early rheumatoid arthritis. Rheumatology 2004;43:906–14.

26. Mottonen T, Hannonen P, Leirisalo-Repo M, et al. Comparison of combination therapy and single drug therapy in early RA. Lancet 1999;353:1568–73.

27. Rantalaiho V, Korpela M, Laasone L, et al. Early combination disease modifying anti-rheumatic therapy and tight control improve long term radiologic outcome in patients with early RA. Arthritis Res Ther 2010;12:R122.

28. Rantaliaho V, Korpela M, Haanonen P, et al. The good initial response to therapy with a combination of traditional disease modifying anti-rheumatic drugs is sustained over time. Arthritis Rheum 2009;60:1222–31.

29. Maini R, Breedveld F, Kalden J, et al. Sustained improvement over two years in physical function structural damage and signs and symptoms among patients with rheumatoid arthritis treated with infliximab and methotrexate. Arthritis Rheum 2004;50:1051–65.

30. Breedveld F, Emery P, Keystone E, et al. Infliximab in active early RA. Ann Rheum Dis 2004;63:149–55.

31. Breedveld F, Weismann M, Kavanaugh A, et al. The PREMIER Study. Arthritis Rheum 2006;54:26–37.

32. Genovese M, Bathon J, Martin R, et al. Etanercept versus methotrexate in patients with early rheumatoid arthritis. Arthritis Rheum 2002;46:1443–50.

33. Baumgartner S, Fleischmann R, Moreland L, et al. Etanercept in patients with rheumatoid arthritis with recent onset versus established disease: improvement in disability. J Rheumatol 2004;31:1532–7.

34. Smolen J, van der Heijde D, St Clair E, et al. Predictors of joint damage in patients treated with high dose methotrexate with or without concomitant infliximab. Arthritis Rheum 2006;54:702–10.

35. Smolen J, Han C, van der Heijde D, et al. Radiographic changes in rheumatoid arthritis patients attaining different disease activity states with methotrexate monotherapy and infliximab with methotrexate. Ann Rheum Dis 2009;68: 323–7.

36. Van der Heijde D, Landewe R, Klareskog L, et al. Presentation and analysis of data on radiographic outcome in clinical trials. Arthritis Rheum 2005;52:49–60.

37. Grigor C, Capell H, Stirling A, et al. Effect of a treatment strategy of tight control for rheumatoid arthritis (the TICORA study). Lancet 2004;364:263–9.

38. Boers M, Verhoeven A, Markusse H, et al. Randomized comparison of combined step down prednisone, methotrexate and sulfasalazine with sulfasalazine alone in early rheumatoid arthritis. Lancet 1997;350:309–18.

39. van Tuyl L, Lems W, Voskuyl A, et al. Tight control and intensified COBRA combination treatment in early RA. Ann Rheum Dis 2008;67:1574–7.

40. Goekoop-Ruiterman Y, deVries-Bouwstra J, Allart C, et al. Comparison of treatment strategies in early RA. Ann Intern Med 2007;146:406–15.

41. van der Bijl A, Goekoop-Ruiterman Y, deVries-Bouwstra J, et al. Infliximab and methotrexate as induction therapy in patients with early rheumatoid arthritis. Arthritis Rheum 2007;56:2129–34.

42. Moreland L, O'Dell J, Paulus C, et al. Two year radiographic results from the TEAR trial [abstract]. Arthritis Rheum 2010;62(Suppl 10):1368.

43. Moreland L, O'Dell J, Paulus C, et al. TEAR: Treatment of Early Aggressive RA: a randomized, double-blind, 2-year trial comparing immediate triple DMARD versus methotrexate plus etanercept to step-up from initial methotrexate monotherapy [abstract]. Arthritis Rheum 2009;60(Suppl 10):1895.

44. van Vollenhoven R, Ernestam S, Geborek P, et al. Addition of infliximab compared with addition of sulfasalazine and hydroxychloroquine in patients with early rheumatoid arthritis. Lancet 2009;374:459–66.
45. Vermeer M, Kuper H, Hoekstra M, et al. Implementation of a treat to target strategy in very early RA. Arthritis Rheum 2011;63:2865–72.
46. von Eijk I, Nielan M, van der Horst-Bruinsma I, et al. Aggressive therapy in patients with early arthritis results in similar outcome compared to conventional care. Rheumatology 2012;51:646–94.
47. van Dongen H, van Aken J, Lard L, et al. Efficacy of methotrexate treatment in patients with probable rheumatoid arthritis. Arthritis Rheum 2007;56:1424–32.
48. van der Linden M, Knevel R, Huizinga T, et al. Classification of rheumatoid arthritis: comparison of the 1987 American College of Rheumatology criteria and the 2010 American College of Rheumatology/European League Against Rheumatism criteria. Arthritis Rheum 2011;63:37–42.
49. Sokka T, Pincus T. Most patients receiving routine care for rheumatoid arthritis in 2001 did not meet inclusion criteria for most recent clinical trials or American College of Rheumatology criteria for remission. J Rheumatol 2003;30:1138–46.
50. Sokka T, Hetland M, Makinen H, et al. Remission and rheumatoid arthritis data in patients receiving usual care in 24 countries. Arthritis Rheum 2008;58:2642–51.
51. Pincus T, Seguardo O. Most visits of most patients with rheumatoid arthritis to most rheumatologist do not include a formal quantitative joint count. Ann Rheum Dis 2007;65:820–2.
52. Pincus T, Swearingen C, Bergman M, et al. RAPID 3 on a MDHAQ: agreement with DAS 28 and CDAI activity categories, scored in 5 versus more than 90 seconds. Arthritis Care Res 2010;62:181–9.
53. Molenaar E, Voskuyl A, Dinant H, et al. Progression of radiologic damage in RA in patients with clinical remission. Arthritis Rheum 2004;50:36–42.
54. Cohen G, Gossec L, Dougados M, et al. Radiologic damage in patients with rheumatoid arthritis on sustained remission. Ann Rheum Dis 2007;66:358–63.
55. Naredo E, Collado P, Cruz A, et al. Longitudinal power Doppler ultrasonographic assessment of joint inflammatory activity in early rheumatoid arthritis: predictive valve in disease activity and radiologic progression. Arthritis Rheum 2007;57:116–24.
56. Hetland M, Ejbjerg B, Horslev-Pertesen K, et al. MRI bone edema is the strongest predictor of subsequent radiographic progression. Ann Rheum Dis 2009;68:384–90.
57. Brown A, Conaghan P, Karim Z, et al. An explanation for the apparent dissociation between clinical remission and continued structural deterioration in rheumatoid arthritis. Arthritis Rheum 2008;58:2958–67.

Evolution of Classification Criteria for Rheumatoid Arthritis: How Do the 2010 Criteria Perform?

Elizabeth C. Ortiz, MD*, Shuntaro Shinada, MD

KEYWORDS

• Rheumatoid arthritis • Classification criteria
• Inflammatory arthritis • Guidelines

Key Points

- The classification criteria for rheumatoid arthritis (RA) have undergone a substantial evolution since the 1950s.

- The 1987 revised criteria for rheumatoid arthritis (RA) lead to improved performance and more confidence in correct classification compared with the 1958 criteria.

- The 2010 criteria were created with a focus to facilitate study of subjects at earlier stages in the disease.

- The data show that the new 2010 American College of Rheumatology-European League Against Rheumatism criteria identify patients with RA at an earlier point in their disease course.

- The new 2010 criteria create a more heterogeneous group of patients now classified as having RA, including patients with self-limiting disease or other arthritides, and can lead to overtreatment.

Disclosures: None for each author.
Funding support: None for each author.
Division of Rheumatology, Keck School of Medicine, University of Southern California, 2011 Zonal Avenue HMR 711, Los Angeles, CA 90033, USA
* Corresponding author.
E-mail address: elizabeo@usc.edu

INTRODUCTION AND HISTORICAL PERSPECTIVE

In the past two decades the identification and management of rheumatoid arthritis (RA) has changed multiple times. Gone are the days of managing end-stage joints and long-term prednisone use complications. Now, early, almost subclinical, identification of RA is sought out and aggressive combination therapy is the norm. RA is a chronic systemic autoimmune disorder that leads to synovial inflammation, progressive joint erosions, and eventual disability. The American Rheumatism Association (ARA), the precursor to the American College of Rheumatology (ACR), first proposed classification criteria for RA in 1956. Eleven criteria with 19 exclusions were proposed and resulted in three categories: definite, probable, and possible RA.[1] Two years later, in an effort to increase specificity, the ARA added the category classic RA, further complicating matters. These criteria were developed from the experiences of five committee members, review of recent epidemiologic data at that time, and analysis of 332 cases provided by interested physicians from around the United States and Canada. In 1966, the New York Criteria were developed at the Third International Symposium on Populations Studies of the Rheumatic Disease. The New York Criteria were more specific; however, they were also more cumbersome and never gained wide acceptance. The 1956 classification criteria were used for almost 30 years, standardizing the vocabulary and allowing research results to be more easily compared. The criteria helped foster better communication between physicians and enabled more effective teaching. The use of the 1956 classification criteria was generally supported; however, there were some observed problems. In practice there was little difference between definite and classic RA and many patients who were labeled probable RA were ultimately found to have a different disease. The various exclusions were though to be burdensome and three of the criteria required invasive procedures, such as mucin clot, nodule biopsy, and synovial biopsy.[1]

Almost 30 years later, the clinical and biochemical knowledge of RA has expanded exponentially. The shortcomings of the 1956 diagnostic criteria became apparent and the criteria were viewed as old-fashioned. The ARA again appointed a subcommittee of the Diagnostic and Therapeutic Criteria to review and revise the criteria. Subjects with RA, as well as subjects without RA (controls), were studied and the then-current ARA classification criteria were dissected. Numerous disease discriminators were studied, such as morning stiffness, pain and swelling of various joints, nodules, and laboratory and radiographic findings, and their sensitivity and specificity were calculated. Shortly thereafter, the 1987 revised criteria were established. The revisions kept five of the original 1958 ARA criteria and provided more precise definitions for several others (**Table 1**).[1] The explicit definitions of criteria that were provided lead to improved performance and ultimately more confidence in a correct classification. These new criteria performed better than both the 1958 ARA and the New York Criteria and simplified classification because it eliminated the need for extensive radiographs and invasive procedures. The classification subcategories were dropped and definite and classic RA were relabeled as simply RA. The term probable RA was exchanged for terms such as undifferentiated polyarthritis, undifferentiated oligoarthritis, or undifferentiated monoarthritis, and the lengthy list of exclusions, previously part of the 1958 criteria, was dropped. Although it was debated that this might lead to misclassification of patients with other diseases, such as systemic lupus erythematosus, polymyalgia rheumatica, Sjögren syndrome, and HLA-B27–associated spondyloarthropathy, the advantage to eliminating this onerous list was felt to outweigh this possible risk.

A NEW AGE

Another 20 years passed and, again, rheumatologists found themselves dealing with out-of-date classification criteria. Although the 1987 criteria were not meant to be

Table 1 Comparison of 1987 and 1958 classification criteria for RA	
1987	**1958**
Morning stiffness in and around joints for at least 1 h	Morning stiffness
Soft tissue joint swelling observed by physician in at least 3/14 joint groups (Right or left: MCP, PIP, wrist, elbow, knee, ankle, MTP)	Swelling of a joint
Symmetric swelling of one joint area	Swelling of another joint
Rheumatoid nodule	Pain on movement or tenderness in a joint
Rheumatoid factor by method positive in <5% normal population	Symmetric swelling
Radiographic changes in wrist or hands: erosions or juxtaarticular osteoporosis	Rheumatoid nodule
—	Rheumatoid factor
—	Radiographic changes
—	Mucin clot
—	Synovial biopsy
—	Nodule biopsy
RA: 4/7	Classical RA: 7/11 Definite RA: 5/11 Probable RA: 3/11

Abbreviations: MCP, metacarpalphalangeal; MTP, metatarsalphlangeal; PIP, proximal inter-phalangeal.
Data from Silman AJ. The 1987 revised American rheumatism association criteria for rheumatoid arthritis. Br J Rheumatol 1988;27(5):341–3.

used for diagnosis, in the rheumatology community these criteria were largely deemed the gold standard for the diagnosis of RA. In the past two decades, rheumatologists again had an exponential growth in their knowledge of RA. Studies emerged, highlighting the effectiveness of early, aggressive, combination therapy. For the first time, remission of disease was a realistic therapeutic goal and the need to uniformly identify patients in the earliest stage became imperative. Korpela and colleagues[2] with the FIN-RACo (Finnish Rheumatoid Arthritis Combination Therapy) Trial Group found that aggressive initial treatment with methotrexate, sulfasalazine, hydroxychloroquine, and prednisolone resulted in more rates of remission and less peripheral joint radiographic damage when compared with disease-modifying antirheumatic drug (DMARD) monotherapy. This group found that aggressive treatment early in a subject's course was key. Verstappen and colleagues[3] confirmed this idea with the CAMERA (Computer Assisted Management in Early Rheumatoid Arthritis) trial. This group demonstrated intensive treatment in early RA (<1 year) resulted in higher rates of remission when compared with more conventional treatment. Verstappen and colleagues[3] used frequent visits and standardized criteria to aggressively titrate medications early in the disease course and found this resulted in lower inflammatory markers and decreased morning stiffness and tender and swollen joints. The BeST (Behandel-Strategieën) Study challenged previous paradigms of treatment algorithms by evaluating the effectiveness of four different treatment strategies: sequential DMARD monotherapy, step-up combination therapy, initial combination therapy with tapered high-dose prednisone, and initial combination therapy with the tumor necrosis factor antagonist infliximab. Goekoop-Ruiterman and colleagues[4] found that initial combination therapy, with either prednisolone or infliximab, was superior to monotherapy and the step-up combination treatment strategy in function and Health Assessment Questionnaire scores. These studies, and others, emphasized the idea of a window of opportunity to drastically alter the course of the disease for a patient with aggressive, early therapy.

As in 1983, at the beginning of the new millennium the pitfalls of the 1987 ARA classification criteria were becoming apparent. One pitfall was that early disease was often not appropriately identified.[5] From France, Saraux and colleagues[6] evaluated at the ability of the 1987 criteria to correctly predict the diagnosis of RA in a cohort of subjects with arthritis followed for 2 years. Using the opinion of a panel of five rheumatologists as the gold standard of an RA diagnosis, they evaluated the specificity and sensitivity of the 1987 criteria at a subject's initial visit as well as 2 years later. They found that the 1987 criteria were not as effective at predicting a diagnosis of RA 2 years later, thus making these criteria limited in identifying early disease.[6] They further evaluated each criterion and how well it performed (**Table 2**). Not surprisingly, criteria such as rheumatoid nodules and radiographic changes had a low sensitivity but high specificity for the diagnosis of RA at the initial visit. This was not unexpected because many patients do not exhibit these findings early in their disease course.

NEW CRITERIA EMERGE

As new therapies were introduced and aggressive approaches were becoming more common, there was a growing need for clinical trials focusing on early RA. However, this was hampered by the lack of validated and accepted uniform criteria that reliably identify RA in the early stages. A joint working group of the ACR and the European League Against Rheumatism (EULAR) was formed to develop new criteria specifically for this reason. The focus was not to develop diagnostic criteria but to formulate new classification criteria to facilitate the study of subjects at earlier stages in the disease. This working group set out to develop a set of rules that would identify the subset of subjects at high risk for chronicity and erosive damage, be used as a basis for initiating DMARDs, and would not exclude those later in the disease course.[7] Through a three-phase approach, the joint working group studied and evaluated data on thousands of subjects, identifying variables and their contribution to a diagnosis of RA. A set of new classification criteria based on a scoring system was produced. The criteria can be used at any point in the patient's disease course. Although there are no exclusion criteria, it is noted that these criteria are meant to be used in the proper clinical setting (ie, when there is objective evidence of joint swelling).

PUTTING THE NEW CRITERIA TO THE TEST

Armed with new criteria, the rheumatology world has set forth to evaluate their performance and compare them to the previous model (**Table 3**). In Amsterdam, Britsemmer and colleagues[8] used the 2010 criteria on a cohort of subjects from the early arthritis cohort at the Jan van Breeman Institute. This cohort was made of up individuals older than 18 years of age with at least two swollen joints for less than 2 years who were DMARD naïve. Patients with osteoarthritis, crystal arthropathy, spondyloarthritis, systemic lupus erythematosus, Sjögren syndrome, and infectious arthritis were not a part of the cohort. The subjects were classified using the 2010 criteria as well as the 1987 criteria and the initiation of methotrexate was considered the gold standard for a diagnosis of RA. The investigators found that the 2010 ACR-EULAR criteria had a high sensitivity when compared with the 1987 ACR criteria, 0.85 versus 0.76,

Table 2
The 2010 ACR-EULAR classification criteria for RA

	Score
Target population (who should be tested?)	—
1. Patients who have at least 1 joint with definite clinical synovitis (swelling)[a]	—
2. Patients with the synovitis not better explained by another disease[b]	
Classification criteria for RA (score-based algorithm: add score of categories A-D; a score of $\geq$6/10 is needed for classification of a patient as having definite RA)[c]	—
A. Joint involvement[d]	
1 large joint[e]	0
2–10 large joints	1
1–3 small joints (with or without involvement of large joints)[f]	2
4–10 small joints (with or without involvement of large joints)	3
>10 joints (at least 1 small joint)[g]	5
B. Serology (at least 1 test result is needed for classification)[h]	
Negative RF and negative ACPA	0
Low-positive RF or low-positive ACPA	2
High-positive RF or high-positive ACPA	3
C. Acute-phase reactants (at least 1 test result is needed for classification)[i]	
Normal CRP and normal ESR 0	0
Abnormal CRP or normal ESR 1	1
D. Duration of symptoms[j]	
<6 wk	0
$\geq$6 wk	1

Abbreviations: ACPA, anticitrullinated protein antibody; CRP, C-reactive protein; ESR, erythrocyte sedimentation rate.

[a] The criteria are aimed at classification of newly presenting patients. In addition, patients with erosive disease typical of RA with a history compatible with prior fulfillment of the 2010 criteria should be classified as having RA. Patients with long-standing disease, including those whose disease is inactive (with or without treatment) who, based on retrospectively available data, have previously fulfilled the 2010 criteria should be classified as having RA.

[b] Differential diagnoses differ in patients with different presentations, but may include conditions such as systemic lupus erythematosus, psoriatic arthritis, and gout. If it is unclear about the relevant differential diagnoses to consider, an expert rheumatologist should be consulted.

[c] Although patients with a score of less than 6 out of 10 are not classifiable as having RA, their status can be reassessed and the criteria might be fulfilled cumulatively over time.

[d] Any swollen or tender joint on examination, which may be confirmed by imaging evidence of synovitis. Distal interphalangeal joints, first carpometacarpal joints and first metatarsophalangeal joints are excluded from assessment. Categories of joint distribution are classified according to the location and number of involved joints, with placement into the highest category possible based on the pattern of joint involvement.

[e] Shoulders, elbows, hips, knees and ankles.

[f] The metacarpophalangeal joints, proximal interphalangeal joints, second to fifth metatarsophalangeal joints, thumb interphalangeal joints and wrists.

[g] At least one of the involved joints must be a small joint; the other joints can include any combination of large and additional small joints, as well as other joints not specifically listed elsewhere (eg, temporomandibular, acromioclavicular, sternoclavicular).

[h] International unit (IU) values that are less than or equal to the upper limit of normal (ULN) for the laboratory and assay. Low-positive are IU values that are higher than the ULN but three or less times the ULN for the laboratory and assay. High positive are IU values that are more than three times the ULN for the laboratory and assay. When rheumatoid factor (RF) information is only available as positive or negative, a positive result should be scored as low-positive for RF.

[i] Normal or abnormal is determined by local laboratory standards.

[j] Patient self-report of the duration of signs or symptoms of synovitis (eg, pain, swelling, tenderness) of joints that are clinically involved at the time of assessment, regardless of treatment status.

Data from Aletaha D, Neogi T, Silman AJ, et al. 2010 Rheumatoid arthritis classification criteria: an American College of Rheumatology/European league against rheumatism collaborative initiative. Ann Rheumatic Dis 2010;69:1580–8.

Table 3
The sensitivity and specificity of the 2010 ACR-EULAR classification criteria for RA

Study	Number of Patients	Gold Standard for RA Diagnosis, Outcomes Used[a]	Sensitivity	Specificity
Van der Linden et al[12,b]	2258	1. Initiation of methotrexate within 1st y 2. Initiation of DMARD within the 1st y 3. Persistence of arthritis in those followed for 5 y	1. 0.84 2. 0.74 3. 0.71	1. 0.60 2. 0.74 3. 0.65
Cader et al[9]	265	1. DMARD use 2. Methotrexate use	1. 0.62 2. 0.68	1. 0.78 2. 0.72
Britsemmer et al[8]	455	1. Methotrexate treatment within first y 2. Expert opinion 3. Erosive disease at 3 y	1. 0.85 2. 0.90 3. 0.91	1. 0.5 2. 0.48 3. 0.21
Varache et al[14]	270	Combination of opinion of office-based rheumatologist and treatment with DMARD or glucocorticoid at 2 y	0.51	0.90
de Hair et al[11]	301	Meeting 1987 criteria after 2 y of follow-up	0.88	0.76

[a] Direct comparison of studies is difficult as there is no true gold standard for the diagnosis of RA and each study used a different method to confirm diagnosis.
[b] Used in the development of the ACR-EULAR 2010 Classification Criteria for Rheumatoid Arthritis.

respectively. The new criteria do carry with it a higher risk of false positives, which could lead to unnecessary exposure to toxic DMARDs.[8]

A second group, from The University of Birmingham, also sought to investigate the criteria. Selecting subjects from the early inflammatory arthritis clinic at Sandwell and West Birmingham Hospitals National Health Service Trust, Cader and colleagues[9] studied subjects with less than 3 months of synovial swelling. The investigators found the 2010 criteria identified more subjects at baseline as RA when compared with the 1987 criteria. The new criteria identified more subjects that would go on to use DMARD therapy, especially methotrexate, with a sensitivity of 0.68 (2010 criteria) versus 0.42 (1987 criteria).[9] Interestingly, this group also showed 26% of those who met only the 2010 criteria at baseline went on to have disease resolution without DMARD therapy over an 18-month follow-up period. This supports the notion that early aggressive treatment in some individuals will lead to over treatment in others.

In Amsterdam, these findings were replicated in a cohort of subjects with early arthritis who were DMARD naïve.[10] The 1987 and the 2010 classification criteria were used with this cohort, using fulfillment of the 1987 criteria at 2 years as the gold standard for an RA diagnosis. Of those subjects that would have been classified as having undifferentiated arthritis using the 1987 criteria, 85% fit the 2010 criteria for RA at baseline. The investigators also found high level subjects who were false positive among those who initially fit the 2010 criteria. These subjects were characterized as having high rates of monoarthritis, negative IgM-rheumatoid factor (RF) and anticitrullinated protein antibody (ACPA), and they had self-limiting disease at 2-year follow-up.[10]

Although many of the subjects in the Leiden Early Arthritis Clinic cohort were used in the development of the 2010 criteria, a larger number from this cohort were studied to determine if the new 2010 criteria could identify subjects in an earlier stage when compared with the 1987 criteria.[11] Over 2000 subjects were studied and outcome measures included use of methotrexate within the first year, use of any DMARD within the first year, and persistence of arthritis at 5 years. Within this cohort, 68% of subjects who did not meet the 1987 criteria at baseline but did 1 year later meet the 2010 criteria at baseline. However, similar to the other studies, using only the 2010 criteria would have misclassified 9.4% of the subjects as having RA.[11] Although this does not validate the use of the 2010 criteria because many of the subjects were the same as those used in the development of the criteria, it does support what other cohort studies have demonstrated. The new criteria do detect disease at an earlier stage with the sacrifice of misclassifying patients with some with milder, self-limiting disease. From South Korea, Jung and colleagues[12] found that when subjects did not fulfill the 2010 criteria it was mostly because of a lack of RF and/or cyclic citrullinated peptide, or too few affected joints.

From Brittany, France, Varache and colleagues[13] sought to evaluate not only the effectiveness of the ACR-EULAR 2010 criteria and compare it to the ACR 1987 criteria, but also attempted to establish whether a scoring system using a combination of factors would improve specificity and sensitivity for an RA diagnosis. This group used a cohort of 270 subjects with greater than one joint synovitis for less than 1 year and followed these subjects for 2 years. As a gold standard for the diagnosis of RA, these investigators used a combination of an office-based rheumatologist's opinion and treatment with a DMARD and/or glucocorticoid after 2-year follow-up. From the original cohort of 270 subjects, there was a large proportion (111) that had an alternate diagnosis at baseline, leaving 143 subjects to be scrutinized. Using the 2010 ACR-EULAR criteria, 42.2% of those who did not meet the new criteria (scores ≤6) went on to have RA at the end of 2 years, whereas 75.6% of those with scores greater than 6 had confirmed RA after 2 years. Although the 2010 criteria did perform slightly better when compared with the 1987 criteria, there was no statistically significant difference in diagnostic accuracy between the two criteria sets. This was true when applied to their overall cohort as well as when applied to a subgroup of subjects having synovitis, no radiographic evidence of RA, and no other likely diagnosis. Varache and colleagues[13] then went on to evaluate each criterion and found that the addition of symmetric joint involvement increased accuracy. It was also found that the most significant difference adding to any improvement seen with the 2010 criteria when compared with the 1987 criteria was the exclusion of subjects with an alternate diagnosis.

A NEW FACE

With the earlier identification of RA it does beg the question, what will undifferentiated arthritis look like? From the Netherlands, Krabben and colleagues[14] studied subjects identified as having undifferentiated arthritis from their Leiden Early Arthritis Clinic and applied the 2010 criteria to them. The 2010 criteria were applied to 1696 subjects with either undifferentiated arthritis or RA and 776 subjects with 2010 undifferentiated arthritis. When compared with the previously labeled subjects with undifferentiated arthritis or the 1987 undifferentiated arthritis patients, the 2010 subjects with undifferentiated arthritis were found to have overall milder disease with fewer swollen and tender joints and less frequent positive autoantibodies (RF and ACPA).[14] After 1 year of follow-up, a DMARD was initiated more often in the 1987 undifferentiated arthritis group and DMARD-free remission was achieved more often in the 2010 undifferentiated arthritis group. This implies that previously labeled undifferentiated arthritis are now being classified as RA using the 2010 criteria. Zeidler[15] reviews the results from six recent studies, evaluates the performance of the 2012 ACR-EULAR RA criteria, and likewise concludes that there is a significant risk for misclassification in early and very early RA.

BEYOND RA

The data show that the 2010 ACR-EULAR criteria identify patients as RA at an earlier point in their disease course. Many of these patients go on to require DMARD or biologic therapy. On the other hand, the new criteria create a more heterogeneous group of patients now classified as RA, including patients with self-limiting disease or other arthritides. Classifying a patient as having RA, who in actuality has a self-limiting disease, can potentially lead the patient to undergo unnecessary exposure to a toxic medication. There exists the possibility of misclassifying a patient as having RA who, in fact, should have a different diagnosis such as systemic lupus erythematosus, spondyloarthropathy, Sjögren syndrome, or a crystal-induced arthropathy. As previously discussed, many studies have been performed to evaluate the performance of the 2010 criteria using early arthritis cohorts that tend to exclude subjects with other inflammatory arthritides. One of the daily dilemmas for a practicing rheumatologist is to identify, then classify the type of inflammatory arthritis occurring in an afflicted patient. Although the 2010 criteria may allow a rheumatologist to identify a patient with RA earlier in the disease course, it is unclear whether these criteria can aid in distinguishing between the various other inflammatory arthritides. It is possible that imaging modalities, such as MRI and musculoskeletal ultrasound, can be used to increase sensitivity and specificity of the criteria.[16] These modalities are already being put to use in clinical practice and are likely to grow in popularity. In Iran, Salehi and colleagues[17] have designed the Iran Criteria for Rheumatoid Arthritis. These criteria include erosions found with MRI as one of its criteria and have found it to be successful. The investigators purport that their criteria is more sensitive in detecting RA patients in the early stages of the disease.

RA is a chronic, inflammatory, autoimmune arthritis that leads to symmetric articular synovitis, articular damage, and physical disability. Not all patients with RA are alike. Patients with RA are a heterogeneous group of people, each with their unique challenges. Classification criteria are created in an attempt to produce a homogenous group of patients that can then be used as subjects for clinical and basic science research. With the development of the new 2010 ACR-EULAR Classification Criteria for Rheumatoid Arthritis, a different population of subjects than those has previously investigated will be studied. Rheumatologists in clinical practice are not limited only to classification criteria for diagnosis of RA. Their clinical acumen and sophisticated imaging modalities guide their judgment. Because the utility of the 2010 criteria will undoubtedly continue to be assessed, the longevity of the 2010 criteria remains to be determined.

REFERENCES

1. Arnett FC, Edworthy SM, Bloch DA, et al. The American Rheumatism Association 1987 revised criteria for the classification of rheumatoid arthritis. Arthritis Rheum 1988;31(3):315–24.
2. Korpela M, Laasonen L, Hannonen P, et al, FIN-RACo Trial Group. Retardation of joint damage in patients with early rheumatoid arthritis by initial aggressive treatment with disease-modifying antirheumatic drugs. Arthritis Rheum 2004;50(7): 2072–81.
3. Verstappen SM, Jacobs JW, van der Veen MJ, et al, Utrecht Rheumatoid Arthritis Cohort study group. Intensive treatment with methotrexate in early rheumatoid

arthritis: aiming for remission. Computer Assisted Management in Early Rheumatoid Arthritis (CAMERA, an open-label strategy trial). Ann Rheum Dis 2007;66:
1443–9.

4. Goekoop-Ruiterman YM, de Vries-Bouwstra JK, Allaart CF, et al. Clinical and
radiographic outcomes of four different treatment strategies in patients with early
rheumatoid arthritis (the BeST Study). Arthritis Rheum 2005;52(11):3381–90.

5. Banal F, Dougados M, Combescure C, et al. Sensitivity and specificity of the
American College of Rheumatology 1987 criteria for the diagnosis of rheumatoid
arthritis according to disease duration: a systematic literature review and meta-
analysis. Ann Rheum Dis 2009;68:1184–91.

6. Saraux A, Berthelot JM, Chales G, et al. Ability of the American College of rheumatology 1987 criteria to predict rheumatoid arthritis in patients with early arthritis
and classification of these patients two years later. Arthritis Rheum 2001;44(11):
2485–91.

7. Aletaha D, Neogi T, Silman AJ, et al. 2010 Rheumatoid arthritis classification
criteria: an American College of Rheumatology/European league against rheumatism collaborative initiative. Ann Rheum Dis 2010;69:1580–8.

8. Britsemmer K, Ursum J, Gerritsen M, et al. Validation of the 2010 ACR/EULAR
classification criteria for rheumatoid arthritis: slight improvement over the 1987
criteria. Ann Rheum Dis 2011;70:1468–70.

9. Cader MZ, Filer A, Hazlehurst J, et al. Performance of the 2010 ACR/EULAR
criteria for rheumatoid arthritis: comparison with 1987 ACR criteria in a very early
synovitis cohort. Ann Rheum Dis 2011;70:949–55.

10. de Hair MJ, Lehmann KA, van de Sande MG, et al. The clinical picture of rheumatoid arthritis according to the 2010 American College of rheumatology/Euro-
pean league against rheumatism criteria: is this still the same disease? Arthritis
Rheum 2012;64(2):389–93.

11. van der Linden MP, Knevel R, Huizinga TW, et al. Classification of Rheumatoid
Arthritis. Arthritis Rheum 2011;63(1):37–42.

12. Jung SJ, Lee SW, Ha YJ, et al. Patients with early arthritis who fulfill the 1987 ACR
classification criteria for rheumatoid arthritis but no the 2010 ACR/EULAR criteria.
Ann Rheum Dis 2012;71(6):1097–8.

13. Varache S, Cornec D, Morvan J, et al. Diagnostic accuracy of ACR/EULAR 2010
criteria for rheumatoid arthritis in a 2-year cohort. J Rheumatol 2011;38(7):
1250–7.

14. Krabben A, Huizinga TW, van der Helm-van Mil AH. Undifferentiated arthritis
characteristics and outcomes when applying the 2010 and 1987 criteria for rheumatoid arthritis. Ann Rheum Dis 2012;71:238–41.

15. Zeidler H. The need to better classify and diagnose early and very early rheumatoid arthritis. J Rheumatol 2012;39(2):212–7.

16. Kawashiri SY, Suzuki T, Okada A, et al. Musculoskeletal ultrasonography assists
the diagnostic performance of the 2010 classification criteria for rheumatoid
arthritis. Mod Rheumatol 2012. [Epub ahead of print].

17. Salehi I, Khazaeli S, Khak M. Early diagnosis of rheumatoid arthritis: an introduction to the newly designed Iran Criteria for Rheumatoid Arthritis. Rheumatol Int
2012. [Epub ahead of print].

Early Juvenile Idiopathic Arthritis

Katherine Anne B. Marzan, MD*, Bracha Shaham, MD

KEYWORDS

- Juvenile idiopathic arthritis • Early • Pediatric
- Biologic therapy • Aggressive treatment

Key Points

- Early juvenile idiopathic arthritis (JIA) may have a subtle presentation and be difficult to diagnose.
- The timely diagnosis and treatment of early JIA improves prognosis.
- Disease activity, even early in the course of JIA, can cause joint damage and long-term consequences. However, control of disease activity in the first 6 months of disease improves long-term prognosis.
- There are predictors of persistent disease and joint erosions early in the disease process of JIA that may identify patients who require more aggressive therapy.
- Early aggressive therapy of JIA for rapid disease control and remission is the goal of treatment.

Juvenile idiopathic arthritis (JIA) is a chronic immunoinflammatory disease defined by the International League of Associations for Rheumatology (ILAR) criteria as arthritis in one or more joints that begins before the 16th birthday, persists for at least 6 weeks, and excludes all other known conditions.[1] Classification criteria rely on the characteristics of the disease at onset and during its course and include seven subgroups (**Table 1**).[2] The early course of JIA influences whether active disease persists into adulthood. In addition, adults whose JIA is in remission suffer the physical and psychosocial consequences that stem not only from the chronicity of their condition and treatment but also from the earliest stages of their disease. Outcome studies have underlined the importance of early diagnosis and early aggressive treatment in improving prognosis.

The authors have nothing to disclose.

Division of Rheumatology, Children's Hospital Los Angeles, Keck School of Medicine of USC, 4650 Sunset Boulevard, MS#60, Los Angeles, CA 90027, USA

* Corresponding author.

E-mail address: kmarzan@chla.usc.edu

Rheum Dis Clin N Am 38 (2012) 355–372

doi:10.1016/j.rdc.2012.04.006

Table 1
ILAR classification criteria for juvenile idiopathic arthritis

Subtype	Criteria	Exclusions
Oligoarthritis Persistent Extended	Arthritis in 4 or fewer joints during first 6 mo of disease Never more than 4 joints affected Greater than 4 joints affected after 6 mo of disease	(A) Psoriasis or history of psoriasis in the patient or first degree relative (B) Arthritis in an HLA-B27–positive male beginning after the sixth birthday (C) AS, ERA, sacroiliitis with IBD, Reiter syndrome, or acute anterior uveitis or a history of 1 of these disorders in a first-degree relative (D) Presence of IgM RF on at least 2 occasions at least 3 mo apart (E) Presence of systemic arthritis
Polyarthritis RF Negative	Arthritis affecting 5 or more joints during first 6 mo of disease RF test is negative	Exclusions A, B, C, D, E
Polyarthritis RF Positive	Arthritis affecting 5 or more joints during first 6 mo of disease 2 or more tests of RF at least 3 mo apart are positive	Exclusions A, B, C, E
Systemic	Arthritis in any number of joints together with a fever of at least 2 wk duration that is documented to be daily (quotidian) for at least 3 d and is accompanied by one or more of the following: Evanescent rash, generalized lymphadenopathy, enlargement of liver or spleen, serositis	Exclusions A, B, C, D
ERA	Arthritis and enthesitis or arthritis or enthesitis with at least two of the following: Sacroiliac joint tenderness and/or inflammatory spinal pain, positive HLA-B27, family history in at least one first or second-degree relative with medically confirmed HLA-B27–associated disease, anterior uveitis that is usually associated with pain, redness, or photophobia, onset of arthritis in a boy after 6 y of age	Psoriasis in at least one first- or second-degree relative Presence of systemic arthritis
Juvenile psoriatic arthritis	Arthritis plus psoriasis, or arthritis plus at least two of the following: dactylitis, nail pits or onycholysis, psoriasis in a first-degree relative	Exclusions B, C, D, E Arthritis fulfilling two JIA categories
Undifferentiated arthritis	Fulfills criteria in no category or in 2 or more categories	—

Abbreviations: AS, ankylosing spondylitis; ERA, enthesitis-related arthritis; IBD, inflammatory bowel disease; RF, rheumatoid factor.
Adapted from Petty RE, Southwood TR, Baum J, et al. Revision of the proposed classification criteria for juvenile idiopathic arthritis: Durban, 1977. J Rheumatol 1998;25:1991–4.

Historically, juvenile arthritis was termed juvenile chronic arthritis, by the European League Against Rheumatism and juvenile rheumatoid arthritis by the American College of Rheumatology (ACR). Although these two classifications had some overlap, there were significant distinctions. However, the ILAR nomenclature of JIA has now been internationally adopted (**Table 2**). It is important to remain cognizant of these differences in definition and classification criteria because they contribute to difficulties in assessing the characteristics and outcome studies of juvenile arthritis.

THE IMPACT OF DISEASE
The Need for Early Aggressive Treatment of JIA

In the last decade there has been an evolution in the understanding of the clinical course and long-term outcomes for JIA. Initially remission rates up to 60% were described in JIA.[3] However, subsequent studies noted much lower rates with 33% at 10 years for JIA in general[4] and 44% at 15 years for enthesitis-related arthritis (ERA).[5] More tellingly, clinical remission off medications at 5 years was sustained in only 6% of JIA patients. Although a significant number of patients diagnosed with JIA achieve periods of inactive disease, this was in the context of a pattern alternating with periods of disease activity.[4,6] This was mirrored by a pattern of fluctuating disability.[7] JIA can have significant consequences with chronic pain, localized growth

Table 2
Comparison of JRA, JCA, and JIA classification criteria

	JRA (ACR, 1986)	JCA (EULAR, 1977)	JIA (ILAR, 1997)
Duration of arthritis	6 wk	3 mo	6 wk

Onset types or classification	1. Pauciarticular: <5 joints	1. Pauciarticular: <5 joints	1. Oligoarticular: <5 joints
			  a. Persistent
			  b. Extended

—	2. Polyarticular: ≥5 joints No distinction of RF positive or negative	2. Polyarticular: RF negative	2. Polyarticular: RF negative
—	No distinction of RF positive or negative	3. Polyarticular: RF positive	3. Polyarticular: RF positive
—	3. Systemic: characteristic fever and rash	4. Systemic: characteristic fever and rash	4. Systemic: characteristic fever and rash
JPsA included	No	5. JPsA	5. JPsA
JAS included	No	6. JAS	6. ERA Includes IBD

—	Excludes IBD	Includes IBD	7. Undifferentiated arthritis
			  a. Fits no other category
			  b. Fits more than one category

Other diseases excluded	Yes	Yes	Yes

Abbreviations: ACR, American College of Rheumatology; ERA, enthesitis-related arthritis; EULAR, European League Against Rheumatism; IBD, inflammatory bowel disease; ILAR, International League of Associations for Rheumatology; JAS, juvenile ankylosing spondylitis; JCA, juvenile chronic arthritis; JRA, juvenile rheumatoid arthritis; JPsA, juvenile psoriatic arthritis.

disturbances, impaired linear growth, joint destruction, osteoporosis, visual loss, and impaired development. Systemic JIA (sJIA) can lead to significant morbidity and death.[3,4,8–11] Contrary to the previous misconception that JIA was a disease that children would ultimately outgrow,[12] studies show sustained resolution of disease only occurs in a minority of patients.[6,8,13] Many patients with JIA go on to become adults with active disease or have sequelae of their JIA.[8,9,13] In addition, some juvenile onset forms of arthritis seem to have worse functional outcomes than their adult onset counterparts.[14] The probability of attaining remission is decreased in proportion to delay to referral to a tertiary care center and proper early treatment.[4] Aggressive treatment early in the disease improves outcomes.[15,16] This new perspective coupled with advances in the knowledge of immune mediators of inflammation and tissue damage and the development of biologic response modifiers has shifted the treatment paradigm and made remission an attainable goal.[8,13]

CLINICAL PRESENTATION OF EARLY JIA

Children with JIA tend to be stoic and manifest symptoms according to their age and developmental level. They may exhibit joint inflammation only by difficulty moving following a period of inactivity or focus on compensatory technique to perform a task.[17–19] In assessing children for arthritis, it is important to review any change in age-appropriate activities. Flexion contracture, weakness, and muscle atrophy may develop early.

The pattern of early joint involvement is characterized by disease subtype. Symmetric large and small joint synovitis is typical of polyarticular JIA and may be found in sJIA. In polyarthritis, constitutional symptoms and early cervical spine and temporomandibular joint (TMJ) involvement are common. Rheumatoid nodules can occur early and confer a worse prognosis.[20] Lower extremity large joint disease is more typical of oligoarticular JIA and ERA. Fifty percent of oligoarthritis patients have only one joint affected at onset,[21,22] with the knee most commonly presenting.[23] Systemic symptoms are absent and laboratory markers of inflammation are normal or minimally elevated. Early hip joint involvement is rare in all but ERA. In contrast to adult seronegative arthritis, ERA presents in peripheral joints with later axial involvement. At diagnosis, only half of juvenile psoriatic arthritis (JPsA) patients have a psoriatic rash and distal interphalangeal joint inflammation is typical. Although any joint may be involved at presentation, early JIA may present with cervical spine, TMJ, middle ear, and cricoarytenoid cartilage involvement with torticollis,[24] asymmetry of oral opening with refusal to chew, conductive hearing loss,[25] or hoarseness.[26] Micrognathia is a hallmark of early onset JIA and is a presenting feature in more than 50% of patients with disease onset before age 4 years.[27,28] Abnormal gait due to leg length discrepancy may be an early clinical presentation.[29]

sJIA differs most from the other subtypes with autoinflammatory characteristics. Fever is typically quotidian, but it can be unremitting and intermittent at onset.[30] Synovitis is present at onset in 88% of patients,[30] though some patients may not develop it until months later.[31] Macrophage activating syndrome (MAS) shares many features with sJIA and may present a diagnostic dilemma in an acutely deteriorating patient.[32] Limited features of MAS occur in some sJIA patients only as serologic markers of active disease.[33]

PATHOGENESIS OF JIA

T cells are important in initiating the immune response in JIA, though some B cell dysregulation has also been postulated.[34–37] Several inflammatory cytokines play a prominent role, including tumor necrosis factor α (TNF-α),[34,38] interleukin (IL)-1,[39,40] and IL-6, resulting in cartilage destruction, joint-space narrowing, and erosions.[41,42]

Similar to adult arthritis, in JIA there is persistent cellular inflammatory infiltrate in the synovium with neovascularization, pannus formation, metalloproteinase release, and subsequent cartilage destruction and bone erosions.[43,44] Significant pathologic joint involvement is seen early in the disease process. The synovial membrane immunohistology in early untreated JIA demonstrates synovial hyperplasia, fibrosis, focal aggregates of T and B cells, marked macrophage populations in the lining and sublining layer, and angiogenesis. The most significant hyperplasia and angiogenesis is seen in polyarticular arthritis regardless of rheumatoid factor (RF) status and in those that later develop extended oligoarticular disease. The significant vascularization seen early in the disease perpetuates inflammation that leads to local growth disturbances and facilitates infiltration of the synovial membrane into the cartilage, development of erosions, and bone destruction.[43]

LABORATORY MARKERS

The diagnosis of JIA is made clinically with established laboratory markers of little diagnostic value, though they play a role in identifying JIA patients at risk for specific complications. The presence of antinuclear antibody (ANA) identifies children at highest risk for eye involvement. ANA-positive patients are primarily female, with early age of disease onset, asymmetric arthritis, lower total joint involvement over time, and at increased risk of chronic iridocyclitis.[4,45,46] RF positivity is associated with erosive disease.[4,47] A positive ANA and RF can be seen in healthy children associated with infections and in children who have musculoskeletal complaints without an autoimmune or rheumatic disease.[4,48] Its presence is not diagnostic and must be interpreted with caution in patients without objective evidence of arthritis. These tests have no diagnostic role in substantiating or excluding a diagnosis of JIA.[49]

Several laboratory markers may have a future role in JIA. Elevated serum osteopontin levels at baseline may signal the need for early use of biologic agents as methotrexate nonresponders in JIA had higher levels compared with responders and to controls.[50] The proinflammatory calcium-binding protein S100A12 has been observed in high concentration in the serum of sJIA patients and may have utility distinguishing from severe systemic infections and childhood leukemia.[51] The MRP-8/MRP-14 complexes that are secreted by activated phagocytes may be a future diagnostic marker. In active sJIA, serum levels are significantly elevated compared with controls, systemic infection, leukemia, and other rheumatologic inflammatory diseases.[52]

IMAGING

Advances in imaging techniques—in particular MRI—allows the ability to detect changes early in the disease course and before observed symptoms making it a useful adjunct in early diagnosis.[53,54] MRI can detect the earliest stages of bone erosions.[55] Systemic gallium scintigraphy has also been suggested to detect early JIA.[56] Ultrasound may be helpful for enthesitis.[57]

EFFECTS OF EARLY DISEASE ACTIVITY

Localized growth disturbances are common[9] and occur in 10% to 48% of JIA patients during the first 2 to 3 years of disease.[47] They are seen primarily at sites of inflammation with overgrowth due to hyperemia and accelerated growth maturation or impaired growth resulting from destruction of the growth center and premature closure of the epiphysis resulting in leg length discrepancies and micrognathia.[9,58,59]

At diagnosis, periarticular osteopenia is the most common radiographic change seen; however, joint-space narrowing and erosions have also been demonstrated even in RF negative polyarthritis.[60] Up to 81% of patients exhibit radiographic abnormalities by 3 years of follow-up with the highest frequency in RF-positive polyarthritis. Predictors of erosions include young age, increased mobility-restricted joints, and radiographic findings of swelling and osteopenia.[47] Erosions have been detected by MRI in patients with JIA who have had disease duration of fewer than or equal to 3 years.[55] MRI evidence of sacroiliitis may be detectable as early as 1 year after disease onset.[61] Furthermore, MRI changes of children with recent-onset JIA revealed synovium with irregular thickness and low-intensity synovial tissue.[53,54] Typical MRI changes of arthritis can even be seen before observed symptoms,[54] indicating insidious disease and damage early in disease course.

Early onset JIA is associated with low total-body bone mineral content and low bone mineral density that is impacted by longer disease duration and increased disease severity.[62] In addition, patients with JIA have moderate reductions in bone mass gains and bone turnover early in the disease course within 2 years of diagnosis.[11]

Growth impairment in JIA is a well-known complication, particularly in systemic and polyarticular JIA, and can be seen even in disease that is not longstanding. Although the use of glucocorticoids plays a role, the metabolic demands of active disease with inflammatory cytokines (TNF-α, IL-1, IL-6) also interferes with the growth hormone–insulin-like growth factor axis resulting in delayed growth and altered body composition. Adults with a history of JIA have reduced final height. Although the lowest median heights are noted in sJIA, evidence for impaired linear growth in comparison with the general population was seen for all subtypes of JIA.[9,58] In an in vitro study, TNF-α and IL-1β suppressed longitudinal bone growth locally.[63]

The effects of early disease activity in JIA extend beyond the musculoskeletal system. Reduced brachial flow-mediated dilation indicating endothelial cell dysfunction has been demonstrated in children and adolescents with all subtypes of JIA as compared with healthy controls. Patients with sJIA had additional increased carotid intima-media thickness.[64] Perimyocarditis is a component of active sJIA.[9]

PROGNOSIS AND OUTCOMES

The course and outcome of JIA cannot be predicted by baseline features. However, disease inactivity within the first 5 years is associated with lower number of restricted joints, less cumulative articular damage, and better functional and radiographic outcome. Targeting remission through aggressive therapeutic interventions provides better outcome.[15]

Therapy and treatment response within the first 6 months of disease is a factor in improved long-term outcome. In a retrospective study of JIA patients treated with methotrexate, an ACR pediatric (Pedi) 70 response at 6 months of therapy predicted a more favorable long-term outcome. They experienced greater and sustained improvement at 5 years in terms of joints with active disease and restricted motion compared with those that had achieved an ACR Pedi 30 or 50.[16] Furthermore, specifically in sJIA, persistent systemic symptoms, thrombocytosis, and the need for corticosteroids at 6 months after disease onset were predictive of joint destruction within 2 years and poor functional outcome. Absence of active arthritis, an ESR less than 26 mm/h and no requirement for corticosteroids at 3 and 6 months were predictive of earlier time to remission.[65–67] The therapeutic response of the disease, regardless of type, seems to be more of a determining factor of long-term outcome than the presenting disease characteristics.[16]

PREDICTORS OF DISEASE ACTIVITY AND PROGNOSIS

Because the response within the first 6 months seems to play a role in long-term outcome, identifying predictors of early inactive disease and risk factors for persistent disease in JIA is paramount. In a prospective study of patients a median of .65 months after diagnosis and 6 months after disease onset, a shorter duration from disease onset to diagnosis, younger age, and patients with oligoarticular JIA (46%) correlated with inactive disease at 6 months. Notably, only 33% of patients achieved inactive disease at 6 months—primarily with the use of nonsteroidal antiinflammatory drugs (NSAIDs), intraarticular corticosteroids, and disease-modifying antirheumatic drugs (DMARDs). Only 0.6% of patients received biologic therapy[68] and its earlier use would likely have increased this number.

Although oligoarticular-onset JIA seems to have the best prognosis (remission rate up to 68%–73%),[6,9] nearly 50% of patients with oligoarthritis can go on to develop polyarticular extension of the disease,[9] RF-positive polyarticular disease,[6] or ERA that confer a worse prognosis (remission rate 12% or less)[9] and the need for more aggressive management. Predictors of persistent disease and joint erosions in oligoarticular and polyarticular arthritis include young age at onset, large numbers of affected joints, long duration of elevated ESR, and IgM RF in first 6 months of disease. The presence of HLA-DRB1*08 predicted persistent disease and, in combination with HLA-B27 (but not HLA-B27 alone), predicted joint erosions.[69]

Patients with ERA have poorer outcomes than those with oligoarticular and polyarticular subtypes of JIA.[5] Persistent disease activity was also associated with HLA-DRB1*08 as well as ankle arthritis in the first 6 months and a first-degree relative with ankylosing spondylitis (AS). Poor physical health status after 23 years was associated with high numbers of affected joints at 6 months.[5] Risk factors for sacroiliitis included a persistently elevated ESR and hip arthritis in the first 6 months. Early predictors of sacroiliitis in ERA were the number of active joints and entheses at onset.[61]

JPsA requires early aggressive therapy.[70] However, the onset of arthritis often precedes the development of psoriasis by many years. The ability to differentiate JPsA from other subtypes of JIA—particularly oligoarticular JIA, a known subtype with better prognosis that typically is treated less aggressively—is vital. Age of disease onset for JPsA (8.2 years ± 3.6) tends to be older than for oligoarticular JIA patients (6 years ± 4.1) and younger than for ERA patients (11.1 years ± 2.8). Predictors of JPsA in a patient presenting with oligoarticular arthritis include a history of psoriasis in the patient or a first degree relative, dactylitis, ankle or toe arthritis, and HLA-DRB1*11/12.[70]

Sacroiliitis and may take 5 to 10 years before becoming evident in JIA. Though early aggressive therapy for sacroiliitis and lumbar inflammation is important to prevent radiographic progression of the disease, physical examination and plain radiography have limited ability to detect early findings. Risk factors for sacroiliitis include male sex, hip arthritis, number of active joints, number of enthesitis, and older age of onset. An MRI of the sacroiliac joints at baseline and periodically may be of value because it demonstrates silent sacroiliitis in individuals with no symptoms or sacroiliac abnormalities on examination.[61,71] Axial involvement does not respond well to traditional DMARDs[72,73] and the early identification of at risk individuals indicates the need for biologic therapy in particular anti-TNF agents.[71]

MANAGEMENT

The goals of JIA management include inactive disease with subsequent clinical remission, normal growth and development, preservation of psychosocial integrity, participation in normal activities, and prevention of long-term complications associated with the disease and its treatment. It is a multidisciplinary approach that includes pharmacologic administration, physical and occupational therapy, and psychological support,[44,74] which should be included in the management as early as possible.

MEDICATIONS

Similar to adult studies, there seems to be a window of opportunity early in the disease course that improves outcomes with the concept that there is a narrow time frame in which resetting of active disease is easiest to achieve. The use of DMARD therapy early in the disease suppresses disease activity with beneficial effects. The advent of biologics has made this even more attainable.[8,13,44,75]

NSAIDs had traditionally been the foundation of therapy. It remains an important initial treatment; however, its limited efficacy precludes its use as monotherapy in all subclasses of JIA except some oligoarthritis. DMARDs are rapidly included in the treatment regimen. Methotrexate (MTX) is effective in active arthritis and is the most used second-line agent. It is given weekly at doses between .5–1 mg/kg or 10–30 mg/m^2. Its use in JIA has been well established and extensively described.[76–78] It is now also recommended as initial therapy for JIA patients with high disease activity or features of poor prognosis, with the exception of those with sJIA and active fever but no arthritis.[79]

INTRAARTICULAR CORTICOSTEROIDS

Intraarticular corticosteroid (IAS) injection has beneficial long-lasting effects with suppression of synovial inflammation and reversion of pannus formation without deleterious effects to the articular cartilage or linear growth.[80] Its early use has also been associated with less leg-length discrepancy.[29] The use of IAS is an effective initial therapeutic modality, particularly in oligoarticular JIA in which there is high-to-moderate joint disease activity and/or poor prognostic factors and in patients who remain with any evidence of disease activity after 2 months of NSAID therapy.[80,81] Triamcinolone hexacetonide is recommended because it is superior to triamcinolone acetonide in terms of response rate and time to flare.[29,82–84] Concomitant use of MTX results in longer disease remission.[85]

BIOLOGIC AGENTS
Anti-TNF Agents

Anti-TNF agents have greatly affected the ability to achieve rapid disease improvement and effective disease control. Etanercept given by subcutaneous (SC) injection at a dose of .8 mg/kg weekly or .4 mg/kg twice weekly is effective and well-tolerated.[86–88] A randomized double-blind placebo-controlled trial of polyarticular JIA patients showed a 74% response rate during the 3 month open label phase with significant difference in disease flare in the double blind portion (81% placebo vs 7% etanercept).[86] Long-term data showed continued efficacy with 78% at an ACR Pedi 70.[87] The use of once weekly .8 mg/kg etanercept was rapidly effective with ACR Pedi 30 reached by 75% of patients in 4 weeks and an ACR Pedi 70 reached by 75% of patients by week 12.[88] Etanercept improves longitudinal growth independent of pubertal growth spurt and may contribute to the restoration of normal growth in JIA patients.[89,90] Infliximab has shown efficacy in combination with MTX.[91,92] The starting dose is usually 6 to 10 mg/kg, though doses as much as 10 to 15 mg/kg have been used.[91] An international trial of MTX-treatment–resistant patients confirmed the efficacy of combination infliximab and MTX with 73%, 70%, and 52% achieving an ACR Pedi 30, 50, and 70, respectively. Although patients had a rapid response within 2 weeks, there were associated infusion reactions and later note of diminished efficacy.[84] It may be more effective in uveitis than the other anti-TNF agents.[91] Adalimumab is given by SC injection at 20 mg or 40 mg every other week for patients less than 30 kg and more than or equal to 30 kg, respectively.[93–96] A randomized trial on the use of adalimumab with or without MTX in polyarticular-course JIA showed efficacy and a rapid response with 67% on monotherapy and 77% on combination MTX and adalimumab achieving an ACR Pedi 30 within 4 weeks. At the end of the 16 week lead-in period, 59% and 82% had achieved an ACR Pedi 70 respectively. Disease flare in the adalimumab-treated group (43%) was significantly lower than the placebo group (71%).[97] Adalimumab may be beneficial in patients who have failed other anti-TNF use and in uveitis.[98–100]

Abatacept

Abatacept, a selective costimulation pathway modulator, has also shown efficacy in achieving disease control within 6 months. It is given at 10 mg/kg (maximum 1000 mg) every 2 weeks for 3 doses, then every 4 weeks by infusion. It has proven to be an effective therapeutic option for juvenile polyarticular-course arthritis, including patients who had failed at least one DMARD and anti-TNF therapy. In the open-label extension phase of a randomized trial, 75% achieved an ACR Pedi 70. Furthermore, an ACR Pedi 90 and 100 were achieved by 57% and 39% patients, respectively, who had uninterrupted abatacept. The response time for abatacept may be as long as 4 to 6 months, though patients continue to show progressive improvement over time.[101,102] Abatacept improves health-related quality of life in JIA. Its use in the first 4 months showed improvements in patient pain, discomfort, global health, and physical function.[103]

IL-1 and IL-6 Inhibition

sJIA has not been found to be as responsive to DMARDs and anti-TNF agents as the other classes of JIA.[104] In particular, in early sJIA in which fever and rash are prominent features, anti-TNF agents have been less effective.[105–107] IL-1 and IL-6 inhibition have emerged as effective therapy for sJIA. IL-1 inhibition, in particular, seems to be promising first line treatment early in the disease course.[35,42,108]

Anakinra, a recombinant human IL-1 receptor antagonist, is given as a daily SC injection at 1 to 2 mg/kg. Younger children may require the higher doses.[109] Anakinra has the most favorable response in sJIA patients in whom its use has shown efficacy and safety.[35,109–112] However, an even greater impact of anakinra in sJIA may be the benefits of its use early in the disease instead of in recalcitrant course. In patients with sJIA who receive anakinra as first-line therapy, fever and rash resolved in more than 95% of patients within 1 month. In addition, with its use, prolonged corticosteroids can be avoided and severe therapy-resistant arthritis prevented.[35]

Canakinumab is a fully human monoclonal antibody with a long half-life that selectively blocks IL-1β. Preliminary data from a phase II multicenter dose-escalation, open-label study in patients with sJIA and active systemic symptoms demonstrated it to be rapid and effective therapy. Within 15 days, 60% achieved an ACR Pedi 50 and four patients had inactive disease with ability to taper corticosteroids. A dose of 4 mg/kg by SC injection every 4 weeks was assessed as most appropriate for maintaining patients free of relapse. Canakinumab also shows promise as a first-line therapy in sJIA. A phase III trial is currently in progress in children with sJIA.[108]

Tocilizumab, a humanized monoclonal antibody that inhibits IL-6 activity,[42,113] is given by infusion every 2 weeks at 12 mg/kg and 8 mg/kg for a weight of less than 30 kg and greater than or equal to 30 kg, respectively.[42,114,115] Though the use of anti–IL-1 therapy predated that of anti–IL-6, tocilizumab is the first biologic approved for the treatment of sJIA.[42] Clinical trials of tocilizumab show an effective rapid response within 2 to 6 weeks with an ACR Pedi 30, 50, and 70 achieved by 91%, 86%, and 68%, respectively.[113,116] Interestingly, patients who did not respond were younger with a shorter disease duration and more severe inflammation than those that did respond.[117] Data at 12 weeks from the phase III TENDER trial (Efficacy and safety of tocilizumab in patients with systemic-onset JIA) showed a significant difference from placebo with 85%, 71%, and 37% of patients at an ACR Pedi of 30, 50, and 70.[114,115] Additionally its use has demonstrated radiographic improvement of joint-space narrowing, subchondral bone cysts, and erosions.[118] It has been proposed that tocilizumab may be most effective when arthritis in sJIA is becoming more prevalent and systemic symptoms less prominent, instead of very early in the disease process when characteristic systemic autoinflammatory symptoms are most evident.[42]

COMBINATION THERAPY

Combination therapy may be more effective than monotherapy.[88,119] Concomitant use of MTX with IAS results in longer disease remission in the injected joint.[85] The Aggressive Combination Drug Therapy in Very Early Polyarticular Juvenile Idiopathic Arthritis (ACUTE-JIA) trial was a multicenter randomized, open-label clinical trial that evaluated aggressive combination therapy in early polyarticular JIA patients who were DMARD naïve and had arthritis for more than 6 months. Patients were randomized into three treatment arms: TNF (infliximab plus MTX), combo (combination MTX, sulfasalazine, and hydroxychloroquine), and MTX (MTX monotherapy). An ACR Pedi 75 was reached by 75%, 65%, and 50% of the TNF, COMBO, and MTX groups, respectively. Those patients on TNF therapy spent 6 months in inactive disease, which was significantly greater than the 3 months of the COMBO therapy and 1 month for the MTX group. Disease control was achieved more rapidly and sustained for a greater length of time in patients on TNF and MTX.[120]

The Trial of Early Aggressive Therapy in Polyarticular JIA (TREAT) study was a multicenter controlled trial of two aggressive treatments. Treatment arms consisted of MTX, etanercept, and prednisolone combination, and MTX placebo etanercept and placebo prednisolone combination. Clinical inactive disease (CID) at 6 months and clinical remission on medication at 12 months were evaluated. No statistical significance was noted between the two treatment arms; however, the achievement of an ACR Pedi 70 by 4 months was a significant predictor of CID at 6 months. More importantly, shorter disease duration at baseline was a significant predictor of achievement of CID at 6 months.[121]

Combination therapy with MTX and adalimumab also showed increased efficacy early in treatment of JIA.[97] At the end of the 16 week open-label period, 94% of the combination MTX and adalimumab group had achieved an ACR Pedi 30 versus 74% on adalimumab monotherapy. Similarly, more patients on combination therapy (82%) achieved an ACR Pedi 70 than those on monotherapy (59%).

Aggressive therapeutic intervention is not without risks of adverse events, particularly infections and the raised concern of malignancy. It is, however, important to be able to initiate early and aggressive therapy in patients with predictors of persistent disease and joint erosions.[14,61,69] Patients who particularly require early aggressive disease control are those who have a large number of affected joints, young age at onset, RF-positive polyarthritis, family history of AS, ankle arthritis, elevated ESR and IgM RF in first 6 months of disease, and presence of HLA-DRB1*08.[5,6,69] In light of the paradoxic need to achieve disease control as quickly and as early in the disease process as possible but limit the use of biologics that have proven so effective due to concerns for infection and malignancy, one treatment strategy advocated is induction and maintenance therapy. A biologic agent would be used early in the course of the disease to induce remission and, after achievement of inactive disease, continue maintenance therapy with a DMARD.[120]

In 2011, the American College of Rheumatology released treatment recommendations for JIA that were to serve as references for care and not meant to preclude individual patient assessment and clinical decision making. These guidelines can be fully reviewed in the 2011 Arthritis Care and Research publication where they are outlined in detail.[79] They reflect the importance of aggressive treatment early in the disease with methotrexate as initial therapy and TNF-α inhibitors as soon as after 3 months of methotrexate therapy. NSAID monotherapy was limited to patients with four or fewer joints with low disease activity, no contractures, and no features of poor prognosis. Regardless of number of joints, continuation of NSAID monotherapy for more than 2 months was deemed inappropriate for patients with active joint disease activity or greater than 1 month in patients with systemic symptoms. MTX as initial therapy was recommended for patients with high disease activity or those with moderate disease activity and features of poor prognosis. A joint injection with triamcinolone hexacetonide was recommended for active joint disease regardless of concurrent therapy, emphasizing that a shorter duration of response indicated the need for escalation of systemic treatment. TNF-α inhibitor therapy was recommended if moderate or high disease activity persisted after 3 months of MTX therapy or low disease activity persisted after 6 months of MTX therapy. Anti-TNF therapy was recommended as initial therapy for patients with sacroiliac disease. For systemic JIA with active systemic symptoms, systemic glucocorticoids were recommended. In addition, initiation of anakinra was recommended in those patients with poor prognosis regardless of current therapy and for all patients who sustained or developed fever while on corticosteroids.

SUMMARY

JIA is an immunoinflammatory disease of childhood that is distinct from adult arthritis but has a burden of disease with significant impact well into the adult years. It is now recognized that a considerable number of JIA patients will have active disease or sequelae of disease that persists into adulthood. Although longstanding disease is a risk factor for irreversible damage and functional disability, the changes begin early in the disease process. In addition, there are several prognosticating and risk factors that are important to recognize to provide appropriate treatment. This is crucial because the disease activity and response to treatment in the first 6 months of disease greatly influences the long-term prognosis. The recognition of early manifestations of JIA to facilitate early referral, diagnosis, and effective aggressive treatment by a pediatric rheumatologist is vital. Advances in treatment options with the advent of biologic therapy and the change in approach to early aggressive intervention have provided the armamentarium to make remission an attainable goal.

REFERENCES

1. Petty RE, Southwood TR, Manners P, et al. International League of Associations for Rheumatology classification of juvenile idiopathic arthritis: second revision, Edmonton, 2001. J Rheumatol 2004;31:390–2.
2. Petty RE, Southwood TR, Baum J, et al. Revision of the proposed classification criteria for juvenile idiopathic arthritis: Durban, 1997. J Rheumatol 1998;25:1991–4.

3. Flato B, Aasland A, Vinje O, et al. Outcome and predictive factors in juvenile rheumatoid arthritis and juvenile spondyloarthropathy. J Rheumatol 1998;25: 366–75.

4. Fantini F, Gerloni V, Gattinara M, et al. Remission in juvenile chronic arthritis: a cohort study of 683 consecutive cases with a mean 10 year followup. J Rheumatol 2003;30:579–84.

5. Flatø B, Hoffmann-Vold AM, Reiff A, et al. Long-term outcome and prognostic factors in enthesitis-related arthritis: a case control study. Arthritis Rheum 2006;54(11):3573–82.

6. Wallace CA, Huang B, Bandeira M, et al. Patterns of clinical remission in select categories of juvenile idiopathic arthritis. Arthritis Rheum 2005;52(11): 3554–62.

7. Magni-Manzoni S, Pistorio A, Labò E, et al. A longitudinal analysis of physical functional disability over the course of juvenile idiopathic arthritis. Ann Rheum Dis 2008;67:1159–64.

8. Minden K. Adult outcomes of patients with juvenile idiopathic arthritis. Horm Res 2009;72(Suppl 1):20–5.

9. Minden K, Niewerth M, Listing J, et al. Long-term outcome in patients with juvenile idiopathic arthritis. Arthritis Rheum 2002;46(9):2392–401.

10. Reiff AO. Treatment update on juvenile arthritis. In: Rakel RE, Bope ET, editors. Conn's current therapy—2006. Philadelphia: Saunders Elsevier; 2006. p. 1188–94.

11. Lien G, Selvaag AM, Flato B, et al. A two-year prospective controlled study of bone mass and bone turnover in children with early juvenile idiopathic arthritis. Arthritis Rheum 2005;52(3):833–40.

12. Wallace CA, Levinson JE. Juvenile rheumatoid arthritis: outcome and treatment for the 1990s. Rheum Dis Clin North Am 1991;17:891–905.

13. Levinson JE, Wallace CA. Dismantling the pyramid. J Rheumatol 1992;19(Suppl 330):6–10.

14. Stone M, Warren RW, Bruckel J, et al. Juvenile-onset ankylosing spondylitis is associated with worse functional outcomes than adult-onset ankylosing spondylitis. Arthritis Rheum 2005;53(3):445–51.

15. Magnani A, Pistori A, Mangi-Manzoni S, et al. Achievement of a state of inactive disease at least once in the first 5 years predicts better outcome of patients with polyarticular juvenile idiopathic arthritis. J Rheumatol 2009; 36(3):628–34.

16. Bartoli M, Tarò M, Magni-Manzoni S, et al. The magnitude of early response to methotrexate therapy predicts long-term outcomes of patients with juvenile idiopathic arthritis. Ann Rheum Dis 2008;67:370–4.

17. Hagglund KJ, Schopp LM, Alberts KR, et al. Predicting pain among children with juvenile rheumatoid arthritis. Arthritis Care Res 1995;8:36–42.

18. Kuis W, Heijnen CJ, Hogeweg JA, et al. How painful is juvenile chronic arthritis? Arch Dis Child 1997;77:451–3.

19. Thastum M, Zachariae R, Scholer M, et al. Cold pressor pain: comparing responses of juvenile arthritis patients and their parents. Scand J Rheumatol 1997;26:272–9.

20. Ansell BM. Juvenile chronic arthritis with persistently positive tests for rheumatoid factor (sero-positive juvenile rheumatoid arthritis). Ann Pediatr (Paris) 1983; 30:545–50.

21. Cassidy JT, Brody GL, Martel W. Monarticular juvenile rheumatoid arthritis. J Pediatr 1967;70:867–75.

22. Schaller J, Wedgwood RJ. Pauciarticular juvenile rheumatoid arthritis. Arthritis Rheum 1969;12:30.
23. Huemer C, Malleson PN, Cabral DA, et al. Patterns of joint involvement at onset differentiate oligoarticular juvenile psoriatic arthritis from pauciarticular juvenile rheumatoid arthritis. J Rheumatol 2002;29:1531–5.
24. Uziel Y, Rathaus V, Pomeranz A, et al. Torticollis as the sole initial presenting sign of systemic onset juvenile rheumatoid arthritis. J Rheumatol 1998;25:166–8.
25. Siamopoulou-Mavridou A, Asimakopoulos D, Mavridis A, et al. Middle ear function in patients with juvenile chronic arthritis. Ann Rheum Dis 1990;49:620–3.
26. Malleson P, Riding K, Petty R. Stridor due to cricoarytenoid arthritis in pauciarticular onset juvenile rheumatoid arthritis. J Rheumatol 1986;13:952–3.
27. Olson L, Eckerdal O, Hallonsten AL, et al. Craniomandibular function in juvenile chronic arthritis: a clinical and radiographic study. Swed Dent J 1991;15:71–83.
28. Ronchezel MV, Hilario MO, Goldenberg J, et al. Temporomandibular joint and mandibular growth alterations in patients with juvenile rheumatoid arthritis. J Rheumatol 1995;22:1956–61.
29. Sherry DD, Stein LD, Reed AM, et al. Prevention of leg length discrepancy in young children with pauciarticular juvenile rheumatoid arthritis by treatment with intraarticular steroids. Arthritis Rheum 1999;42(11):2330–4.
30. Beherens EM, Beukelman T, Gallo L, et al. Evaluation of the presentation of systemic onset juvenile rheumatoid arthritis: data from the Pennsylvania Systemic Onset Juvenile Arthritis Registry (PASOJAR). J Rheumatol 2008;35:343–8.
31. Schneider R, Laxer RM. Systemic onset juvenile rheumatoid arthritis. Baillieres Clin Rheumatol 1998;12:245–71.
32. Ravelli A, Magni-Manzoni S, Pistorio A, et al. Preliminary diagnosis guidelines for macrophage activation syndrome complicating systemic juvenile idiopathic arthritis. J Pediatr 2005;146:598–604.
33. Henter JI, Horne A, Arico M, et al. HLH -2004: diagnostic and therapeutic guidelines for hemophagocytic lymphohistiocytosis. Pediatr Blood Cancer 2007;48:127–31.
34. Wilkinson N, Jackson G, Gardner-Medwin J. Biologic therapies for juvenile arthritis. Arch Dis Child 2003;88:186–91.
35. Nistala K, Moncrieffe H, Newton KR, et al. Interleukin-17 producing T cells are enriched in the joints of children with arthritis, but have a reciprocal relationship to regulatory T cell numbers. Arthritis Rheum 2008;58:875–87.
36. Wehrens EJ, van Wijk F, Roord ST, et al. Treating arthritis by immunomodulation: is there a role for immunomodulatory T cells? Rheumatology 2010;49:1632–44.
37. Prakken BJ, Albani S. Using biology of disease to understand and guide therapy of JIA. Best Pract Res Clin Rheumatol 2009;23:599–608.
38. Ou LS, See LC, Wu CJ, et al. Association between serum inflammatory cytokines and disease activity in juvenile idiopathic arthritis. Clin Rheumatol 2002;21:52–6.
39. Nigrovic PA, Mannion M, Prince FH, et al. Anakinra as first-line disease-modifying therapy in systemic juvenile idiopathic arthritis. Report of forty-six patients from an international multicenter series. Arthritis Rheum 2011;63:545–55.
40. Reiff A. The use of anakinra in juvenile arthritis. Curr Rheumatol Rep 2005;7:434–40.
41. Yokota S, Miyamae T, Imagawa T, et al. Clinical study of tocilizumab in children with systemic-onset juvenile idiopathic arthritis. Clin Rev Allergy Immunol 2005;28:231–7.
42. Reiff A. Treatment of systemic juvenile idiopathic arthritis with tocilizumab—the role of anti-interleukin-6 therapy after a decade of treatment. Biol Ther 2012;2:001.

43. Finnegan S, Clarke S, Gibson D, et al. Synovial membrane immunohistology in early untreated juvenile idiopathic arthritis: differences between clinical subgroups. Ann Rheum Dis 2011;70:1842–50.

44. Ravelli A, Martini A. Juvenile idiopathic arthritis. Lancet 2007;369:767–78.

45. Ravelli A, Varnier GC, Oliveira S, et al. Antinuclear antibody-positive patients should be grouped as a separate category in the classification of juvenile idiopathic arthritis. Arthritis Rheum 2011;63:267–75.

46. Avcin T, Cimaz R, Falcini F, et al. Prevalence and clinical significance of anti-cyclic citrullinated peptide antibodies in juvenile idiopathic arthritis. Ann Rheum Dis 2002;61:608–11.

47. Selvaag AM, Flato B, Dale K, et al. Radiographic and clinical outcome in early juvenile rheumatoid arthritis and juvenile spondyloarthropathy: a 3-year prospective study. J Rheumatol 2006;33:1382–91.

48. Periloux BC, Shetty AK, Leiva LE, et al. Antinuclear antibody (ANA) and ANA profile tests in children with autoimmune disorders: a retrospective study. Clin Rheumatol 2000;19:200–3.

49. McGhee JL, Kikingbird LM, Jarvis JN. Clinical utility of antibody tests in children. BMC Pediatr 2004;4:13.

50. Masi L, Ricci L, Zulian F, et al. Serum osteopontin as a predictive marker of responsiveness to methotrexate in juvenile idiopathic arthritis. J Rheumatol 2009;36:2308–13.

51. Wittkowski H, Frosch M, Wulffraat N, et al. S100A12 is a novel molecular marker differentiating systemic-onset juvenile idiopathic arthritis from other causes of fever of unknown origin. Arthritis Rheum 2008;58:3924–31.

52. Frosch M, Ahlmann M, Vogl T, et al. The myeloid-related proteins 8 and 14 complex, a novel ligand of toll-like receptor 4, and interleukin-1beta form a positive feedback mechanism in systemic-onset juvenile idiopathic arthritis. Arthritis Rheum 2009;60:883–91.

53. Kirkhus E, Flato B, Riise O, et al. Differences in MRI findings between subgroups of recent-onset childhood arthritis. Pediatr Radiol 2011;41:432–40.

54. Gardner-Medwin JM, Killeen OG, Ryder CA, et al. Magnetic resonance imaging identifies features in clinically unaffected knees predicting extension of arthritis in children with monoarthritis. J Rheumatol 2006;33(11):2337–43.

55. Malattia C, Damasio MB, Magnaguagno F, et al. Magnetic resonance imaging, ultrasonography and conventional radiography in the assessment of bone erosions in juvenile idiopathic arthritis. Arthritis Care Res 2008;59(12):1764–72.

56. Yamazaki S, Okano M, Toita N, et al. Early diagnosis for polyarthritis of juvenile idiopathic arthritis using systemic gallium scintigraphy. Pediatr Int 2009;51(4):587–90.

57. Kamel M, Eid H, Mansour R. Ultrasound detection of heel enthesitis: a comparison with magnetic resonance imaging. J Rheumatol 2003;30:774–8.

58. Bechtold S, Roth J. Natural history of growth and body composition in juvenile idiopathic arthritis. Horm Res 2009;72(Suppl 1):13–9.

59. Petty RE, Cassidy JT. Chronic arthritis in childhood. In: Cassidy JT, Petty RE, Laxer RM, et al, editors. Textbook of pediatric rheumatology. 6th edition. Philadelphia: Saunders Elsevier; 2010. p. 211–35.

60. Mason T, Reed AM, Nelson AM, et al. Frequency of abnormal hand and wrist radiographs at time of diagnosis of polyarticular juvenile rheumatoid arthritis. J Rheumatol 2002;29:2214–8.

61. Pagnini I, Savelli S, Matucci-Cerinic M, et al. Early predictors of juvenile sacroiliitis in enthesitis-related arthritis. J Rheumatol 2010;37:2395–401.

62. Lien G, Flato B, Haugen M, et al. Frequency of osteopenia in adolescents with early-onset juvenile idiopathic arthritis. A long-term outcome study of one hundred five patients. Arthritis Rheum 2003;48:2214–23.
63. Mårtensson K, Chrysis D, Sävendahl L. Interleukin-1beta and TNF-alpha act in synergy to inhibit longitudinal growth in fetal rat metatarsal bones. J Bone Miner Res 2004;19(11):1805–12.
64. Vlahos AP, Theocharis P, Bechlioulis A, et al. Changes in vascular function and structure in juvenile idiopathic arthritis. Arthritis Care Res 2011;63(12): 1736–44.
65. Singh-Grewal D, Schneider R, Bayer N, et al. Predictors of disease course and remission in systemic juvenile idiopathic arthritis. Arthritis Rheum 2006;54: 1595–601.
66. Spiegel LR, Schneider R, Lang BA, et al. Early predictors of poor functional outcome in systemic onset juvenile rheumatoid arthritis: a multicenter cohort study. Arthritis Rheum 2000;43:2402–9.
67. Schneider R, Lang BA, Reilly BJ, et al. Prognostic indicators of joint destruction in systemic juvenile rheumatoid arthritis. J Pediatr 1992;12:200–5.
68. Oen K, Tucker L, Huber AM, et al. Predictors of early inactive disease in juvenile idiopathic arthritis: results of a Canadian mulitcenter, prospective inception cohort study. Arthritis Care Res 2009;61(8):1077–86.
69. Flato B, Lien G, Smerdel A, et al. Prognostic factors in juvenile rheumatoid arthritis: a case-control study revealing early predictors and outcome after 14.9 years. J Rheumatol 2003;30:386–93.
70. Flato B, Lien G, Smerdel-Ramoya A, et al. Juvenile psoriatic arthritis: longterm outcome and differentiation from other subtypes of juvenile idiopathic arthritis. J Rheumatol 2009;36:642–50.
71. Stoll ML, Bhore R, Dempsey-Robertson M, et al. Spondyloarthritis in a pediatric population: risk factors for sacroiliitis. J Rheumatol 2010;37:2402–8.
72. Chen J, Liu C. Is sulfasalazine effective in ankylosing spondylitis? A systematic review of randomized controlled trials. J Rheumatol 2006;33:722–31.
73. Haibel H, Brandt HC, Song IH, et al. No efficacy of subcutaneous methotrexate in active ankylosing spondylitis: a 16-week open label trial. Ann Rheum Dis 2007;66:419–21.
74. Wallace CA. Current management of juvenile idiopathic arthritis. Best Pract Res Clin Rheumatol 2006;20:279–300.
75. van Rossum MAJ, van Soesbergen RM, Boers M, et al. Long-term outcome of juvenile idiopathic arthritis following a placebo-controlled trial: sustained benefits of early sulfasalazine treatment. Ann Rheum Dis 2007;66: 1518–24.
76. Giannini EH, Brewer EJ, Kuzmina N, et al. Methotrexate in resistant juvenile rheumatoid arthritis. Results of the USA-USSR double-blind, placebo-controlled trial. The pediatric rheumatology collaborative study group and the cooperative children's study group. N Engl J Med 1992;326(16):1043–9.
77. Ravelli A, Martini A. Methotrexate in juvenile idiopathic arthritis: answers and questions. J Rheumatol 2000;27:1830–3.
78. Ruperto N, Murray KJ, Gerloni V. A randomized trial of parenteral methotrexate comparing an intermediate dose with a higher dose in children with juvenile idiopathic arthritis who failed to respond to standard doses of methotrexate. Arthritis Rheum 2004;50(7):2191–201.
79. Beukelman T, Patkar NM, Saag KG, et al. 2011 American College of Rheumatology recommendations for the treatment of juvenile idiopathic arthritis: initiation

and safety monitoring of therapeutic agents for treatment of arthritis and systemic features. Arthritis Care Res 2011;63(4):465–82.

80. Huppertz HI, Tschammler A, Horwitz AE, et al. Intraarticular corticosteroids for chronic arthritis in children: efficacy and effects on cartilage and growth. J Pediatr 1995;127:317–21.

81. Ravelli A, Manzoni SM, Viola S, et al. Factors affecting the efficacy of intraarticular corticosteroid injection of knees in juvenile idiopathic arthritis. J Rheumatol 2001;28:2100–2.

82. Eberhard BA, Sison MC, Gottlieb BS, et al. Comparison of the intraarticular effectiveness of triamcinolone hexacetonide and triamcinolone acetonide in treatment of juvenile rheumatoid arthritis. J Rheumatol 2004;31:2507–12.

83. Zulian F, Martini G, Gobber D, et al. Triamcinolone acetonide and hexacetonide intra-articular treatment of symmetrical joints in juvenile idiopathic arthritis: a double-blind trial. Rheumatology 2004;43:1288–91.

84. Beukelman T, Guevara JP, Albert DA, et al. Optimal treatment of knee monoarthritis in juvenile idiopathic arthritis: a decision analysis. Arthritis Rheum 2008; 59:1580–8.

85. Marti P, Molinari L, Bolt IB, et al. Factor influencing the efficacy of intra-articular steroid injections in patients with juvenile idiopathic arthritis. Eur J Pediatr 2008; 167:425–30.

86. Lovell DJ, Giannini EH, Reiff A, et al. Etanercept in children with polyarticular juvenile rheumatoid arthritis. N Engl J Med 2000;342:763–9.

87. Lovell DJ, Reiff A, Jones OY, et al. Long-term safety and efficacy of etanercept in children with polyarticular-course juvenile rheumatoid arthritis. Arthritis Rheum 2006;54(6):1987–94.

88. Horneff G, Ebert A, Fitter S. Safety and efficacy of once weekly etanercept 0.8 mg/kg in a multicentre, 12 week trial in active polyarticular course juvenile idiopathic arthritis. Rheumatology 2009;48:916–9.

89. Vojvodich PF, Hansen JB, Andersson U, et al. Etanercept treatment improves longitudinal growth in prepubertal children with juvenile idiopathic arthritis. J Rheumatol 2007;34:2481–5.

90. Giannini EH, Ilowite NT, Lovell DJ, et al. Effects of long-term etanercept treatment on growth in children with selected categories of juvenile idiopathic arthritis. Arthritis Rheum 2010;62:3259–64.

91. Gerloni V, Pontikaki I, Gattinara M, et al. Efficacy of repeated intravenous infusions of an anti-tumor necrosis factor α monoclonal antibody, infliximab, in persistently active, refractory juvenile idiopathic arthritis. Arthritis Rheum 2005;52:548–53.

92. Ruperto N, Lovell DJ, Cuttica R, et al. Long-term efficacy and safety of infliximab plus methotrexate for the treatment of polyarticular-course juvenile rheumatoid arthritis: findings from an open-label treatment extension. Ann Rheum Dis 2010;69:718–22.

93. Marzan KA, Reiff AO. Adalimumab in juvenile rheumatoid arthritis/juvenile idiopathic arthritis. Expert Rev Clin Immunol 2008;4:549–58.

94. Keystone E, Haraoui B. Adalimumab therapy in rheumatoid arthritis. Rheum Dis Clin North Am 2004;30:349–64.

95. Weisman MH, Moreland LW, Furst DE, et al. Efficacy, pharmacokinetic, and safety assessment of adalimumab, a fully human anti-tumor necrosis factor-alpha monoclonal antibody, in adults with rheumatoid arthritis receiving concomitant methotrexate: a pilot study. Clin Ther 2003;25:1700–21.

96. Humira® (adalimumab). [package insert]. North Chicago (IL): Abbott Laboratories; 2011.

97. Lovell DJ, Ruperto N, Goodman S, et al. Adalimumab with or without metho-trexate in juvenile rheumatoid arthritis. N Engl J Med 2008;359:810–20.
98. Katsicas MM, Russo RA. Use of adalimumab in patients with juvenile idiopathic arthritis refractory to etanercept and/or infliximab. Clin Rheumatol 2009;28: 985–8.
99. Trachana M, Pratsidou-Gertsi P, Pardalos P, et al. Safety and efficacy of adalimu-mab treatment in Greek children with juvenile idiopathic arthritis. Scand J Rheu-matol 2011;40:101–7.
100. Vazquez-Cobian LB, Flynn T, Lehman TJ. Adalimumab therapy for childhood uveitis. J Pediatr 2006;149:572–5.
101. Ruperto N, Lovell DJ, Quartier P, et al. Long-term safety and efficacy of abatacept in children with juvenile idiopathic arthritis. Arthritis Rheum 2010;62:1792–802.
102. Ruperto N, Lovell DJ, Quartier P, et al. Abatacept in children with juvenile idio-pathic arthritis: a randomised, double-blind, placebo-controlled withdrawal trial. Lancet 2008;372:383–91.
103. Ruperto N, Lovell DJ, Li T, et al. Abatacept improves health-related quality of life, pain, sleep quality, and daily participation in subjects with juvenile idiopathic arthritis. Arthritis Care Res 2010;62:1542–51.
104. Prakken B, Albani S, Martini A. Juvenile idiopathic arthritis. Lancet 2011;377: 2138–49.
105. Russo RA, Katsicas MM. Clinical remission in patients with systemic juvenile idiopathic arthritis treated with anti-tumor necrosis factor agents. J Rheumatol 2009;36(5):1078–82.
106. Quartier P, Taupin P, Bourdeaut F, et al. Efficacy of etanercept for the treatment of juvenile idiopathic arthritis according to the onset type. Arthritis Rheum 2003; 48:1093–101.
107. Kimura Y, Pinho P, Walco G, et al. Etanercept treatment in patients with re-fractory systemic onset juvenile rheumatoid arthritis. J Rheumatol 2005;32: 935–42.
108. Ruperto N, Quartier P, Wulffraat N, et al. A phase II, multicenter, open-label study evaluating dosing and preliminary safety and efficacy of canakinumab in systemic juvenile idiopathic arthritis with active systemic features. Arthritis Rheum 2012;64:557–67.
109. Reiff A, Porras O, Rudge S, et al. Preliminary data from a study of Kineret TM (anakinra) in children with juvenile rheumatoid arthritis. Arthritis Rheum 2002; 46(Suppl):S496.
110. Quartier P, Allantaz F, Cimaz R, et al. A multicentre, randomised, double-blind, placebo controlled trial with interleukin-1 receptor antagonist anakinra in patients with systemic onset juvenile idiopathic arthritis (ANAJIS trial). Ann Rheum Dis 2011;70:747–54.
111. Gattorno M, Piccini A, Lasiglie D, et al. The patterns of response to anti-interleukin-1 treatment distinguishes two subsets of patients with systemic-onset juvenile idiopathic arthritis. Arthritis Rheum 2008;58:1505–15.
112. Ilowite N, Porras O, Reiff A, et al. Anakinra in the treatment of polyarticular-course juvenile rheumatoid arthritis: safety and preliminary efficacy results of a randomized multicenter study. Clin Rheumatol 2009;28:129–37.
113. Yokota S, Miyamae T, Imagawa T, et al. Therapeutic efficacy of humanized re-combinant anti-interleukin-6 receptor antibody in children systemic-onset juve-nile idiopathic arthritis. Arthritis Rheum 2005;52:818–25.
114. De Benedetti F, Brunner H, Allen R, et al. Tocilizumab is efficacious in patients with systemic juvenile idiopathic arthritis across baseline demographic and

disease characteristics and prior/baseline treatments: 52 week data from a phase 3 clinical trial. Arthritis Rheum 2011;63(Suppl 10):abstract 2621.

115. De Benedetti F, Brunner H, Ruperto N, et al. Efficacy and safety of tocilizumab in patients with systemic juvenile idiopathic arthritis: 2 year data from a phase III clinical trial. Arthritis Rheum 2011;63(Suppl 10):abstract L111.

116. Woo P, Wilkinson N, Prieur AM, et al. Open label phase II trial of single, ascending doses of MRA in Caucasian children with severe systemic juvenile idiopathic arthritis: proof of principle of the efficacy of IL-6 receptor blockade in this type of arthritis and demonstration of prolonged clinical improvement. Arthritis Res Ther 2005;7:R1281.

117. Yokota S, Imagawa T, Mori M, et al. Efficacy and safety of tocilizumab in patients with systemic-onset juvenile idiopathic arthritis: a randomized, double- blind, placebo- controlled, withdrawal phase III trial. Lancet 2008;371:998–1006.

118. Inaba Y, Ozawa R, Imagawa T, et al. Radiographic improvement of damaged large joints in children with systemic juvenile idiopathic arthritis following tocilizumab treatment. Ann Rheum Dis 2011;70:1693–5.

119. Horneff G, De Bock F, Foeldvari I, et al. Safety and efficacy of combination etanercept and methotrexate compared to treatment with etanercept only in patients with juvenile idiopathic arthritis (JIA): preliminary data from the German JIA registry. Ann Rheum Dis 2009;68(4):519–25.

120. Tynjälä P, Vähäsalo P, Tarkiainen M, et al. Aggressive combination drug therapy in very early polyarticular juvenile idiopathic arthritis (ACUTE-JIA): a multicentre randomized open-label clinical trial. Ann Rheum Dis 2011;70:1605–12.

121. Wallace CA, Giannini EH, Spalding SJ, et al. Trial of early aggressive therapy in polyarticular juvenile idiopathic arthritis. Arthritis Rheum 2012;64(6):2012–21.

Early Psoriatic Arthritis

Dafna D. Gladman, MD, FRCPC*

KEYWORDS

- Psoriasis • Psoriatic arthritis • Prognosis • Treatment
- Early disease

Key Points

- Psoriatic arthritis is an inflammatory musculoskeletal disease associated with psoriasis that is usually seronegative for rheumatoid factor.[1]
- Psoriatic arthritis affects men and women equally, usually during the fourth decade, although it may affect children and octogenarians.
- Psoriatic arthritis may lead to deformities, joint damage, reduced quality of life and function.
- Early detection and treatment may prevent untoward outcomes.

WHAT IS PSORIATIC ARTHRITIS?
Psoriatic Arthritis: The Entity

Psoriatic arthritis is an inflammatory musculoskeletal disease associated with psoriasis that is usually seronegative for rheumatoid factor.[1] Although the occurrence of arthritis among patients with psoriasis has been known since the nineteenth century, psoriatic arthritis was initially considered a variant of rheumatoid arthritis. It was defined as an entity separate from rheumatoid arthritis primarily because of the efforts of Wright in the late 1950s and 1960s, and Moll and Wright in the 1970s.[2] It was accepted as an entity by the American Rheumatology Association (now the American College of Rheumatology) in 1964.[3]

Psoriatic arthritis affects men and women equally, usually during the fourth decade, although it may affect children and octogenarians. Most (70%) patients with psoriatic arthritis develop their arthritis after the onset of psoriasis. About 15% develop the skin and joint manifestations simultaneously. However, in some 15% of cases, the arthritis precedes the onset of psoriasis.[4] Although it is possible that in many of these cases the psoriasis were missed because a careful search for hidden lesions was not performed, there are patients whose arthritis begins long before the onset of psoriasis.[5] In these cases, the diagnosis becomes difficult, and physicians rely on the clinical features unique to psoriatic arthritis (discussed later) to make the diagnosis.

No financial disclosures.
Psoriatic Arthritis Program, Centre for Prognosis Studies in the Rheumatic Diseases, Toronto Western Hospital, University Health Network, 399 Bathurst Street 1E-410B, Toronto, Ontario, Canada
* Corresponding author.
E-mail address: dafna.gladman@utoronto.ca

Prevalence of Psoriatic Arthritis

The prevalence of psoriatic arthritis is unknown.[6] Estimates from population studies have ranged from 0.01% in China to 0.47% in Australian Aborigines (**Table 1**).[7–11] It is difficult to compare these prevalence data because the methodologies in studies are varied, from small population areas to large administrative databases. Some are based on patient report, others on physician observation. Moreover, the diagnosis of psoriatic arthritis may be difficult, and classification criteria have not been universally accepted until the recent Classification of Psoriatic Arthritis (CASPAR) criteria.[1]

The prevalence of psoriatic arthritis among patients with psoriasis has also varied, from 6.25% in a study from the Mayo Clinic to 48% from a Swedish study (**Table 2**).[6,12–22] Because it is estimated that psoriasis occurs in 1% to 3% of the population, and the frequency of psoriatic arthritis is about 30%, it is possible that the frequency of psoriatic arthritis is between 0.3% and 1%.

CAUSE AND PATHOGENESIS OF PSORIATIC ARTHRITIS

The cause of psoriatic arthritis remains unknown. However, there is evidence to support genetic, environmental, and immunologic factors in both cause and pathogenesis of the disease.

Genetic Factors

There is strong evidence for familial clustering of both psoriasis and psoriatic arthritis.[23] Twin studies show a higher concordance rate for psoriasis among monozygotic than dizygotic twins, and family studies have shown that there is a recurrence risk ratio of 4 to 10. Although a higher concordance rate was seen for psoriatic arthritis, the number of twins with this disease was low, and it was not statistically significant. Recurrence risk ratio for psoriatic arthritis is higher than for psoriasis alone, with λ_1 of 30.[24] Linkage studies have identified several susceptibility loci for psoriasis, including the human leukocyte antigen (HLA) locus on chromosome 6p (PSORS1), and loci on 17q (PSORS2), 4q (PSORS2), 1q (PSORS 4), 3q (PSORS5), 19p (PSORS6), 1p (PSROS7), 16q (PSORS8), 4q (PSROS9), and 18p (PSROS10). The strongest association is with a locus within the major histocompatibility complex (MHC). Only 1 genome-wide linkage scan has been reported for psoriatic arthritis identifying a locus on 16q close to the PSORS8 locus.[25] Genome-wide association scans in psoriatic arthritis revealed associations with HLA-C, IL12B, and TNIP1, as well as with a locus on chromosome 2p.[26–28] The differences between psoriasis and psoriatic arthritis have been difficult to interpret from genome-wide scans because not all patients with psoriasis were reviewed to ascertain the absence of psoriatic arthritis.

A comparison of HLA alleles between patients with psoriasis confirmed by a rheumatologist not to have psoriatic arthritis and patients with psoriatic arthritis identified

Table 1
Prevalence of psoriatic arthritis: population-based studies

Geographic Location	Year	Number of Subjects	Estimate (%)
Australia (Aborigines)[11]	2004	847	0.47
Greece[8]	2005	14,233	0.17
United States[10]	2005	27,229	0.25
Italy[9]	2007	2155	0.42
China[7]	2008	241,169	0.01–0.1

Table 2
Prevalence of psoriatic arthritis among patients with psoriasis

Author, Year	Center	No. Patients with Psoriasis	% Psoriatic Arthritis
Leczinsky,[12] 1948	Sweden	534	7
Little et al,[13] 1975	Toronto	100	32
Scarpa et al,[14] 1984	Napoli	180	34
Stern,[15] 1985	Boston	1285	20
Barisic-Drusko et al,[16] 1994	Osijek region	553	10
Salvarani et al,[17] 1995	Regio Emilia	205	36
Shbeeb et al,[18] 2000	Mayo Clinic	1056	6.25
Brockbank,[19] 2001	Toronto	126	31
Alenius et al,[20] 2002	Sweden	276	48
Gelfand et al,[10] 2002	United States	672	11
Zachariae,[21] 2003	Denmark	5795	30
Reich et al,[22] 2009	Germany	1511	20.6

that HLA-B*08, HLA-B*38, and HLA*B-27 were increased among patients with psoriatic arthritis, whereas HLA-C*0602 was higher among patients with psoriasis without arthritis.[29]

Environmental Factors

There is also evidence that environmental factors are important in the development of psoriatic arthritis among patients with psoriasis. A recent study that compared patients with psoriatic arthritis with those with psoriasis who were confirmed not to have psoriatic arthritis by a rheumatologist revealed that infections requiring antibiotics, and trauma, were associated with the presence of psoriatic arthritis, suggesting that these factors are important in the development of psoriatic arthritis.[30] Smoking was found to be protective, and the mechanism for that is currently under investigation.

Immunologic Factors

Several immunologic abnormalities have been detected among patients with psoriasis and psoriatic arthritis. The presence and activated state of both CD8+ T cells and natural killer (NK) cells in the psoriatic synovium and the response of the disease to immunomodulatory therapy indicate that the immune system, especially the lymphocytes, play an important role in the pathogenesis of psoriatic arthritis.[31] It has been suggested that that autoimmunity directed against a common skin and joint autoantigen(s) leads to chronic autoreactive T-cell driven inflammation. Prior response to exogenous ligands encoded by pathogens, as well as prior episodes of inflammation, result in expansion of memory effector CD8+ T cells that recognize stress-related self-antigens and initiates and maintains pathways of inflammation mediated by the expression of transcription factors such as nuclear factor-κB and activator protein-1, resulting in skin and synovial inflammation. This model combines the genetic factors as well as possible environmental factors. Again, whether the same or different mechanisms operate in the development of joint versus skin disease is unclear.

Whatever the mechanism, the inflammation leads to synovial proliferation, release of cytokines, and subsequent joint destruction.

THE CLINICAL PICTURE OF PSORIATIC ARTHRITIS

Wright and Moll[32] described 5 clinical patterns of psoriatic arthritis. These include distal arthritis involving the distal interphalangeal joints of the hands and feet; oligoarthritis, affecting fewer than 5 joints; polyarthritis affecting 5 or more joints that is indistinguishable from rheumatoid arthritis; arthritis mutilans, a very destructive form of arthritis; and a spondyloarthritis, affecting the axial skeleton. Although these patterns clearly occur in psoriatic arthritis, they are not mutually exclusive. Patients may switch pattern over time, and more than 1 pattern may occur in an individual patient.[33] Therefore, recent descriptions of psoriatic arthritis tend to concentrate on the presence of peripheral arthritis, with or without spinal involvement.[34]

Peripheral Arthritis

Psoriatic arthritis affects the peripheral joints of the hands and feet in most patients. The arthritis is inflammatory in nature, and there is prolonged morning stiffness in about half the patients (**Fig. 1**). There is improvement of the pain and stiffness with activity and worsening with rest. Unlike rheumatoid arthritis, the inflamed joints in psoriatic arthritis have a purplish discoloration. At onset, the arthritis tends to be oligoarticular, involving 4 or fewer joints, and asymmetric. Although all joints may be affected by psoriatic arthritis, at least 53% of patients have distal joint involvement. As the disease progresses it may become more polyarticular. As more joints are accrued it becomes more symmetric. Therefore patients with long-standing disease are more likely to have polyarticular and symmetric disease.[35] Patients with psoriatic arthritis do not complain of as much pain as patients with rheumatoid arthritis, the prototype inflammatory form of arthritis. Thus, the diagnosis of psoriatic arthritis is often missed among patients with psoriasis.

Axial Disease

Half of the patients with psoriatic arthritis have inflammatory spinal disease as well. As in ankylosing spondylitis, the apophyseal joints of the spine and the sacroiliac joints are affected (**Fig. 2**). In a small minority, the axial disease occurs without any peripheral arthritis. In these cases, it is difficult to determine whether the patient has ankylosing spondylitis with psoriasis, or axial psoriatic arthritis. As noted for the peripheral joints, patients with axial psoriatic arthritis do not have as much pain as patients with ankylosing spondylitis, and the condition is often missed, especially if radiographs are not performed.[36]

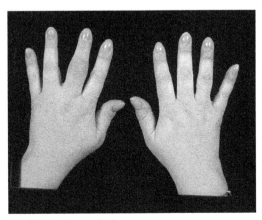

Fig. 1. Inflammatory arthritis, oligoarticular.

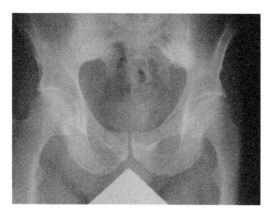

Fig. 2. Sacroiliitis.

Enthesitis

Inflammation at insertion of tendons into bones (enthesitis) is a feature common to the seronegative spondyloarthropathies (**Fig. 3**). It is more common in patients with psoriatic arthritis than in patients with ankylosing spondylitis. It most commonly affects the plantar fascia and Achilles tendon, but several enthesitis sites have been recognized and grouped in different indices.[37] Enthesitis may be the only musculoskeletal manifestation among patients with psoriasis.

Dactylitis

Dactylitis, or sausage digit, results from inflammation of a whole digit, including the joints and tendons (**Fig. 4**). It is another typical manifestation of psoriatic arthritis occurring in close to 50% of patients. Dactylitis is an important feature of psoriatic arthritis because it is associated with greater joint damage.[38]

DIAGNOSING PSORIATIC ARTHRITIS

As noted earlier, the diagnosis of psoriatic arthritis may be difficult. When a patient with psoriasis presents with inflammatory arthritis, it is important to determine that this is not rheumatoid arthritis with psoriasis. The clinical picture described earlier is helpful

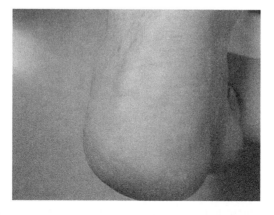

Fig. 3. Enthesitis.

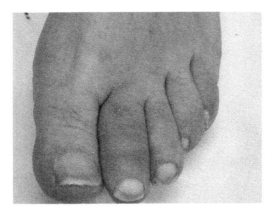

Fig. 4. Dactylitis.

because, if there is distal joint involvement, which is uncommon in rheumatoid arthritis, then the diagnosis of psoriatic arthritis is more likely. Likewise, the presence of dactylitis, enthesitis, or back involvement facilitate the diagnosis of psoriatic arthritis. Patients with psoriatic arthritis also tend to have a purplish discoloration over their joints, which is helpful in making the diagnosis. The presence of nail lesions is more common in psoriatic arthritis than in psoriasis without psoriatic arthritis. Several classification criteria have been proposed.[39] The CASPAR criteria have been internationally accepted and have high sensitivity and specificity for the disease.[1]

What is Early Psoriatic Arthritis?

Most drug trials and observational cohort studies included patients with long disease duration, on average between 7 and 9 years.[40] The concept of early psoriatic arthritis is recent, and has become more relevant since the advent of new therapies that seem to prevent disease progression and may even lead to healing of erosions and restoration of cartilage.[41] Nonetheless, there is still no widely accepted definition of early disease. Should only patients with recent onset of joint symptoms be included? Should it be a short duration from the time of diagnosis? Because patients with psoriatic arthritis often do not complain of pain, it is difficult to rely only on onset of symptoms. It is more appropriate to consider the duration from the time of diagnosis. Most investigators consider early disease within 1 or 2 years of the diagnosis of psoriatic arthritis.

Why Should Psoriatic Arthritis be Identified Early?

Wright[42] described psoriatic arthritis as milder than rheumatoid arthritis, an observation supported by another study from the United Kingdom.[43] However, in the past few decades, it has become clear that the disease is more common and more severe than was previously appreciated. Psoriatic arthritis causes deformities and joint damage leading to impaired quality of life and function, and is associated with an increased mortality risk.[44,45] Moreover, psoriatic arthritis is associated with important comorbidities that add to the disease burden.[46]

Psoriatic arthritis is now recognized as a major health issue with important consequences. Most studies reporting on outcome in patients with psoriatic arthritis include patients with long-standing disease. One study included patients with psoriatic arthritis within 2 years of onset of symptoms, with a mean duration of disease from onset of symptoms of 5 months.[47] Of the 129 patients identified as having psoriatic arthritis among the more than 1000 patients seen in the early arthritis clinic, 27%

had at least 1 joint erosion at presentation to the early arthritis clinic, suggesting that the disease may be aggressive at an early stage. At their 2-year follow-up, 47% of these patients were found to have erosive disease despite most having been treated with disease-modifying antirheumatic drugs (DMARDs). A recent study showed that disease progression is more marked in those patients presenting with established disease of more than 2 years' duration.[48]

Until 2000, there were no treatments that led to reduction in progression of joint damage.[49] However, with the advent of anti–tumor necrosis factor (TNF) agents, it is now possible to arrest progression of damage in these patients.[50–53] Because it has been shown that the degree of inflammation predicts progression of both clinical and radiological damage, both as a global feature and in the individual joint, clinicians and patients should obtain appropriate therapy in a timely fashion to prevent joint damage progression.[54,55]

HOW CAN PSORIATIC ARTHRITIS BE IDENTIFIED EARLY?
The CASPAR Criteria

Having established that psoriatic arthritis should be identified early so that it can be treated appropriately, the question is how to do it. Because most patients with psoriatic arthritis develop their arthritis after the onset of psoriasis, it is appropriate to screen patients with psoriasis for the development of psoriatic arthritis.

The CASPAR criteria were developed to address the issue of identification of psoriatic arthritis. The criteria were derived from an international dataset of 588 patients with psoriatic arthritis and 536 patients with other inflammatory forms of arthritis seen consecutively in the participating institutions. Using both classification and regression tree analysis and a logistic regression, the result was the same: in a patient with an inflammatory musculoskeletal disease (peripheral arthritis, spondylitis or enthesitis), the presence of psoriasis (either current, past, or by family history), nail lesions, negative rheumatoid factor, dactylitis, and fluffy periosteal reaction on radiographs of hands or feet were identified as important features, and, if a patient had 3 or more points, the sensitivity was 90% and the specificity was 98% (**Table 3**).[1] The patients included in the derivation dataset had established disease with an average disease duration of 13 years. It was questioned whether the criteria would work as well in early disease, and whether they would distinguish patients seen in an early

Table 3
CASPAR criteria for psoriatic arthritis. Patient must have an inflammatory musculoskeletal disease (peripheral arthritis, enthesitis, or spondylitis) to be considered

Item	Score	Definition
Psoriasis[a]		
Current	2	Observed on current examination
Past	1	History of psoriasis
Family history	1	Family history, first-degree or second-degree relatives
Nail lesions	1	Observed on current examination
Dactylitis	1	Observed on current examination or by history by a rheumatologist
Negative rheumatoid factor	1	Using enzyme-linked immunosorbent assay or nephelometry
Fluffy periostitis	1	Ill defined, not osteophytes

[a] Only 1 of the 3 options may be scored.

arthritis clinic, or in a family medicine clinic. Several studies have now confirmed that the CASPAR criteria function well regardless of the setting. Thus, in early psoriatic arthritis of less than 2 years' duration, the sensitivity was 99%,[56] although it was lower at 77% for patients seen within 12 months of onset of symptoms in Italy.[57] Among British patients with early arthritis, the sensitivity was 78% and the specificity 97%,[58] although among patients with early arthritis in Leiden, the sensitivity of the CASPAR criteria was 88%.[59] In a family medicine clinic, the sensitivity was 100% and the specificity was 98%.[60] However, the CASPAR criteria were applied by rheumatologists in all these settings.

Screening Questionnaires

The difficulty with the CASPAR criteria is that they require a rheumatologist to determine the stem of the criteria; that is, whether the patient has an inflammatory musculoskeletal disease. Because it is impractical to expect all patients with psoriasis to be seen by a rheumatologist, several screening questionnaires that are completed by patients have been developed (**Table 4**). The first attempt to develop a screening tool for psoriatic arthritis was from Canada, and although the sensitivity and specificity were high, 85% and 88% respectively for a score of 7 or higher, it was published only in abstract form.[61] Subsequent modifications of the Psoriatic Arthritis Questionnaire (PAQ) have been published. The first was from Sweden, where the modification of the PAQ achieved only 60% sensitivity and 62.2% specificity with a cutoff of 4 of 8 (best cutoff).[20] The Leeds group used the PAQ as a substrate but added additional questions on back disease, as well as a mannequin for patients to show their affected areas. The resultant Psoriasis Epidemiologic Screening Trial (PEST) showed high sensitivity (92%) and good specificity (78%).[62] They also used Alenius modification of the PAQ, which provided only 63% sensitivity and 72% specificity. More recently, another Canadian group further developed the PAQ into the PASQ (psoriatic arthritis screening questionnaire). This instrument also has a mannequin and provided a high sensitivity of 97% and a specificity of 75% for a cutoff of 7.[63] In Boston, a joint effort by dermatologists and rheumatologists resulted in the development of the Psoriatic Arthritis Screening Evaluation (PASE).[64] This version provided a sensitivity of 82% and a specificity of 73% with a cutoff of 47. An updated version provides a sensitivity of 70% with improved specificity at 80% with a cutoff of 47, and both sensitivity and specificity of 76% with a cutoff of 44.[65] This instrument includes a functional questionnaire as well. The screening tools mentioned earlier were developed specifically for patients with psoriasis. The Toronto Psoriatic Arthritis Screen (ToPAS) was developed to identify psoriatic arthritis in patients with or without psoriasis. It has high sensitivity

Table 4				
Comparison of screening questionnaires for psoriatic arthritis				
Item	**PEST[62]**	**PASQ[63]**	**PASE[65]**	**ToPAS[66]**
Derivation	PAQ	PAQ	Physicians and patients	Physicians and patients
Pictures/drawings	Yes	Yes	No	Yes
Tested in Psoriasis	Yes	Yes	Yes	Yes
General population	No	No	No	Yes
Sensitivity (%)	92	97	76	87
Specificity (%)	78	75	76	93

Abbreviations: PAQ, Psoriatic Arthritis Questionnaire; PASE, Psoriatic Arthritis Screening Evaluation; PASQ, Psoriatic Arthritis Screening Questionnaire; PEST, Psoriasis Epidemiologic Screening Trial; ToPAS, Toronto Psoriatic Arthritis Screen.

(87%) and specificity (93%) for patients with psoriasis as well as patients seen in general dermatology clinics, general rheumatology clinics, and family medicine clinics.[66] The PASE and ToPAS were compared in a Dutch psoriasis cohort and, although the area under the curve was greater for the ToPAS (ToPAS 0.85 [0.76–0.93], PASE 0.75 [0.65–0.86]) the confidence intervals suggest that there is no significant difference between the instruments.[67] These instruments are currently being studied in trials to identify patients with psoriatic arthritis. Thus there are screening tools that can identify patients with psoriatic arthritis early, and these should perhaps be incorporated in dermatology clinics to identify patients with psoriatic arthritis.

Risk Factors for Psoriatic Arthritis Among Patients with Psoriasis

There are several risk factors for the development of psoriatic arthritis among patients with psoriasis. The clinical features that distinguish patients with psoriatic arthritis from those who have psoriasis without arthritis include nail lesions and severity and site of the skin lesions, including scalp and intergluteal areas.[10,68] Several genetic markers that differentiate patients with psoriatic arthritis from those with psoriasis without arthritis have been identified. These include HLA-B*27, HLA-B*08, and HLA-B*38, which occur more commonly among patients with psoriatic arthritis, and HLA-C*06, which occurs more frequently among patients with psoriasis without arthritis.[29] Soluble biomarkers may also help identify patients with psoriasis who may develop psoriatic arthritis. These biomarkers include high-sensitivity C-reactive protein, osteoprotegerin, matrix metalloproteinase-3, and the ratio of C-propeptide of type II collagen (CPII) to collagen fragment neoepitopes Col2-3/4(long mono) (C2C) (CPII/C2C).[69] Thus it is possible that, in the next few years, a panel of biomarkers will be developed that will identify patients with psoriasis destined to develop psoriatic arthritis, and thus patients will be diagnosed earlier and treated appropriately. Whether these biomarkers will be helpful in identifying patients destined to develop psoriatic arthritis beyond the clinical features and the genetic markers that have been identified remains to be determined.

Identifying Early Psoriatic Arthritis

There are few studies that address the issue of identifying patients with psoriatic arthritis early. A recent study from Italy highlights that early identification is possible if there is good collaboration between rheumatologists and dermatologists. That study identified 33 patients with early psoriatic arthritis that was defined as presence of symptoms for 1 year or less.[70] Although most of these patients had polyarticular disease, their function was not markedly impaired. Radiographs did not show structural change but ultrasound examinations did document the presence of inflammation. Gisondi and colleagues[71] also highlight that radiographic assessment is insufficient in early psoriatic arthritis, whereas magnetic resonance imaging (MRI) and ultrasound assessments can detect disease early among patients with psoriasis. Similar conclusions were reached by Anandarajah and Ritchlin.[72]

A Swedish registry for patients with early psoriatic arthritis defined as less than 2 years' duration was established in 2000. In their first report in 2002, they included 92 patients of whom 60 were diagnosed with definite psoriatic arthritis, whereas 32 were considered possible psoriatic arthritis. The average disease duration was 9 months.[73] Despite the early stage of the disease, most patients had polyarticular disease and had been treated with DMARDs. By 2007, more than 300 patients were entered into the Swedish Early Psoriatic Arthritis registry, with 2-year follow-up available for 184 of these patients.[74] Of these, 156 were considered to have psoriatic arthritis, and 130 fulfilled CASPAR criteria. The report published in 2008 included

135 patients with mean disease duration of 11 months. They noted that patients changed pattern over the 2-year follow-up, with patients initially presenting as oligoarthritis progressing to polyarticular disease or achieving remission, and those beginning with polyarticular disease becoming oligoarthritis or monoarthritis at follow-up. At 2 years, 32% of the patients had radiographic changes of psoriatic arthritis; however, only 120 patients had radiographs at baseline and only 79 had repeat radiographs at 2 years. Baseline factors associated with remission included a low number of inflamed joints and the presence of nail lesions, which have been reported in the past. A lower actively inflamed joint count at baseline was found to be associated with remission in a previous study.[75] Nail lesions seemed to be protective of mortality in 1 study.[76] As was noted earlier, patients who present to clinic with disease duration of less than 2 years have less disease progression than those presenting after 2 years.[48]

The definition of early arthritis therefore requires validation. There are clinical features, genetic and other biomarkers, as well as imaging features that help identify patients with psoriasis who might develop psoriatic arthritis. Further work is required to produce algorithms that would be helpful in the clinic to achieve the goal of identifying patients with psoriatic arthritis early.

How Should Patients with Early Psoriatic Arthritis be Treated?

Although traditional DMARDs have not shown prevention of progression of damage in psoriatic arthritis, anti-TNF agents have led to a reduction of radiographic progression.[49–53] These agents have all shown the ability to improve quality of life and function. Therefore, it is most appropriate to treat patients with medications that are clearly disease modifying. These medications include the anti-TNF agents, but there are several drugs that are currently being investigated that may have similar properties. However, there are no specific trials of the treatment of early disease in psoriatic arthritis to determine whether early treatment arrests disease progression.

Do Clinicians Make a Difference?

Although there are no specific randomized trials in early psoriatic arthritis, there is evidence from observational studies that treating early may make a difference. Chandran and colleagues[77] reappraised the response to methotrexate and found that, compared with an earlier trial,[78] patients are now treated earlier in the course of their disease and with a higher dose, and the clinical response is better. There was also less damage progression. Further studies are needed to prove that treatment in early disease prevents the untoward outcomes highlighted in this article.

REFERENCES

1. Taylor WJ, Gladman DD, Helliwell PS, et al. Classification criteria for psoriatic arthritis: development of new criteria from a large international study. Arthritis Rheum 2006;54:2665–73.
2. Gladman DD. Psoriatic arthritis from Wright's era till today. J Rheumatol Suppl 2009;83:4–8.
3. Blumberg BS, Bunim JJ, Calkins E, et al. ARA nomenclature and classification of arthritis and rheumatism (tentative). Arthritis Rheum 1964;7:93–7.
4. Gladman DD, Shuckett R, Russell ML, et al. Psoriatic arthritis - clinical and laboratory analysis of 220 patients. Q J Med 1987;62:127–41.
5. Gorter S, van der Heijde DM, van der LS, et al. Psoriatic arthritis: performance of rheumatologists in daily practice. Ann Rheum Dis 2002;61:219–24.

6. Chandran V, Raychaudhuri SP. Geoepidemiology and environmental factors of psoriasis and psoriatic arthritis. J Autoimmun 2010;34:J314–21.
7. Zeng QY, Chen R, Darmawan J, et al. Rheumatic diseases in China. Arthritis Res Ther 2008;10:R17.
8. Trontzas P, Andrianakos A, Miyakis S, et al. Seronegative spondyloarthropathies in Greece: a population-based study of prevalence, clinical pattern, and management. The ESORDIG study. Clin Rheumatol 2005;24:583–9.
9. De Angelis R, Salaffi F, Grassi W. Prevalence of spondyloarthropathies in an Italian population sample: a regional community-based study. Scand J Rheumatol 2007;36:14–21.
10. Gelfand JM, Gladman DD, Mease PJ, et al. Epidemiology of psoriatic arthritis in the population of the United States. J Am Acad Dermatol 2005; 53:573–7.
11. Minaur N, Sawyers S, Parker J, et al. Rheumatic disease in an Australian Aboriginal community in North Queensland, Australia. A WHO-ILAR COPCORD survey. J Rheumatol 2004;31:965–72.
12. Leczinsky CG. The incidence of arthropathy in a ten-year series of psoriasis cases. Acta Derm Venereol 1948;28:483–7.
13. Little H, Harvie JN, Lester RS. Psoriatic arthritis in severe psoriasis. Can Med Assoc J 1975;112:317–9.
14. Scarpa R, Oriente P, Pucino A, et al. Psoriatic arthritis in psoriatic patients. Br J Rheumatol 1984;23:246–50.
15. Stern RS. The epidemiology of joint complaints in patients with psoriasis. J Rheumatol 1985;12:315–20.
16. Barisic-Drusko V, Dobric I, Pasic A, et al. Frequency of psoriatic arthritis in general population and among the psoriatics in Department of Dermatology. Acta Derm Venereol Suppl (Stockh) 1994;186:107–8.
17. Salvarani C, Lo Scocco G, Macchioni P, et al. Prevalence of psoriatic arthritis in Italian psoriatic patients. J Rheumatol 1995;22:1499–503.
18. Shbeeb M, Uramoto KM, Gibson LE, et al. The epidemiology of psoriatic arthritis in Olmsted County, Minnesota, USA, 1982-1991. J Rheumatol 2000; 27:1247–50.
19. Brockbank JE, Schentag C, Rosen C, et al. Psoriatic arthritis (PsA) is common among patients with psoriasis and family medical clinic attendees [abstract]. Arthritis Rheum 2001;44(Suppl 9):S94.
20. Alenius GM, Stenberg B, Stenlund H, et al. Inflammatory joint manifestations are prevalent in psoriasis: prevalence study of joint and axial involvement in psoriatic patients, and evaluation of a psoriatic and arthritic questionnaire. J Rheumatol 2002;29:2577–82.
21. Zachariae H. Prevalence of joint disease in patients with psoriasis: implications for therapy. Am J Clin Dermatol 2003;4:441–7.
22. Reich K, Kruger K, Mossner R, et al. Epidemiology and clinical pattern of psoriatic arthritis in Germany: a prospective interdisciplinary epidemiological study of 1511 patients with plaque-type psoriasis. Br J Dermatol 2009;160:1040–7.
23. Chandran V. The genetics of psoriasis and psoriatic arthritis. Clin Rev Allergy Immunol 2012. [Epub ahead of print].
24. Chandran V, Schentag CT, Brockbank JE, et al. Familial aggregation of psoriatic arthritis. Ann Rheum Dis 2009;68:664–7.
25. Karason A, Gudjonsson JE, Upmanyu R, et al. A susceptibility gene for psoriatic arthritis maps to chromosome 16q: evidence for imprinting. Am J Hum Genet 2003;72:125–31.

26. Liu Y, Helms C, Liao W, et al. A genome-wide association study of psoriasis and psoriatic arthritis identifies new disease loci. PLoS Genet 2008;4:e1000041.
27. Nair RP, Duffin KC, Helms C, et al. Genome-wide scan reveals association of psoriasis with IL-23 and NF-kappaB pathways. Nat Genet 2009;41:199–204.
28. Ellinghaus E, Stuart PE, Ellinghaus D, et al. Genome-wide meta-analysis of psoriatic arthritis identifies susceptibility locus at REL. J Invest Dermatol 2012;132: 1133–40.
29. Eder L, Chandran V, Pellet F, et al. Human leukocyte antigen risk alleles for psoriatic arthritis among psoriasis patients. Ann Rheum Dis 2012;71:50–5.
30. Eder L, Law T, Chandran V, et al. The association between environmental factors and onset of psoriatic arthritis in patients with psoriasis. Arthritis Care Res 2011; 63:1091–7.
31. Fitzgerald O, Winchester R. Psoriatic arthritis: from pathogenesis to therapy. Arthritis Res Ther 2009;11:214.
32. Wright V, Moll JM. Psoriatic arthritis. In: Wright V, Moll JM, editors. Seronegative polyarthritis. Amsterdam: North-Holland; 1976. p. 169–223.
33. Khan M, Schentag C, Gladman D. Clinical and radiological changes during psoriatic arthritis disease progression: working toward classification criteria. J Rheumatol 2003;30:1022–6.
34. Helliwell P, Marchesoni A, Peters M, et al. A re-evaluation of the osteoarticular manifestations of psoriasis. Br J Rheumatol 1991;30:339–45.
35. Helliwell PS, Hetthen J, Sokoll K, et al. Joint symmetry in early and late rheumatoid and psoriatic arthritis: comparison with a mathematical model. Arthritis Rheum 2000;43:865–71.
36. Gladman DD. Axial disease in psoriatic arthritis. Curr Rheumatol Rep 2007;9: 455–60.
37. Gladman DD, Inman R, Cook R, et al. International spondyloarthritis interobserver reliability exercise – the INSPIRE study: II. Assessment of peripheral joints, enthesitis and dactylitis. J Rheumatol 2007;34:1740–5.
38. Brockbank J, Stein M, Schentag CT, et al. Dactylitis in psoriatic arthritis (PsA): a marker for disease severity? Ann Rheum Dis 2005;62:188–90.
39. Taylor WJ, Marchesoni A, Arreghini M, et al. A comparison of the performance characteristics of classification criteria for the diagnosis of psoriatic arthritis. Semin Arthritis Rheum 2004;34:575–84.
40. Gladman DD, Antoni C, Clegg D, et al. Psoriatic arthritis – epidemiology and clinical features. Ann Rheum Dis 2005;64(Suppl 2):ii14–7.
41. Eder L, Chandran V, Gladman DD. Repair of radiographic joint damage following treatment with a TNF inhibitor in psoriatic arthritis is demonstrable by three radiographic methods. J Rheumatol 2011;38:1066–70.
42. Wright V. Psoriatic arthritis: a comparative study of rheumatoid arthritis, psoriasis and arthritis associated with psoriasis. AMA Arch Derm 1959;80:27–35.
43. Coulton BL, Thomson K, Symmons DP, et al. Outcome in patients hospitalised for psoriatic arthritis. Clin Rheumatol 1989;2:261–5.
44. Gladman DD. Disability and quality of life considerations. Psoriatic arthritis. In: Gordon GB, Ruderman E, editors. Psoriasis and psoriatic arthritis: an integrated approach. Heidelberg (Germany): Springer-Verlag; 2005. p. 118–23.
45. Gladman DD. Mortality in psoriatic arthritis. Clin Exp Rheumatol 2008;26(Suppl 5): s62–5.
46. Rosen CF, Mussani F, Chandran V, et al. Patients with psoriatic arthritis have worse quality of life than those with psoriasis alone. Rheumatology (Oxford) 2012;51:571–6.

47. Kane D, Stafford L, Bresniham B, et al. A prospective, clinical and radiological study of early psoriatic arthritis: an early synovitis clinic experience. Rheumatology 2003;42:1460–8.
48. Gladman DD, Thavaneswaran A, Chandran V, et al. Do patients with psoriatic arthritis who present early fare better than those presenting later in the disease? Ann Rheum Dis 2011;70:2152–4.
49. Prasad R, Gladman D. Current and investigational treatment of psoriatic arthritis. Expert Opin Investig Drugs 2004;13:139–50.
50. Mease PJ, Kivitz AJ, Burch FX, et al. Etanercept treatment of psoriatic arthritis: safety, efficacy, and effect on disease progression. Arthritis Rheum 2004;50:2264–72.
51. Gladman DD, Mease PJ, Ritchlin CT, et al. Adalimumab for long-term treatment of psoriatic arthritis: 48–week data and subanalysis from ADEPT. Arthritis Rheum 2007;56:476–88.
52. van der Heijde D, Kavanaugh A, Gladman DD, et al. Infliximab inhibits progression of radiographic damage in patients with active psoriatic arthritis through one year of treatment: results from the induction and maintenance psoriatic arthritis clinical trial 2. Arthritis Rheum 2007;66:2698–707.
53. Kavanaugh A, van der Heijde D, McInnes I, et al. Golimumab, a human TNF-alpha antibody, administered every 4 weeks as a subcutaneous injection in psoriatic arthritis: clinical efficacy, radiographic, and safety findings through 1 year of the randomized, placebo-controlled, Go-REVEAL Study. Arthritis Rheum 2012. [Epub ahead of print].
54. Bond SJ, Farewell VT, Schentag CT, et al. Predictors for radiological damage in psoriatic arthritis. Results from a Single centre. Ann Rheum Dis 2007;66:370–6.
55. Cresswell L, Chandran V, Farewell VT, et al. Inflammation in an individual joint predicts damage to that joint in psoriatic arthritis. Ann Rheum Dis 2011;70:305–8.
56. Chandran V, Schentag CT, Gladman DD. Sensitivity of the classification of psoriatic arthritis (CASPAR) criteria in early psoriatic arthritis. Arthritis Rheum 2007;57:1560–3.
57. D'Angelo S, Mennillo GA, Cutro MS, et al. Sensitivity of the classification of psoriatic arthritis criteria in early psoriatic arthritis. J Rheumatol 2009;36:368–70.
58. Coates L, Conaghan PG, Emery P, et al. The CASPAR criteria can be used to identify early psoriatic arthritis. Arthritis Rheum 2010;62(Suppl 10):S916.
59. van den Berg R, van Gaalen F, van der Helm-van Mil A, et al. Performance of classification criteria for peripheral spondyloarthritis and psoriatic arthritis in the Leiden early arthritis cohort. Ann Rheum Dis 2012. [Epub ahead of print].
60. Chandran V, Schentag CT, Gladman DD. Sensitivity and specificity of the CASPAR criteria for psoriatic arthritis when applied to patients attending a family medicine clinic. J Rheumatol 2008;35:2069–70.
61. Peloso PM, Hull P, Reeder B. The psoriasis and arthritis questionnaire (PAQ) in detection of arthritis among patients with psoriasis. Arthritis Rheum 1997;40:S64.
62. Ibrahim GH, Buch MH, Lawson C, et al. Evaluation of an existing screening tool for psoriatic arthritis in people with psoriasis and the development of a new instrument: the Psoriasis Epidemiology Screening Tool (PEST) questionnaire. Clin Exp Rheumatol 2009;27:469–74.
63. Khraishi M, Mong J, Mugford G, et al. The electronic Psoriasis and Arthritis Screening Questionnaire (ePASQ): a sensitive and specific tool to diagnose psoriatic arthritis patients. J Cutan Med Surg 2011;15:143–9.
64. Husni ME, Meyer KH, Cohen DS, et al. The PASE questionnaire: pilot-testing a psoriatic arthritis screening and evaluation tool. J Am Acad Dermatol 2007;57:581–7.

65. Dominguez PL, Husni ME, Holt EW, et al. Validity, reliability, and sensitivity-to-change properties of the psoriatic arthritis screening and evaluation questionnaire. Arch Dermatol Res 2009;301:573–9.

66. Gladman DD, Schentag CT, Tom BD, et al. Development and initial validation of a screening questionnaire for psoriatic arthritis: the Toronto Psoriatic Arthritis Screen (ToPAS). Ann Rheum Dis 2009;68:497–501.

67. Diaconu-Popa DA, Driessen RJB, Kerkhof PCM, et al. Performance of two screening instruments, ToPAS and PASE, for detecting psoriatic arthritis in patients with psoriasis. Ann Rheum Dis 2009;68(Suppl 3):656.

68. Wilson FC, Icen M, Crowson CS, et al. Incidence and clinical predictors of psoriatic arthritis in patients with psoriasis: a population-based study [Erratum appears in Arthritis Rheum 2010;62:574]. Arthritis Rheum 2009;61:233–9.

69. Chandran V, Cook RJ, Edwin J, et al. Soluble biomarkers differentiate patients with psoriatic arthritis from those with psoriasis without arthritis. Rheumatology (Oxford) 2010;49:1399–405.

70. Bonifati C, Elia F, Francesconi F, et al. The diagnosis of early psoriatic arthritis in an outpatient dermatological centre for psoriasis. J Eur Acad Dermatol Venereol 2012;26:627–33.

71. Gisondi P, Tinazzi I, Del GM, et al. The diagnostic and therapeutic challenge of early psoriatic arthritis. Dermatology 2010;221(Suppl 1):6–14.

72. Anandarajah AP, Ritchlin CT. The diagnosis and treatment of early psoriatic arthritis. Nat Rev Rheumatol 2009;5:634–41.

73. Svensson B, Holmstrom G, Lindqvist U. Development and early experiences of a Swedish psoriatic arthritis register. Scand J Rheumatol 2002;31:221–5.

74. Lindqvist UR, Alenius GM, Husmark T, et al. The Swedish early psoriatic arthritis register – 2-year followup: a comparison with early rheumatoid arthritis. J Rheumatol 2008;35:668–73.

75. Gladman DD, Ng Tung Hing E, Schentag CT, et al. Remission in psoriatic arthritis. J Rheumatol 2001;28:1045–8.

76. Gladman DD, Farewell VT, Husted J, et al. Mortality studies in psoriatic arthritis. Results from a single centre. II. Prognostic indicators for mortality. Arthritis Rheum 1998;41:1103–10.

77. Chandran V, Schentag CT, Gladman DD. Reappraisal of the effectiveness of methotrexate in psoriatic arthritis: results from a longitudinal observational cohort. J Rheumatol 2008;35:469–71.

78. Abu-Shakra M, Gladman DD, Thorne JC, et al. Longterm methotrexate therapy in psoriatic arthritis: clinical and radiologic outcome. J Rheumatol 1995;22:241–5.

Early Spondyloarthritis

Denis Poddubnyy, MD[a], Martin Rudwaleit, MD[b],*

KEYWORDS

- Spondyloarthritis • Ankylosing spondylitis • Early diagnosis
- ASAS

Key Points

- Spondyloarthritis (SpA) is a common group of interrelated inflammatory rheumatic conditions with a prevalence of 1% to 2%.

- MRI of the sacroiliac joints and the spine has substantially improved making an early diagnosis of nonradiographic axial SpA and ankylosing spondylitis.

- New criteria developed by the Assessment of SpondyloArthritis international Society (ASAS) that include MRI help to better classify patients with early predominant axial disease or predominant peripheral disease.

- Programs targeting chronic back patients with young age at onset and referral to the rheumatologists if either inflammatory back pain or HLA-B27 is present have been proven effective in identifying patients with axial SpA in primary care.

- International recommendations for the management of ankylosing spondylitis and the use of anti-TNF agents have recently been updated by ASAS/European League Against Rheumatism (EULAR).

The term spondyloarthritis (SpA) is an umbrella term for a group of diseases sharing common clinical and genetic features, including involvement of the axial skeleton (sacroiliac joints and spine), peripheral arthritis, enthesitis, dactylitis, acute anterior uveitis, associated psoriasis or inflammatory bowel disease, and presence of the HLA-B27 antigen. Depending on the predominant clinical manifestations, SpA can be classified either as axial SpA (characterized by predominant involvement of the spine and/or sacroiliac joints as in ankylosing spondylitis (AS) and nonradiographic axial SpA, or as peripheral SpA (peripheral arthritis, enthesitis, and/or dactylitis).

Nonradiographic (ie, without definite sacroiliitis on radiography) axial SpA and AS are now considered as different stages of one disease continuum referred to as axial SpA

The authors have nothing to disclose in relation to the content of this article.
[a] Rheumatology, Medical Department I, Campus Benjamin Franklin, Charité Universitätsmedizin Berlin, Hindenburgdamm 30, Berlin 12203, Germany; [b] Endokrinologikum Berlin, and Charité University Medicine, Jägerstr. 61 (Q207), Berlin 10117, Germany
* Corresponding author.
E-mail address: martin.rudwaleit@endokrinologikum.com

rheumatic.theclinics.com

(**Fig. 1**).[1] The rate of progression from nonradiographic (without radiographic sacroiliitis) to radiographic (with definite radiographic sacroiliitis; ie, AS) stage was recently estimated to be about 12% over 2 years,[2] yet there are probably patients who remain at the nonradiographic stage during the entire course of their disease without progression to established AS. Although in AS sacroiliac joints are normally involved ahead of the spine in an estimated 10% of patients with AS or axial SpA, syndesmophytes can be found in the absence of definite radiographic sacroiliitis.[3]

HOW OFTEN IS SPONDYLOARTHRITIS IN THE GENERAL POPULATION?

AS—the prototype disease of the SpA group—has an estimated prevalence of about 0.5%[4,5] in the general white population (including the United States), while the estimated prevalence for the whole group of SpA is about 1.5% to 2%.[4,5] The prevalence of AS and the whole group of SpA is related to the frequency of HLA-B27 in a given population. HLA-B27 is most prevalent in northern countries and is highest in the Haida Indian population (up to 50%),[6] giving a high prevalence of AS of about 6%.[6] In the central European population, the HLA-B27 is as common as 6% to 9%[4,7,8]; whereas, in Japanese or Central and South African antigen populations its prevalence is 1% or less with a resulting low SpA prevalence.[9,10]

In most patients, the first symptoms of SpA (usually back pain) start in the third or fourth decade of life. Males are about 2.5 times more often affected than females and have, in general, more severe disease (more radiographic damage). In up to 40% of AS patients, significant functional impairment occurs with a close relationship

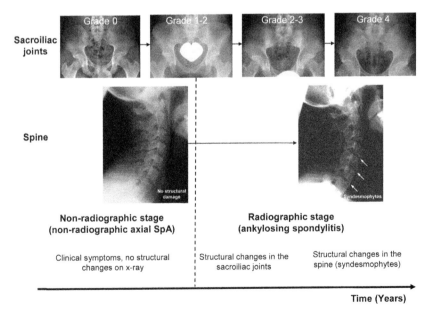

Fig. 1. Continuum of axial spondyloarthritis. At the early disease stage no or very little radiographic damage of the sacroiliac joints and the spine can be visualized on radiograph (nonradiographic stage). The radiographic stage refers to the presence on radiographs of structural damage of the sacroiliac joints (radiographic sacroiliitis grade 2–4) and/or spine (syndesmophytes—bony bridges between vertebral bodies, spondylodiscitis, and arthritis-ankylosis of the facet joints).

between the grade of impairment and disease duration.[11,12] The diagnosis of AS is commonly delayed by 8 to 10 years after the first symptom onset,[13] which represents a major unsolved problem in this area.

WHAT ARE THE REASONS FOR THE LATE DIAGNOSIS IN SPONDYLOARTHRITIS?

There are several factors contributing to the long diagnostic delay in AS. One of the most obvious is the usual application of the modified New York criteria for classification and diagnosis of AS,[14] which require the presence of radiographic sacroiliitis for definite AS diagnosis (**Box 1**). Published in 1984, these criteria still remain a basis for AS diagnosis in clinical practice in many countries. Because radiographic sacroiliitis usually develops rather late (after years) in AS, in many patients these criteria are obviously useless in patients with early disease.

In contrast to many other rheumatic diseases, early axial SpA with back pain as the most prominent clinical symptom often has no clinical manifestation that is readily recognizable by the clinician, such as swollen joints or skin rash, and that could aid in making a diagnosis. Lack of SpA-awareness among primary care physicians is another reason for the long diagnostic delay. Back pain is extremely prevalent in the general population and SpA accounts for only about 5% of causes of chronic back pain.[15] A simple and effective screening strategy in primary care and subsequent referral to the rheumatologist of those back pain patients with a higher probability of axial SpA is needed to effectively diagnose patients earlier.

WHY IS EARLY DIAGNOSIS IMPORTANT?

Recent data from an early SpA cohort demonstrated that patients with early (nonradiographic) axial SpA have the same level of pain and stiffness in comparison with patients with more advanced disease (established AS)[3] and, therefore, require also effective treatment. Early diagnosis would lead to early initiation of the most appropriate and effective therapy[16,17] and reassures the patient. Moreover, short disease duration and a good functional status were among predictors of a good clinical response to the tumor necrosis factor α (TNF-α) blocking agents.[18–20]

Box 1
The modified New York criteria for AS

Clinical criteria

- Low back pain and stiffness for more than 3 months that improves with exercise, but is not relieved by rest.
- Limitation of motion of the lumbar spine in both the sagittal and frontal planes.
- Limitation of chest expansion relative to normal values corrected for age and sex.

Radiological criterion

- Sacroiliitis grade $\geq$2 bilaterally, or grade 3 to 4 unilaterally.

Definite AS is present if the radiological criterion is associated with at least one clinical criterion.

Data from van der Linden S, Valkenburg HA, Cats A. Evaluation of diagnostic criteria for ankylosing spondylitis. A proposal for modification of the New York criteria. Arthritis Rheum 1984;27(4):361–8.

WHICH CLINICAL MANIFESTATIONS ARE RELEVANT FOR EARLY DIAGNOSIS?

The principal features of SpA that are relevant for early diagnosis are presented in **Fig. 2**.

The leading clinical symptom of AS or axial SpA is back pain. Back pain in general is extremely prevalent: at least two-thirds of the people in the world experience back pain during their lives.[21] Back pain in SpA has several typical features distinguishing it to some degree from pain of other origin and has been termed inflammatory back pain. Inflammatory back pain is a chronic back pain (duration >3 months), that often starts insidiously and usually before 45 years of age, often has a peak intensity in the second half of the night and early morning hours, improves with exercise but does not improve (even worsens) at rest, and is accompanied by morning stiffness (usually lasting more than 30 minutes). A less frequent but more specific feature of inflammatory back pain is an alternating buttock pain (**Box 2**).

Currently, three sets of criteria for inflammatory back pain exist (Calin criteria,[22] Berlin criteria,[23] and the most recent criteria by the Assessment of SpondyloArthritis international Society (ASAS) experts[24]), all combining the features listed in **Box 2**.

Of note, inflammatory back pain can be observed in 20% to 25% of patients with noninflammatory (mechanical) causes of chronic back pain.[22,23] Although the presence of inflammatory back pain alone does not suffice to make a diagnosis of axial SpA, the presence of inflammatory back pain is an important symptom that should prompt further diagnostic tests for axial SpA.

In addition to inflammatory back pain, other aspects of the patient's medical history provide diagnostic clues in early SpA. These include (1) a major reduction in back pain within 48 hours in response to a full dose of a nonsteroidal antiinflammatory drug (NSAID), (2) a positive family history of spondyloarthritis, and (3) a history of psoriasis or inflammatory bowel disease, or uveitis.

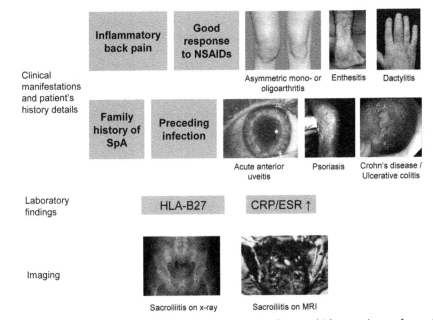

Fig. 2. Clinical, laboratory and imaging manifestations of SpA, which are relevant for early diagnosis. (*Courtesy of* ASAS: Assessment of Spondyloarthritis International Society, Maastricht, The Netherlands. Available at: www.asas-group.org; with permission.)

Box 2
Typical clinical features of inflammatory back pain

- Insidious onset
- Morning stiffness in the spine for more than 30 minutes
- Improvement of pain and stiffness with exercise and not with rest
- Pain at night, usually in the second half with improvement on getting up
- Alternating buttock pain

The back pain in AS and nonradiographic axial SpA typically starts before 45 years of age and runs a chronic or relapsing course (duration of more than 3 months).

Limitation of the spinal mobility is a feature of rather advanced SpA, and, on the other hand, pain-mediated reduction of mobility might occur also in other back pain conditions.

Other SpA manifestations (ie, peripheral arthritis, enthesitis, dactylitis, uveitis, psoriasis, and inflammatory bowel disease) may or may not be present at disease onset of axial SpA and may develop later. If present, these manifestations significantly increase the probability of axial SpA.[25,26]

In peripheral SpA, the presence of peripheral arthritis plays a major role in the diagnosis. Of diagnostic importance is the pattern of joint involvement, which in SpA is usually asymmetric, oligoarticular ($\leq$4 joints) and affects predominantly the lower limbs. Enthesitis (especially heel) and dactylitis are typical for peripheral SpA. The medical history regarding a urogenital or gastrointestinal infection within 1 to 4 weeks before symptom onset also has a diagnostic value in SpA (reactive arthritis, a subset of peripheral spondyloarthritis).

ARE THERE ANY SPECIFIC LABORATORY TESTS FOR SpA?

In contrast to rheumatoid arthritis or connective tissues disease, no disease-specific autoantibodies were found in SpA until now. However, there is a genetic marker (HLA-B27) that is strongly associated with this disease. More than 80% of the patients with AS[3,27] and more than 70% of the patients with axial SpA[3] are positive for HLA-B27 as opposed to about 8% in the general white population,[27] which makes this marker relevant as a diagnostic tool. However, despite the strong association between AS and HLA-B27, AS develops only in a minority (about 5%) of HLA-B27 positive subjects.[7] Twin studies demonstrated that HLA-B27 contributes less than 40% of the genetic susceptibility to AS.[28] Therefore, attempts to identify other genes within and outside the major histocompatibility complex associated with AS and SpA are still ongoing. Recently, two new loci related to AS, ERAP1 (ARTS1) and IL23R, have been identified.[29]

Acute phase reactants (C-reactive protein [CRP] and erythrocyte sedimentation rate) have a limited value in the early SpA diagnosis because about 50% of patients with SpA have normal values of these tests.[30] Yet, CRP is relevant for disease assessment because it indicates active inflammation; correlates, albeit weakly, with clinical parameters such as spinal pain[30]; and predicts radiographic progression in the sacroiliac joints and in the spine.[2,31]

In suspected reactive arthritis with a history of a preceding infection, bacterial serology and testing the morning urine for *Chlamydia trachomatis* by polymerase chain reaction or using a urethral or cervical swab can be of diagnostic value. In a preceding gastrointestinal infection, stool cultures are usually negative once the arthritis develops.

CAN IMAGING HELP IN THE EARLY SpA DIAGNOSIS?

Imaging is essential for early SpA diagnosis. A diagnosis of definite AS requires the presence of definite sacroiliitis (at least grade 2 bilaterally or grade 3 unilaterally) on the radiographs (**Fig. 3**). Radiographs of sacroiliac joints are still the first imaging procedure in suspected axial SpA. In case of unequivocal sacroiliitis on radiographs (see **Fig. 3**), no further diagnostic imaging is needed. However, normal radiographs or suspicious abnormalities only require further diagnostic imaging in the context of suggestive clinical symptoms or findings because structural change visible on radiographs can take months or years to occur. Moreover, the interpretation of radiographs of the sacroiliac joints can be challenging and depends on many factors, including quality of the image, chosen radiograph technique, individual variation of the sacroiliac anatomy, and the reader's experience.[2,32] These all decrease the reliability of this method. Spinal radiographs should normally not be considered as a first diagnostic procedure in case of suspicion of early SpA, because structural changes in the spine (eg, syndesmophytes) develop usually later than radiographic sacroiliitis.

CT scan of sacroiliac joints detects structural changes (sclerosis, erosions, joint space width alteration, and ankylosis) more reliably than conventional radiography and is, therefore, considered the gold standard of detection of bony damage (**Fig. 4**). However, CT cannot visualize active inflammation and is associated with relatively high radiation exposure and costs. As mentioned previously, structural damage cannot be considered as an early sign, which also limits the diagnostic value of CT scan in early SpA, Thus, CT scan is indicated rather in cases of differential diagnosis of SpA with degenerative changes, osteitis condensans ilii, fractures, and so forth.

Recently, MRI became almost the standard imaging method for the early identification of patients with sacroiliitis due to axial SpA. The main reason for this is the ability of MRI to visualize not only structural damage of sacroiliac joints (eg, erosions, sclerosis, and ankylosis) but also active inflammatory lesions occurring before any structural changes visible on radiographs or CT scan. MRI has both an estimated sensitivity and specificity of about 90%,[26] is not associated with ionizing radiation, and has very few contraindications. However, MRI is not available in all places in the world and is associated with relatively high costs in comparison to conventional radiographs, for instance. The diagnostic value of MRI in the detection of structural damage lesions (erosions, sclerosis, joint space changes, and ankylosis) is not entirely clear and needs further studies.

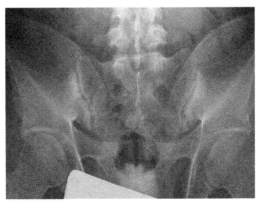

Fig. 3. Radiograph of the sacroiliac joints of a 26-year-old male patient with a history of back pain over the previous 6 years. Subchondral sclerosis and multiple erosions are evident, corresponding to definite bilateral radiographic sacroiliitis of grade 2.

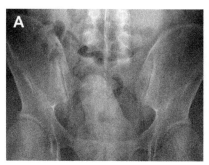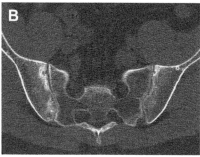

Fig. 4. Sacroiliac joints of a 31-year-old male patient with a history of back pain over the previous 8 years. (*A*) Radiograph: definite subchondral sclerosis of both sacroiliac joints with suspicious erosions and possible joint space narrowing on the left side and definite erosions on the right side. (*B*) CT scan: the structural changes (erosions and sclerosis) are clearly visualized and better seen as compared with plain radiograph.

For the diagnosis of axial SpA, two MRI sequences are of importance: short tau inversion recovery (STIR) and T1-weighted sequences. T2-weighted sequence (with or without fat suppression) and T1-weighted postcontrast fat-suppressed sequence are supplementary and usually do not provide additional information to the previously mentioned sequences. STIR is a method of visualization of active inflammatory lesions (**Fig. 5**B), which is important for early SpA diagnosis. In T1-weighted images, several kinds of postinflammatory changes providing supportive information (eg, relevant for the differential diagnosis), can be recognized: fatty lesions (fat depositions), erosions, and, to a lesser extent, sclerosis and ankylosis (see **Fig. 5**C).

Recently the ASAS developed a definition of an active sacroiliitis on MRI.[33] According to this consensus the following types of active inflammatory lesions are considered as compatible with SpA: bone marrow edema or osteitis, synovitis, enthesitis, and capsulitis (**Table 1**). Importantly, only bone marrow edema or osteitis is essential for defining active sacroiliitis. The presence of synovitis, enthesitis, and capsulitis without bone marrow edema or osteitis is compatible with SpA but is not sufficient for making a diagnosis of active sacroiliitis. The same applies to structural lesions in the sacroiliac joints reflecting past inflammation: sclerosis, erosions, fatty lesions, and bony bridges or ankylosis—these changes are compatible with SpA, but their sensitivity and specificity regarding SpA diagnosis is not totally clear, particularly if the lesions are minor.

The diagnostic value of other imaging methods (such as quantitative scintigraphy,[34] contrast-enhanced Doppler-ultrasonography,[35] and PET[36]) is limited in axial SpA, and these methods are not recommended for routine imaging if MRI is available. Nonetheless, ultrasonography plays an important role in the diagnosis of arthritis and, especially, enthesitis, that is particularly relevant in peripheral SpA.[37]

WHAT IS THE ROLE OF THE NEW ASAS CLASSIFICATION CRITERIA FOR SPONDYLOARTHRITIS?

In general, classification criteria, in contrast to diagnostic criteria, are developed for the classification of patients in clinical trials and are not intended for use as diagnosis-making tools in clinical practice. Nonetheless, in the absence of true diagnostic criteria, classification criteria are often used for diagnostic purposes. Two historical sets of criteria for SpA in general (Amor criteria[38] and the European Spondyloarthropathy Study Group criteria[39]) have been widely used in the past decades but have several

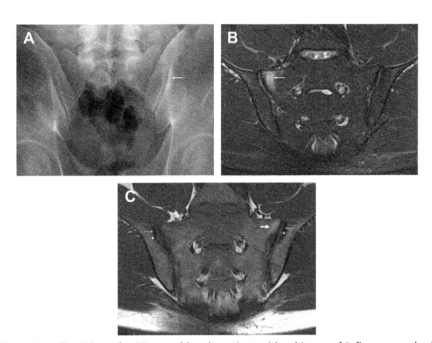

Fig. 5. Sacroiliac joints of a 27-year-old male patient with a history of inflammatory back pain over the previous 12 months. (*A*) Conventional radiograph: no definite structural changes on the right side and only suspicious changes (small localized area with subchondral sclerosis) on the left side (*arrow*) without clear erosions or joint space width changes; sacroiliitis grade I left side. (*B*) MRI (STIR sequence): large area of hyperintense signals (*arrow*) corresponding to bone marrow edema located subchondrally and highly compatible with active sacroiliitis. (*C*) MRI (T1-weighted sequence): erosions (*arrowheads*), fatty lesion and fat deposition (*thick arrow*), and subchondral sclerosis (hypointense in both STIR and T1 sequences, *thin arrows*).

limitations (eg, absence of MRI as an imaging tool, no differentiation between axial and peripheral SpA, and no possibility to classify patients with enthesitis without synovitis as SpA), which resulted in the development of new classification criteria for axial[40,41] and peripheral SpA[42] by the ASAS group (**Fig. 6**).

The set of criteria to be applied in clinical trials and studies depends on the leading clinical manifestation. In case of axial manifestations (back pain >3 months and onset <45 years), the axial SpA criteria should be applied. These criteria include two arms: (1) the imaging arm—patients should have sacroiliitis on radiographs or MRI and at least one additional SpA parameter and (2) the clinical arm—patients without sacroiliitis on imaging or lack of imaging information must be positive for HLA-B27 and have at least two more SpA parameters. The sensitivity of the axial SpA criteria was 82.9%, specificity—84.4% in the ASAS study population.[41]

In patients with peripheral manifestations only (peripheral arthritis compatible with SpA—usually predominantly affecting lower limbs and/or asymmetric; enthesitis or dactylitis) one or two SpA features (depending on the features being positive; see **Fig. 6**) must be present to fulfill the peripheral SpA criteria. The sensitivity of these criteria was 77.8% and specificity was 82.2%.[42]

The development of the SpA criteria by ASAS was an important step toward a better definition of the early disease stage particularly in axial SpA. Therefore, the criteria can

Table 1
ASAS- Outcome Measures in Rheumatoid Arthritis Clinical Trials (OMERACT) definition of active inflammatory lesions on MRI compatible with active sacroiliitis

Active Inflammatory Lesion	Definition
Bone marrow edema or osteitis	Hyperintense signal on STIR images and usually as a hypointense signal on T1 images. The more intense the signal the more likely that it reflects active inflammation. A strong hyperintense signal is similar to that of blood vessels or spinal fluid. Hyperintense signals on contrast-enhanced, T1-weighted, fat-saturated images (T1 after gadolinium) reflect increased vascularization and are referred to as osteitis
	Bone marrow edema or osteitis is an indicator of active sacroiliitis but may be found in other diseases as well
	Affected bone marrow areas are typically located periarticularly (subchondral bone marrow)
	Bone marrow edema may be associated with signs of structural damage such as sclerosis or erosions
Synovitis	Synovitis is best detected as a hyperintense signal on contrast-enhanced, T1-weighted, fat-saturated images in the synovial part of the sacroiliac joints (intensity similar to blood vessels). STIR sequences do not differentiate between synovitis and physiologic joint fluid
	Synovitis on MRI as a single feature (without bone marrow edema) is very rare and does not suffice for making a diagnosis of sacroiliitis for classification purposes
Enthesitis	Depicted as a hyperintense signal on STIR images and/or on contrast-enhanced, T1-weighted, fat-saturated images at sites where ligaments and tendons attach to bone, including the retroarticular space (interosseous ligaments). The signal may extend to bone marrow and soft tissue
Capsulitis	Capsulitis has similar signal characteristics to those of synovitis but these changes involve the anterior and posterior capsule. Anteriorly, the joint capsule gradually continues into the periosteum of the iliac and sacral bones and thus corresponds to an enthesis. Capsulitis may, therefore, extend far medially and laterally into the periosteum

The presence of definite subchondral bone marrow edema/osteitis highly suggestive of sacroiliitis is mandatory for defining of active sacroiliitis. The presence of synovitis, capsulitis, or enthesitis only without subchondral bone marrow edema/osteitis is compatible with but not sufficient for making a diagnosis of active sacroiliitis.

Data from Rudwaleit M, Jurik AG, Hermann KG, et al. Defining active sacroiliitis on magnetic resonance imaging (MRI) for classification of axial spondyloarthritis: a consensus approach by the ASAS/OMERACT MRI group. Ann Rheum Dis 2009;68(10):1520–7.

be used for the conduct of studies but also help establish a diagnosis by pointing out features that are highly relevant in SpA. In the most recent update of the international ASAS recommendations on the use of anti-TNF agents, the fulfillment of ASAS classification criteria for axial SpA was included as an alternative to fulfillment of the modified New York criteria for AS.[17] There are several ongoing clinical trials investigating the efficacy of anti-TNF agents in patients with axial SpA, including nonradiographic axial SpA, and in patients fulfilling the peripheral SpA criteria. Positive results of these trials would not only increase the number of treatment options for patients with early SpA but also provide important support for the SpA concept.

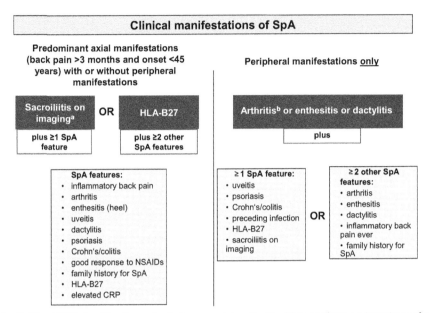

Fig. 6. The ASAS classification criteria for spondyloarthritis. ([a]) Sacroiliitis on imaging refers to definite radiographic sacroiliitis according to the modified New York criteria[14] or sacroiliitis on MRI according to the ASAS consensus definition.[33] ([b]) Peripheral arthritis: usually predominantly lower limb and/or asymmetric arthritis. (*Adapted from* Rudwaleit M, van der Heijde D, Landewe R, et al. The Assessment of SpondyloArthritis International Society classification criteria for peripheral spondyloarthritis and for spondyloarthritis in general. Ann Rheum Dis 2011;70(1):29; with permission.)

IS THERE A DIAGNOSTIC APPROACH FOR CLINICAL PRACTICE?

All clinical, laboratory, and imaging manifestations described above have different diagnostic values as reflected in their sensitivity and specificity regarding SpA diagnosis (**Table 2**). Both sensitivity and specificity of each parameter can be combined in the so-called likelihood ratio (LR). The positive LR (LR+) can be calculated as: LR+ = sensitivity/(1−specificity); and the negative LR (LR−) as: LR− = (1−sensitivity)/specificity. The higher LR+, the better the diagnostic test, and the higher the probability of axial SpA being the present if the test is positive.[1,26,27]

Multiplication of LR+ or LR− of all test results gives an LR product, which can be converted into the individual probability of axial SpA (assuming a pretest probability of axial SpA in patients with chronic low back pain as 5%) using the diagram presented in **Fig. 7**. For the LR product calculation, however, it is recommended to ignore the absence of some clinical manifestations (peripheral arthritis, enthesitis, dactylitis, uveitis, psoriasis, and inflammatory bowel disease) at the time of evaluation because these manifestations may not be present at disease onset but may develop later.[26]

For example, in a patient with inflammatory back pain, HLA-B27 positivity, and psoriasis, the LR product equals $3.1 \times 9.0 \times 2.5 = 69.8$ with posttest SpA probability of about 79% (axial SpA is probable). In case of the presence of active inflammatory lesions in the sacroiliac joints as detected by MRI, the LR product is $3.1 \times 9.0 \times 2.5 \times 9.0 = 627.8$, which gives a nearly 100% probability of axial SpA. However, absence of sacroiliitis on MRI would give an LR product = $3.1 \times 9.0 \times 2.5 \times 0.11 = 7.7$, making the diagnosis of axial SpA rather unlikely.

Table 2
Sensitivity, specificity, and likelihood ratios of single parameters that are relevant for early axial SpA diagnosis

Parameter	Sensitivity, %	Specificity, %	LR +	LR −
Inflammatory back pain	75	76	3.1	0.33
Peripheral arthritis	40	90	4.0	0.67[a]
Enthesitis (heel)	37	89	3.4	0.71[a]
Dactylitis	18	96	4.5	0.85[a]
Anterior uveitis	22	97	7.3	0.80[a]
Psoriasis	10	96	2.5	0.94[a]
Crohn disease/ulcerative colitis	4	99	4.0	0.97[a]
Positive family history for SpA	32	95	6.4	0.72
Good response to NSAIDs	77	85	5.1	0.27
HLA-B27 positivity	90	90	9.0	0.11
Elevated ESR or CRP	50	80	2.5	0.63
Sacroiliitis on MRI	90	90	9.0	0.11

Abbreviations: ESR, erythrocyte sedimentation rate; LR, likelihood ratio.
[a] Because peripheral arthritis, enthesitis, dactylitis, uveitis, psoriasis, and inflammatory bowel disease are not always present at disease onset, it is recommended to ignore their absence on evaluation of the disease probability.
Adapted from Rudwaleit M, Feldtkeller E, Sieper J. Easy assessment of axial spondyloarthritis (early ankylosing spondylitis) at the bedside. Ann Rheum Dis 2006;65(9):1251.

In contrast to classification criteria, the diagnostic algorithm operates with the probability of diagnosis and, therefore, is more suitable for clinical probability practice.

WHICH PATIENTS SHOULD BE REFERRED TO A RHEUMATOLOGIST FOR A DIAGNOSTIC WORK-UP?

Early referral of patients with chronic low back pain to the rheumatologist is essential for early SpA diagnosis. However, as it was already mentioned above, SpA accounts

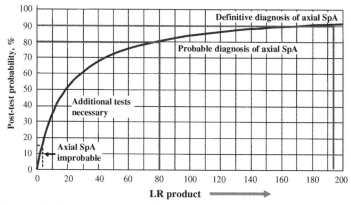

Fig. 7. Relationship between the LR product and the resulting posttest probability of axial SpA, based on an assumed pretest probability of 5% (chronic back pain). (*Adapted from* Rudwaleit M, Feldtkeller E, Sieper J. Easy assessment of axial spondyloarthritis [early ankylosing spondylitis] at the bedside. Ann Rheum Dis 2006;65(9):1252; with permission.)

for about 5% of all causes of chronic back pain. Therefore, a kind of easy-to-apply preselection strategy is required in primary care to increase the probability of axial SpA among patients selected for referral to the rheumatologist. In 2005, a referral strategy (**Fig. 8**) for primary care physicians was proposed which aims at identifying and referring chronic back pain patients with a relatively high probability of axial SpA.[43]

This strategy was subsequently evaluated in the Berlin, Germany, area. Patients were referred by an orthopedist (representing the primary care level for most patients with back pain in Germany) or by primary care physicians to one rheumatology center specialized in SpA. A definite diagnosis of axial SpA has been made in 45.4% of 350 referred patients.[44] Later, this strategy was validated in a multicenter study, which revealed a diagnosis of definite axial SpA in 41.8% of 318 referred patients, thereby confirming the validity of this referral approach. The study also showed that a further increase of the number of SpA parameters required before referral did not improve the performance.[45]

Use of inflammatory back pain as a single referral parameter is a very useful option for countries, in which HLA-B27 testing are also not available in the primary care setting. As shown in two recent studies, about one-third of the patients referred to rheumatologists because of inflammatory back pain were diagnosed with axial SpA.[46,47] However, it is recommended to use HLA-B27 as an alternative to inflammatory back pain, if possible, because it increases the number of SpA cases diagnosed. It is not recommended to perform advanced imaging in primary care because of costs and difficulties in interpretation.

WHICH TREATMENT OPTIONS ARE CURRENTLY AVAILABLE FOR PATIENTS WITH SpA?

The currently available treatment options according to the ASAS/EULAR management recommendations[16,17] are summarized in **Fig. 9**. NSAIDs and nonpharmacologic methods of treatment (eg, physiotherapy) are considered a cornerstone of SpA treatment irrespective of the predominant involvement (axial or peripheral). However, NSAIDs are especially effective in patients with axial involvement, substantially reducing pain and stiffness in most patients.[48,49] Moreover, there are some data indicating that NSAIDs also retard radiographic spinal progression in patients with AS.[50,51] Judgment on the efficacy of an NSAID taken continuously in the maximally

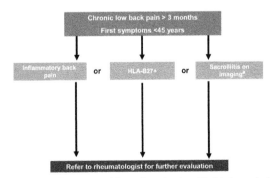

Fig. 8. Early referral strategy for recognition of patients with high probability of axial spondyloarthritis on the primary care level. (ª) Only if available, not recommended routinely for screening in primary care. (*Adapted from* Sieper J, Rudwaleit M. Early referral recommendations for ankylosing spondylitis [including pre-radiographic and radiographic forms] in primary care. Ann Rheum Dis 2005;64(5):661; with permission.)

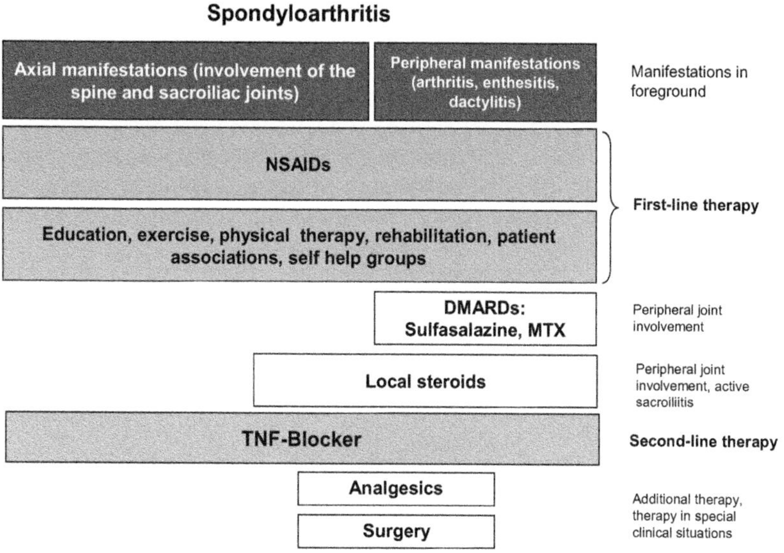

Spondyloarthritis

Fig. 9. Summary of the ASAS-EULAR recommendations for the treatment of axial SpA. DMARDs, disease-modifying antirheumatic drugs, MTX, methotrexate.

recommended or tolerated dose for at least two weeks, unless contraindicated can be made after 2 weeks. In case of inefficacy of the first NSAID, it is recommended to try at least one other NSAID in a full therapeutic dose.

Classic disease-modifying antirheumatic drugs (DMARDs), such as methotrexate, sulfasalazine, or leflunomide, are normally not effective in axial disease, but might be beneficial in peripheral arthritis.[52–54] Therefore, DMARDs are currently reserved for patients with predominant peripheral arthritis. Local steroid injections are also recommended for treatment of peripheral manifestation (arthritis, enthesitis, and dactylitis) but can be also effective (CT scan-guided) in the treatment of active sacroiliitis.[55]

High disease activity (defined as the Bath Ankylosing Spondylitis Disease Activity Index [BASDAI] ≥4) despite adequate NSAIDs treatment in patients with predominant axial involvement and despite local steroids or DMARD treatment in patients with predominant peripheral manifestations is usually considered to be an indication for TNF-α blockers.[17] A positive opinion of a rheumatologist based on the assessment of acute phase reactants, MRI, radiographic data, and radiographic progression of AS is also required.

The currently approved TNF-α blockers infliximab, etanercept, adalimumab, and golimumab demonstrated similarly high efficacy (with major reduction of symptoms as measured by the percentage of patients who achieved the ASAS 40 response, about 40% to 50%) in patients who did not respond to previous NSAID therapy.[56–59] Efficacy of TNF-α blocking agents AS should be assessed after at least 12 weeks of treatment using clinical improvement (BASDAI improvement by ≥50% or by ≥2 absolute points, 0–10 scale).[17] Despite good clinical efficacy, TNF-α blockers were not able to retard radiographic spinal progression in AS over a period of 2 years in recent clinical trials.[60–62] From this point of view, a combination of a TNF-α blocker with an NSAID might provide additional therapeutic benefits.

There are several predictors of a good treatment response to TNF-α blockers. The most important of them are: young age, short disease duration, low level of functional disability, elevated acute phase reactants, and signs of active inflammation on MRI.[18–20] Thus, patients with early and active disease show generally more often a good response to anti–TNF-α treatment in comparison with patients with more advanced disease. It cannot be excluded that early initiation of anti–TNF-α therapy might prevent progression of spinal damage in a long-tem perspective.

Currently, there are nearly no further therapeutic options available for patients who do not respond to anti–TNF-α therapy. However, several promising drugs, including monoclonal antibodies against interleukin (IL)-17 and IL-12/23, are under investigation.

Use of analgesics can be recommended for patients in whom pain cannot be effectively reduced with other treatment modalities.[16]

Surgery might be of benefit for patients with peripheral disease requiring synovectomy, severe hip arthritis (hip arthroplasty), axial disease, and severe spinal deformities or ankylosis with a serious impact on functional status and quality of life (spinal corrective osteotomy).[16]

SUMMARY

In recent years, important steps toward standardizing an early diagnosis of SpA have been made, including development of the new SpA concept (axial vs peripheral), introduction of MRI as one of the key diagnostic imaging tools, development of the new classification criteria for SpA, and application of referral strategies. Further dissemination of these achievements and their consecutive application in clinical practice will contribute to shorten the long diagnostic delay and is likely to improve long-term outcome.

REFERENCES

1. Rudwaleit M, Khan MA, Sieper J. The challenge of diagnosis and classification in early ankylosing spondylitis: do we need new criteria? Arthritis Rheum 2005; 52(4):1000–8.
2. Poddubnyy D, Rudwaleit M, Haibel H, et al. Rates and predictors of radiographic sacroiliitis progression over 2 years in patients with axial spondyloarthritis. Ann Rheum Dis 2011;70(8):1369–74.
3. Rudwaleit M, Haibel H, Baraliakos X, et al. The early disease stage in axial spondyloarthritis: results from the German spondyloarthritis inception cohort. Arthritis Rheum 2009;60(3):717–27.
4. Braun J, Bollow M, Remlinger G, et al. Prevalence of spondylarthropathies in HLA-B27 positive and negative blood donors. Arthritis Rheum 1998;41(1):58–67.
5. Helmick CG, Felson DT, Lawrence RC, et al. Estimates of the prevalence of arthritis and other rheumatic conditions in the United States. Part I. Arthritis Rheum 2008;58(1):15–25.
6. Gofton JP, Robinson HS, Trueman GE. Ankylosing spondylitis in a Canadian Indian population. Ann Rheum Dis 1966;25(6):525–7.
7. van der Linden SM, Valkenburg HA, de Jongh BM, et al. The risk of developing ankylosing spondylitis in HLA-B27 positive individuals. A comparison of relatives of spondylitis patients with the general population. Arthritis Rheum 1984;27(3): 241–9.
8. Khan MA. HLA-B27 and its subtypes in world populations. Curr Opin Rheumatol 1995;7(4):263–9.
9. Hukuda S, Minami M, Saito T, et al. Spondyloarthropathies in Japan: nationwide questionnaire survey performed by the Japan Ankylosing Spondylitis Society. J Rheumatol 2001;28(3):554–9.

10. Belachew DA, Sandu N, Schaller B, et al. Ankylosing spondylitis in sub-Saharan Africa. Postgrad Med J 2009;85(1005):353–7.
11. Zink A, Braun J, Listing J, et al. Disability and handicap in rheumatoid arthritis and ankylosing spondylitis–results from the German rheumatological database. German Collaborative Arthritis Centers. J Rheumatol 2000;27(3):613–22.
12. Feldtkeller E, Bruckel J, Khan MA. Scientific contributions of ankylosing spondylitis patient advocacy groups. Curr Opin Rheumatol 2000;12(4):239–47.
13. Feldtkeller E, Khan MA, van der Heijde D, et al. Age at disease onset and diagnosis delay in HLA-B27 negative vs. positive patients with ankylosing spondylitis. Rheumatol Int 2003;23(2):61–6.
14. van der Linden S, Valkenburg HA, Cats A. Evaluation of diagnostic criteria for ankylosing spondylitis. A proposal for modification of the New York criteria. Arthritis Rheum 1984;27(4):361–8.
15. Underwood MR, Dawes P. Inflammatory back pain in primary care. Br J Rheumatol 1995;34(11):1074–7.
16. Braun J, van den Berg R, Baraliakos X, et al. 2010 update of the ASAS/EULAR recommendations for the management of ankylosing spondylitis. Ann Rheum Dis 2011;70(6):896–904.
17. van der Heijde D, Sieper J, Maksymowych WP, et al. 2010 Update of the international ASAS recommendations for the use of anti-TNF agents in patients with axial spondyloarthritis. Ann Rheum Dis 2011;70(6):905–8.
18. Rudwaleit M, Claudepierre P, Wordsworth P, et al. Effectiveness, safety, and predictors of good clinical response in 1250 patients treated with adalimumab for active ankylosing spondylitis. J Rheumatol 2009;36(4):801–8.
19. Vastesaeger N, van der Heijde D, Inman RD, et al. Predicting the outcome of ankylosing spondylitis therapy. Ann Rheum Dis 2011;70(6):973–81.
20. Rudwaleit M, Listing J, Brandt J, et al. Prediction of a major clinical response (BASDAI 50) to tumour necrosis factor alpha blockers in ankylosing spondylitis. Ann Rheum Dis 2004;63(6):665–70.
21. Deyo RA, Weinstein JN. Low back pain. N Engl J Med 2001;344(5):363–70.
22. Calin A, Porta J, Fries JF, et al. Clinical history as a screening test for ankylosing spondylitis. JAMA 1977;237(24):2613–4.
23. Rudwaleit M, Metter A, Listing J, et al. Inflammatory back pain in ankylosing spondylitis: a reassessment of the clinical history for application as classification and diagnostic criteria. Arthritis Rheum 2006;54(2):569–78.
24. Sieper J, van der Heijde D, Landewe R, et al. New criteria for inflammatory back pain in patients with chronic back pain: a real patient exercise by experts from the Assessment of SpondyloArthritis International Society (ASAS). Ann Rheum Dis 2009;68(6):784–8.
25. Rudwaleit M, Sieper J. A case of axial undifferentiated spondyloarthritis diagnosis and management. Nat Clin Pract Rheumatol 2007;3(5):298–303.
26. Rudwaleit M, Feldtkeller E, Sieper J. Easy assessment of axial spondyloarthritis (early ankylosing spondylitis) at the bedside. Ann Rheum Dis 2006;65(9):1251–2.
27. Rudwaleit M, van der Heijde D, Khan MA, et al. How to diagnose axial spondyloarthritis early. Ann Rheum Dis 2004;63(5):535–43.
28. Brown MA, Kennedy LG, MacGregor AJ, et al. Susceptibility to ankylosing spondylitis in twins: the role of genes, HLA, and the environment. Arthritis Rheum 1997;40(10):1823–8.
29. Burton PR, Clayton DG, Cardon LR, et al. Association scan of 14,500 nonsynonymous SNPs in four diseases identifies autoimmunity variants. Nat Genet 2007;39(11):1329–37.

30. Poddubnyy DA, Rudwaleit M, Listing J, et al. Comparison of a high sensitivity and standard C reactive protein measurement in patients with ankylosing spondylitis and non-radiographic axial spondyloarthritis. Ann Rheum Dis 2010;69(7):1338–41.

31. Poddubnyy D, Haibel H, Listing J, et al. Baseline radiographic damage, elevated acute phase reactants and cigarette smoking status predict radiographic progression in the spine in early axial spondyloarthritis. Arthritis Rheum 2012; 64(5):1388–98.

32. van Tubergen A, Heuft-Dorenbosch L, Schulpen G, et al. Radiographic assessment of sacroiliitis by radiologists and rheumatologists: does training improve quality? Ann Rheum Dis 2003;62(6):519–25.

33. Rudwaleit M, Jurik AG, Hermann KG, et al. Defining active sacroiliitis on magnetic resonance imaging (MRI) for classification of axial spondyloarthritis: a consensual approach by the ASAS/OMERACT MRI group. Ann Rheum Dis 2009;68(10): 1520–7.

34. Song IH, Carrasco-Fernandez J, Rudwaleit M, et al. The diagnostic value of scintigraphy in assessing sacroiliitis in ankylosing spondylitis: a systematic literature research. Ann Rheum Dis 2008;67(11):1535–40.

35. Klauser A, Halpern EJ, Frauscher F, et al. Inflammatory low back pain: high negative predictive value of contrast-enhanced color Doppler ultrasound in the detection of inflamed sacroiliac joints. Arthritis Rheum 2005;53(3):440–4.

36. Strobel K, Fischer DR, Tamborrini G, et al. 18F-fluoride PET/CT for detection of sacroiliitis in ankylosing spondylitis. Eur J Nucl Med Mol Imaging 2010;37(9):1760–5.

37. D'Agostino MA, Aegerter P, Bechara K, et al. How to diagnose spondyloarthritis early? Accuracy of peripheral enthesitis detection by power Doppler ultrasonography. Ann Rheum Dis 2011;70(8):1433–40.

38. Amor B, Dougados M, Mijiyawa M, et al. Rev Rhum Mal Osteoartic 1990;57(2):85–9.

39. Dougados M, van der Linden S, Juhlin R, et al. The European Spondyloarthropathy Study Group preliminary criteria for the classification of spondylarthropathy. Arthritis Rheum 1991;34(10):1218–27.

40. Rudwaleit M, Landewe R, van der Heijde D, et al. The development of Assessment of SpondyloArthritis International Society classification criteria for axial spondyloarthritis (part I): classification of paper patients by expert opinion including uncertainty appraisal. Ann Rheum Dis 2009;68(6):770–6.

41. Rudwaleit M, van der Heijde D, Landewe R, et al. The development of Assessment of SpondyloArthritis International Society classification criteria for axial spondyloarthritis (part II): validation and final selection. Ann Rheum Dis 2009; 68(6):777–83.

42. Rudwaleit M, van der Heijde D, Landewe R, et al. The Assessment of SpondyloArthritis International Society classification criteria for peripheral spondyloarthritis and for spondyloarthritis in general. Ann Rheum Dis 2011;70(1):25–31.

43. Sieper J, Rudwaleit M. Early referral recommendations for ankylosing spondylitis (including pre-radiographic and radiographic forms) in primary care. Ann Rheum Dis 2005;64(5):659–63.

44. Brandt HC, Spiller I, Song IH, et al. Performance of referral recommendations in patients with chronic back pain and suspected axial spondyloarthritis. Ann Rheum Dis 2007;66(11):1479–84.

45. Poddubnyy D, Vahldiek J, Spiller I, et al. Evaluation of 2 screening strategies for early identification of patients with axial spondyloarthritis in primary care. J Rheumatol 2011;38(11):2452–60.

46. Hermann J, Giessauf H, Schaffler G, et al. Early spondyloarthritis: usefulness of clinical screening. Rheumatology (Oxford) 2009;48(7):812–6.

47. Braun A, Saracbasi E, Grifka J, et al. Identifying patients with axial spondyloarthritis in primary care: how useful are items indicative of inflammatory back pain? Ann Rheum Dis 2011;70(10):1782–7.
48. van der Heijde D, Baraf HS, Ramos-Remus C, et al. Evaluation of the efficacy of etoricoxib in ankylosing spondylitis: results of a fifty-two-week, randomized, controlled study. Arthritis Rheum 2005;52(4):1205–15.
49. Sieper J, Klopsch T, Richter M, et al. Comparison of two different dosages of celecoxib with diclofenac for the treatment of active ankylosing spondylitis: results of a 12-week randomised, double-blind, controlled study. Ann Rheum Dis 2008; 67(3):323–9.
50. Wanders A, Heijde D, Landewe R, et al. Nonsteroidal antiinflammatory drugs reduce radiographic progression in patients with ankylosing spondylitis: a randomized clinical trial. Arthritis Rheum 2005;52(6):1756–65.
51. Poddubnyy D, Rudwaleit M, Haibel H, et al. Effect of non-steroidal anti-inflammatory drugs on radiographic spinal progression in patients with axial spondyloarthritis: results from the German Spondyloarthritis Inception Cohort. Ann Rheum Dis 2012. [Epub ahead of print].
52. Braun J, Zochling J, Baraliakos X, et al. Efficacy of sulfasalazine in patients with inflammatory back pain due to undifferentiated spondyloarthritis and early ankylosing spondylitis: a multicentre randomised controlled trial. Ann Rheum Dis 2006;65(9):1147–53.
53. Haibel H, Brandt HC, Song IH, et al. No efficacy of subcutaneous methotrexate in active ankylosing spondylitis: a 16-week open-label trial. Ann Rheum Dis 2007; 66(3):419–21.
54. Haibel H, Rudwaleit M, Braun J, et al. Six months open label trial of leflunomide in active ankylosing spondylitis. Ann Rheum Dis 2005;64(1):124–6.
55. Braun J, Bollow M, Seyrekbasan F, et al. Computed tomography guided corticosteroid injection of the sacroiliac joint in patients with spondyloarthropathy with sacroiliitis: clinical outcome and followup by dynamic magnetic resonance imaging. J Rheumatol 1996;23(4):659–64.
56. van der Heijde D, Dijkmans B, Geusens P, et al. Efficacy and safety of infliximab in patients with ankylosing spondylitis: results of a randomized, placebo-controlled trial (ASSERT). Arthritis Rheum 2005;52(2):582–91.
57. van der Heijde D, Kivitz A, Schiff MH, et al. Efficacy and safety of adalimumab in patients with ankylosing spondylitis: results of a multicenter, randomized, double-blind, placebo-controlled trial. Arthritis Rheum 2006;54(7):2136–46.
58. Davis JC, van der Heijde DM, Braun J, et al. Sustained durability and tolerability of etanercept in ankylosing spondylitis for 96 weeks. Ann Rheum Dis 2005; 64(11):1557–62.
59. Inman RD, Davis JC Jr, Heijde D, et al. Efficacy and safety of golimumab in patients with ankylosing spondylitis: results of a randomized, double-blind, placebo-controlled, phase III trial. Arthritis Rheum 2008;58(11):3402–12.
60. van der Heijde D, Landewe R, Einstein S, et al. Radiographic progression of ankylosing spondylitis after up to two years of treatment with etanercept. Arthritis Rheum 2008;58(5):1324–31.
61. van der Heijde D, Landewe R, Baraliakos X, et al. Radiographic findings following two years of infliximab therapy in patients with ankylosing spondylitis. Arthritis Rheum 2008;58(10):3063–70.
62. van der Heijde D, Salonen D, Weissman BN, et al. Assessment of radiographic progression in the spines of patients with ankylosing spondylitis treated with adalimumab for up to 2 years. Arthritis Res Ther 2009;11(4):R127.

Environmental and Gene-Environment Interactions and Risk of Rheumatoid Arthritis

Elizabeth W. Karlson, MD[a],*, Kevin Deane, MD, PhD[b]

KEYWORDS

- Rheumatoid arthritis • Environmental risk factors
- Gene-environment interactions

Key Points

- Individuals with inherited genetic risk factors who are exposed to environmental triggers are at higher risk of rheumatoid arthritis (RA).

- Multiple environmental factors, including exposure to tobacco smoke, occupational exposures, hormones, infections and dietary factors, are associated with RA risk.

- Circulating RA-related autoimmunity is evident in some patients before the appearance of the first joint symptoms and clinical findings of RA. This asymptomatic phase of disease development suggests that important gene and environmental interactions leading to initiation of RA-related autoimmunity occur long before the onset of clinically apparent disease.

- Natural history studies of the asymptomatic phase of RA development are needed to determine the mechanistic role(s) that environmental factors play in the initiation of RA.

- Animal studies link autoantibodies to RA pathogenesis, and going forward may provide insight to the mechanisms of environmental and genetic factors in the pathogenesis of RA.

Dr Karlson's work was supported by NIH grants AR049880, AR052403, and AR047782. Dr Deane's work was supported by NIH grants AR051394, AR07534, AR051461, AI50864, the American College of Rheumatology Research and Education Foundation's Within Our Reach Program, and the Walter S. and Lucienne Driskill Foundation.
The authors have no conflicts of interest to disclose.
[a] Section of Clinical Sciences, Division of Rheumatology, Allergy and Immunology, Department of Medicine, Brigham and Women's Hospital, 75 Francis Street, Boston, MA 02115, USA;
[b] Division of Rheumatology, Department of Medicine, University of Colorado School of Medicine, 1775 Aurora Court, Mail Stop B-115, Aurora, CO 80045, USA
* Corresponding author.
E-mail address: ekarlson@partners.org

INTRODUCTION

Although the etiology of rheumatoid arthritis (RA) is unknown, a growing body of evidence suggests that it develops in individuals with inherited genetic risk factors after exposure to environmental triggers. The identification of autoantibodies and cytokines in the serum many years before the diagnosis of RA led to conceptualization of the development of RA as occurring in phases (**Fig. 1**).[1–8] In this model of RA development there is an asymptomatic period of genetic risk in which environmental exposures are encountered, followed by an asymptomatic immune-activation phase in which autoantibodies and inflammatory markers are found, likely followed by a phase of articular symptoms in the absence of clearly definable arthritis, which is finally followed by the phase with signs of inflammatory arthritis (IA) that is perhaps initially unclassifiable but over time evolves to the point at which it is classifiable as RA by established criteria such as the 1987 American College of Rheumatology (ACR) criteria or the 2010 ACR/European League Against Rheumatism (EULAR) criteria.[9,10] Similar phases of development have been proposed in other autoimmune diseases such as type 1 diabetes and systemic lupus erythematosus (SLE).[11,12] This pattern suggests a complex series of events in which a genetically susceptible host is exposed to environmental risk factors that trigger autoimmunity with autoantibody production, and a second or more event(s) or exposure(s) that might drive further immune dysregulation and eventual development of symptomatic IA. The interaction between genetic and environmental factors such as cigarette smoking within the subtype of anticitrullinated protein antibody (ACPA)-positive RA[13] provides clues to disease pathogenesis, but much of the complexity of RA etiopathogenesis has yet to be delineated.

Epidemiologic research has produced convincing evidence for strong environmental risk factors for RA, including cigarette smoking,[14–27] exogenous hormone

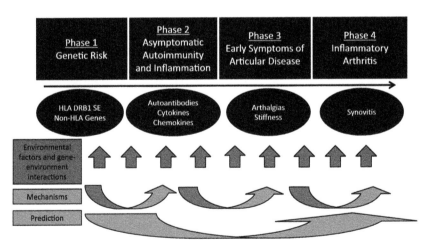

Fig. 1. Phases in the development of rheumatoid arthritis (RA). Phase 1, asymptomatic phase of genetic risk; phase 2, asymptomatic immune-activation phase with autoantibodies and elevated biomarkers such as cytokines and chemokines; phase 3, preclinical phase with abnormal biomarkers of inflammation and perhaps arthralgias; phase 4, clinically apparent inflammatory arthritis (defined as symptomatic joint disease including pain, stiffness and swelling, and identifiable synovitis on examination) that may be undifferentiated arthritis, or fulfill classification for RA. Identifying the environmental factors associated with transitions between phases, key exposure windows leading to transition between phases, and the biological mechanisms involved in these transitions is a challenge for the field.

use,[28–36] and female reproductive factors.[28,37–41] Other exposures have also been identified as risk factors for RA including silica,[42–46] air pollution,[47] and periodontitis,[48] and some exposures such as alcohol have been reported as protective factors[49,50] although these studies have not been widely replicated. Other factors are also associated with increased risk for RA, including higher birth weight.[51,52] Furthermore, having a first-degree relative (FDR) with RA increases RA risk 3- to 9-fold compared with that in the general population, suggesting the influence of shared genetic and/or environmental factors.[53] Recent whole-genome association studies in RA have identified more than 30 novel risk loci confirmed by meta-analysis in addition to well-established associations with the *HLA-DRB1* "shared epitope" (HLA-SE) alleles.[54] Gene-environment interactions between HLA-SE and other potential risk alleles may contribute to RA pathogenesis.[13,55–57] Models that incorporate genetic, biomarker, and lifestyle/environmental factors can now predict the risk of developing RA with greater precision than any of these factors alone.[56,58] This review focuses on validated environmental, lifestyle, and dietary exposures in the pre-RA phases before the appearance of objective signs of IA.

DEFINING THE PHASES OF DEVELOPMENT OF AUTOIMMUNITY, INFLAMMATORY ARTHRITIS, AND EARLY RHEUMATOID ARTHRITIS

Multiple studies have shown that RA-related autoantibodies may be elevated up to[12–15] years before the onset of clinically apparent IA. Some of these studies were performed in a prospective fashion, with careful joint evaluations in currently asymptomatic individuals.[59–61] However, most of these studies are somewhat limited in their conclusions about the precise timing of elevations of RA-related autoantibodies before the onset of clinically apparent IA because they were not performed as part of rigorous prospective evaluations of individuals at risk for future RA.[2–8,59,62–66] Regardless, in sum these studies strongly suggest that RA develops in 4 distinct phases: (1) an asymptomatic phase of genetic risk; (2) an asymptomatic immune-activation phase in which abnormalities of autoantibodies and biomarkers such as cytokines and chemokines are documented up to 14 years before RA[1–5,7,8,66,67]; (3) a preclinical phase with abnormal biomarkers of inflammation and perhaps arthralgias[68,69]; and (4) clinically apparent IA (symptomatic joint disease including pain, stiffness and swelling, and identifiable synovitis on examination) that may be undifferentiated arthritis, or fulfill[7] classification for RA (see **Fig. 1**).[70,71] Identifying the environmental factors associated with transitions between phases, key exposure windows leading to transition between phases, and the biological mechanisms involved in these transitions is a challenge for the field.

EPIDEMIOLOGIC STUDY DESIGN

Studies of the environmental factors associated with RA are often conducted through a case-control design whereby cases with RA and healthy controls are surveyed retrospectively for environmental, lifestyle, and behavioral factors occurring before disease onset in cases and before a matched date (or age) for controls. This study design can be limited by recall bias whereby cases recall and report exposures differentially than do controls.[72] Also, in case-control studies results are reported as odds ratios, which can approximate relative risk in settings where the sample size is high, but do not provide estimates of population risk. The prospective cohort design is considered less biased, as nondiseased subjects can be followed prospectively for exposure assessment while asymptomatic before the development of RA. Examples of prospective cohort studies of RA include the US Nurses' Health Study (NHS),[21] the

Iowa Women's Health Study (IWHS),[24,73] the Malmo Diet and Cancer Study,[39,41] and more recently, Lifelines in the Netherlands. In the Norfolk Arthritis Register (NOAR, United Kingdom) cohort study, risk factors for the development of IA and RA that meet ACR criteria have been studied.[74] The advantages of prospective designs are analyses that produce relative risks, the ability to estimate population-attributable risks, the ability assess repeated time-varying exposures, and the ability to study exposure windows before disease onset.

An alternative approach to understanding both timing of environmental exposures and their influence at points of transition in the phases of RA is prospective cohort studies of high-risk individuals followed for the development of autoantibodies and immune markers. Two groups have led the field in studies of high-risk FDRs: (1) the Studies of the Etiology of RA (SERA) in the United States[75] and (2) studies of North American Natives (NAN) in central Canada.[76] In each of these studies, FDRs are followed annually for environment, lifestyle, and behavioral risk factors and the development of RA-related autoantibodies (rheumatoid factor [RF] and ACPA) and immune markers, as well as signs and symptoms of IA (**Table 1**). Similar studies of FDRs are being launched in Europe.

CIGARETTE-SMOKING EXPOSURE

Modifiable environmental factors contribute substantially to population risk of RA. Multiple case-control and prospective cohort studies have demonstrated that cigarette smoking is the strongest environmental factor linked with RA,[14,15,17–22,24–27,77] and its population-attributable risk is 25% for all RA and 35% for seropositive RF (RF+) and ACPA-positive (ACPA+) RA.[23,27] Relative risks for cigarette smoking range from 1.6 for risk of all RA to 1.8 for risk of seropositive RA.[27] The association appears to be stronger for men than for women.[17,18,22,25,78] Furthermore, several studies demonstrate a dose response between heavier smoking and RA, particularly seropositive RA with persistence of RA risk for 20 years after smoking cessation.[13,21,23,26,27,77] The specific mechanisms by which smoking may be related to the generation of RA-related autoimmunity are unknown; however, there are several clues to pathogenesis. Smoking was shown to be associated with an increased levels of citrullinated proteins as well as expression of peptidyl arginine deiminase 2 (PADI2) in pulmonary cells obtained by bronchoalveolar lavage.[79] In addition, the risk of seropositive RA associated with smoking has been reported to be highest and in those who carry the *HLA-DRB1* shared epitope (*HLA-SE*).[13,77] Recent observations indicate that certain DRB1 alleles, in particular 0401 and 0404, are associated with a strong immunity to citrullinated peptides, such as vimentin or enolase peptides.[57,80–82] The specific time point in the development of RA that smoking acts to increase risk is unknown; however, in the prospective SERA project, smoking was associated with RF positivity in subjects enriched with *HLA-SE* but no RA symptoms, suggesting that smoking may act early in immune dysregulation and may lead to future RA.[83] Smoking has been also been associated with more generalized immune abnormalities including alterations in T-cell function,[84,85] reduction in natural killer cells,[86] impairment of humoral immunity,[86,87] and elevated levels of inflammatory markers such as interleukin (IL)-6 and C-reactive protein[88,89] as well as elevations of RF in the absence of RA.[90] Although some of these effects associated with smoking such as impaired humoral immunity are somewhat paradoxical when trying to understand the relationship between smoking and development of RA, especially seropositive RA, in sum these findings suggest that smoking may lead to autoantigen generation and alteration of other inflammatory factors that in a permissive genetic background lead to the

Table 1
Environmental, behavioral, and lifestyle risk factors for rheumatoid arthritis, inflammatory arthritis, or autoimmunity in prospective cohort studies

Site	Population	Cohort	Smoking	Silica	Air Pollution	Reproductive Factors	Birth Weight	Alcohol	Diet	Periodontal Disease
Boston	Nurses	NHS	X		X	X	X	X	X	X[a]
Iowa	Women	IWHS	X			X			X	
Sweden	General	MDCS	X			X		X		
Netherlands	General	Lifelines	X	X		X	X	X	X	X[b]
UK	General	NOAR	X			X			X	
Colorado	FDR	SERA	X	X		X		X	X	X[a]
Manitoba	FDR	NAN	X	X		X		X		X[b]
Geneva	FDR	Geneva	X	X		X	X	X	X	X[a]

X indicates exposure ascertained by survey.

Abbreviations: FDR, first-degree relative; IWHS, Iowa Women's Health Study; MDCS, Malmo Diet and Cancer Study; NAN, North American Natives; NHS, Nurses' Health Study; NOAR, Norfolk Arthritis Register; SERA, Studies of the Etiology of RA.

[a] Subjects complete survey regarding periodontitis symptoms.
[b] Subjects undergo dental examination for periodontitis.

development of RA-related autoimmunity. However, the specific mechanistic details of how smoking triggers RA, including at what anatomic site smoking may drive RA-related autoimmunity, need further exploration, especially in prospective studies of preclinical RA. Furthermore, recent data suggesting decreased responsiveness to therapy in patients with established RA who are smokers suggests some relationship between disease development and smoking even after the onset of symptomatic IA, although the specific mechanisms of these relationships also need further exploration.[91,92]

OCCUPATIONAL EXPOSURES

A case-control study from Sweden, the Epidemiologic Investigation of RA (EIRA),[42] reported an association between occupational silica exposure and RA among 276 male RA cases and 276 healthy controls with evidence for silica-smoking interaction. Silica dust exposure was a risk factor only for RF+ and ACPA+ RA and not for seronegative RA. Exposure to silica dust through the respiratory tract in occupations such as rock drilling, mining, and sand blasting has been linked to RA risk in other epidemiologic studies.[43–46] High-level exposure to silica dust can cause chronic inflammation and fibrosis in the lung and other organs, and it may be that such inflammation leads to humoral immune responses and hence greater risk for seropositive RA. Furthermore, occupational exposure to other factors such as mineral oils (exposure pathways through the lung and skin) was also investigated in EIRA,[93] and exposure was associated with an increased risk of RF+/ACPA+ RA but not of seronegative RA. Mineral oil can also act as an adjuvant capable of inducing experimental arthritis in rodent models, and may have a similar action in humans.[94,95] Substantial exposure to inhaled organic solvents in occupations such as upholstering, hair-dressing, and concrete work was associated with an increased risk of RA.[96] As with smoking, the specific details of how occupational exposures lead to the generation of RA-related autoimmunity, especially seropositive disease, need further study.

REPRODUCTIVE AND HORMONAL FACTORS

Abundant epidemiologic, clinical, and experimental evidence implicates hormones in the incidence and clinical expression of RA. Women are 2 to 4 times more likely than men to develop RA.[97,98] In women, RA frequently develops at times when sex steroid hormone levels are in flux, such as in the postpartum and perimenopausal periods.[99–102] In most,[28–35,103] but not all studies,[16,38,39,104–107] use of oral contraceptives is protective against the development of RA. Studies such as the NHS demonstrated a strong trend of decreasing risk of RA with increasing total duration of breast feeding,[38] with inverse findings for breast feeding and RA confirmed in 2 studies,[39,108] whereas another study showed a positive association.[40] In the NHS, irregular menstrual cycles and age at menarche of 10 years or younger were associated with increased RA risk[38]; another study demonstrated that both age at menarche of 12 years and younger and early menopause were inversely associated with RA risk.[41] Studies suggest that RA incidence rises with age,[97,109] with a peak incidence at menopause.[38,99,110] However, exogenous estrogen therapy among postmenopausal women did not reduce RA risk.[36,38] In the SERA cohort, among subjects enriched with *HLA-SE* alleles, use of oral contraceptives was associated with a decreased risk for RF positivity, independent of age, education, and smoking. This finding may indicate that hormones or factors related to use of oral contraceptives are acting early in RA-related immune dysregulation to reduce risk for formation of autoantibodies.

INFECTION AND MUCOSAL INFLAMMATION AND THE INITIATION OF RA-RELATED AUTOIMMUNITY

RA-related autoimmunity has been associated with multiple organisms as well as tissue inflammation and injury at sites other than the joints, including the lungs, genitourinary tract, and oral cavity/periodontal region. It has been typically thought that such infections and tissue inflammation are secondarily due to immunosuppression or autoimmune-related injury. However, the growing understanding of the preclinical phases of RA development[71] as well as recent findings show that circulating RF and ACPA elevations are present in the absence of synovitis on knee synovial biopsy, providing support for the concept that RA may be generated outside of the joints.[111] Therefore, it may be that the infections that are associated with autoantibody formation, and inflammation at these extra-articular sites, are providing clues as to etiologic factors and sites that are driving the generation of initial RA-related autoimmunity.

As a specific example of infection and mucosal inflammation in association with RA, recent data have shown an association between established RA and periodontal disease.[112–115] The causal direction remains uncertain, but recent discoveries suggest that gum inflammation and, in particular, infection with organisms such as *Porphyromonas gingivalis* may be important in the pathophysiology of RA development.[113–115] The current hypothesis is that *P gingivalis*–mediated citrullination of human peptides may be responsible for the initial breakdown in self-tolerance that leads to the development of RA-related autoimmunity.[112,116] This intriguing concept needs further exploration, however, as do the roles of multiple other infectious organisms and inflammation at other mucosal sites (including the respiratory tract, gut, and genitourinary tract) that have been implicated in the pathogenesis of RA.[117–125] It is important that investigation of the roles of infectious and mucosal factors in RA is performed in prospective study of the preclinical phases of RA development, to identify the true temporal as well as mechanistic relationships between infections and mucosal inflammation in the early pathogenesis of RA.

DIETARY FACTORS

Dietary intake of vitamin D, antioxidants, fish, protein, and iron may be inversely associated with RA risk, although the data are mixed.[73,126–137] Vitamin D has been implicated as an etiologic and therapeutic factor in several autoimmune diseases including multiple sclerosis,[138,139] type 1 diabetes,[140] and SLE.[141] Vitamin D has pleiotropic effects on the immune system, inhibiting proinflammatory cytokines, upregulating anti-inflammatory cytokines,[142] and regulating the innate and adaptive immune system through the vitamin D receptor.[140] Vitamin D prevents the development of IA in collagen-induced mouse models.[143] One study found a strong protective effect of high vitamin D intake in diminishing RA risk, showing inverse associations for dietary and supplemental vitamin D[73]; another study revealed no association.[136] Furthermore, in a study of approximately 1200 healthy individuals at risk for future RA because of genetic factors (HLA DR4 allele enrichment and/or family history of RA), 76 of whom were positive for the RA-related autoantibodies anti–cyclic citrullinated peptide and/ or RF, there was no association of autoantibody positivity with plasma vitamin D levels.[144] Studies show an inverse relationship between higher vitamin D and lower disease activity in RA after diagnosis.[145,146]

Marine omega-3 fatty acids exert effects through the leukotriene and prostaglandin pathways, decreasing inflammatory mediators, and have multiple known anti-inflammatory properties.[147] Case-control and cohort studies reported a modest protective effect of fish intake on RA risk.[127,128,133,148] Consumption of fish has also been shown to improve RA symptoms and delay RA progression.[149,150]

Antioxidants

Observational case-control and cohort studies suggest that antioxidants may protect against the development of RA, but the results for individual antioxidants are conflicting.[128–132,137,151–153] The IWHS demonstrated an inverse association for β-cryptoxanthin and supplemental zinc and risk of RA, but only a weak inverse association for vitamin C, and no association for vitamin E and risk of RA.[129] In NOAR, vitamin C was inversely associated with the risk of IA, but β-cryptoxanthin and zeaxanthin antioxidants showed only weak inverse associations after adjustment for vitamin C.[130,131] Data from the NHS did not support any prospective association for antioxidants including vitamin C, vitamin E, and β-cryptoxanthin.[137] Furthermore, data from a case-control study[128] and a randomized controlled trial[135] did not support an effect of vitamin E on RA risk.

Protein and Iron

In NOAR, higher intakes of red meat and protein were associated with a risk of IA whereas iron, another nutrient component of meat, showed no association.[130,132] However, no clear associations were observed between dietary protein, iron, or meats, including red meat, and risk of RA in the NHS cohort.[134]

Alcohol

Case-control studies have suggested that alcohol consumption may decrease the risk for RA and RA progression.[49,50,154] Any alcohol versus no alcohol use was associated with lower odds of seropositive RA in several case-control studies.[17,50,155] A dose-dependent protective effect was demonstrated in 2 case-control studies where alcohol consumption was based on patient questionnaires regarding alcohol consumption in the previous week, previous habitual consumption before RA onset, or consumption 10 years before inclusion.[49] Furthermore, there was evidence for alcohol–HLA-SE interaction. However, there was no association between alcohol and RA in the IWHS, a prospective cohort study.[156] In the NHS, moderate alcohol intake (3–6 drinks per week) was associated with reduction in plasma biomarkers of inflammation, including C-reactive protein, soluble tumor necrosis factor receptor 2, and IL-6, among women with pre-RA from whom blood was collected up to 12 years before first symptoms of RA, suggesting an effect of alcohol on inflammation during the asymptomatic phases.[157]

There are several possible mechanisms for the inverse association of alcohol consumption with RA. Moderate alcohol consumption may be associated with reduced levels of inflammatory biomarkers reflective of underlying improved alterations of inflammatory pathways.[158] Alcohol has also been shown to diminish the response to antigens in animals as well as in humans,[159,160] and to suppress the synthesis of proinflammatory cytokines and chemokines, such as tumor necrosis factor α, IL-6, and IL-8, both in vivo and in vitro, in alveolar macrophages and human blood monocytes.[161,162]

INHALED PARTICULATE AIR POLLUTION

Although the first cases of RA may date back thousands of years, the prevalence of RA appears to have increased in Europe in the 1800s.[163,164] This time period is associated with the introduction of tobacco from the New World and increased popularity of smoking, and also coincides with the Industrial Revolution and the advent of air pollution in Europe.[165] In the EIRA cohort, lower socioeconomic status is associated with an increased risk of RA.[166] This association remains strong after adjustment for cigarette smoking, suggesting the existence of an important environmental or lifestyle factor associated with lower socioeconomic status. This finding is particularly interesting given that exposure to air pollution is often much higher for those in lower socioeconomic classes.[167,168] Our evolving understanding of RA pathogenesis suggests that inhaled particulate matter may induce local lung inflammation as well as through systemic inflammation. Indirect support of this hypothesis comes from the observation that air pollution has been clearly linked with other diseases of local lung and systemic inflammation, including asthma[169] and chronic bronchitis,[170,171] cardiovascular disease,[172–174] lung[172,175,176] and laryngeal[177] cancers, and increased all-cause mortality.[178–180] Data from the NHS reported a higher relative risk of RA in the Northeast and upper Midwest regions of the United States, regions with high levels of air pollution.[181,182] Further data suggest a higher risk of RA in women who live closest to a major road, a proxy for traffic pollution.[47]

FAMILY HISTORY

Twin studies demonstrate a high concordance of RA between monozygotic and dizygotic twins.[183] In a Swedish study involving 47,361 subjects with RA, standardized incidence ratios (SIRs) were calculated as relative risk of RA in family members of RA patients as compared with relative risk in those with no affected family members.[53] SIRs for RA were 3.0 in offspring of RA-affected parents, 4.6 in siblings, 9.3 in multiplex families (both parent and sibling), and 6.5 in twins. The 3- to 9-fold increased familial risk of RA suggests strong influence of genetic or shared environmental effects, or both.

INTERACTIONS BETWEEN ENVIRONMENTAL AND GENETIC FACTORS AND RA RISK

There are several potential mechanisms by which gene-environment interactions may trigger RA-related autoimmunity. A gene-environment interaction between HLA-SE and smoking was first described in landmark studies led by Klareskog and colleagues.[13,77] This work has demonstrated that interaction between these 2 factors was strongly associated with specific phenotypes of ACPA+ and RF+, whereas no such association was seen for the risk of developing seronegative RA. Furthermore, the additive nature of the interaction suggested a biological pathway to disease onset. Subsequent studies replicated and expanded on these findings using 2 different methods: case-control analyses comparing RA cases stratified according to autoantibody phenotype with healthy controls,[56] and case-only analyses comparing autoantibody-positive RA cases with autoantibody-negative RA cases, without involving healthy controls.[184,185] Gene-environment interaction between HLA-SE in a case-control study was strongest for autoantibody-positive RA with significant multiplicative interaction.[56] Furthermore, there was a dose response in the gene-environment interactions for both allele dose and smoking dose, with highest risk among heavy smokers with double-copy HLA-SE. Gene-environment interactions between GSTT1 or GSM1 null polymorphisms (resulting in absence of the GSTT1 or GSTM1 enzymes that detoxify cigarette smoke), and the drug-metabolizing enzyme N-acetyletransferase-2 (NAT2) and smoking, further support the synergistic effect smoking and genetics on risk for RA.[186–189]

In an attempt to identify specific mechanistic pathways by which exposure to tobacco smoke may induce RA-related autoimmunity, investigators have also examined bronchoalveolar lavage (BAL) fluid from healthy nonsmokers, healthy smokers, and smokers with concomitant inflammatory lung diseases (such as sarcoidosis and Langerhans cell histiocytosis).[13,79] The investigators found that smoking increases

PAD2 enzyme expression in human lungs and was associated with an increased proportion of citrulline-positive BAL cells (mainly alveolar macrophages), whereas citrullinated cells were not found in nonsmokers.

Overall, this research has led to the hypothesis that smoking induces citrullination, with subsequent immune reactions to citrullinated antigens occurring in *HLA-SE*–positive individuals. This hypothesis is strengthened by the demonstration in *HLA-DRB1*0401* transgenic mice that citrullination of certain peptides renders them more prone to bind to HLA class II molecules with the *HLA-SE*, and to trigger a strong immune response to citrullinated self-antigens.[190] If similar mechanisms are occurring humans to drive the development of RA, based on the phased model of RA development (see **Fig. 1**), the gene-environmental interactions that may lead to RA-related autoimmunity are likely occurring some time before the onset of symptomatic joint disease. However, the mechanisms as well as the specific sequence of gene-environment interactions such as smoking, the generation of citrullinated proteins, and subsequent autoimmunity to those proteins that lead to symptomatic RA are unknown. For example, it may be that some factor other than smoking initially interacts with HLA alleles to generate autoantibodies to citrullinated proteins, and that smoking is a permissive factor that later drives the development of symptomatic RA rather than the initiation of autoimmunity. To fully understand these issues, the development of RA needs to be explored in prospective studies that can in real time evaluate the relationships between gene-environment interactions and the development of RA-related autoimmunity.

PATHOLOGIC ROLES FOR AUTOANTIBODIES IN RA

Despite their strong association with RA, the precise roles of autoantibodies, including RF and ACPAs, in the pathogenesis of RA are unclear, although it will be important to define these roles, especially given the aforementioned data associating the development of seropositive RA with gene-environmental interactions.[13,55–57,191] However, numerous studies suggest that autoantibodies are likely a key aspect of the development of RA.[192,193] In particular, the association of RF and ACPAs with more severe RA (or arthritis in non-RA conditions such as SLE) suggests that these autoantibodies are important contributors to joint disease.[63,192–195] Also, in animal models of arthritis, infusion of antibodies to citrullinated proteins leads to more severe arthritis, suggesting that these autoantibodies play a direct pathogenic role in disease development.[196] In addition, recent work demonstrating in both animal models and humans that circulating immune complexes containing ACPAs and citrullinated fibrinogen activate inflammation through interactions with Toll-like receptor 4 provides a potential mechanism by which circulating ACPAs may induce joint-specific inflammation, a process that is enhanced if RF is also present.[197,198] Finally, as already discussed, the findings in multiple human studies of elevated RF and ACPAs before the onset of RA suggest that autoimmunity to citrullinated proteins is an important factor in the development of RA in the period before the appearance of symptomatic synovitis. In sum, these data suggest that autoantibodies are an important aspect of the pathogenesis of RA; therefore, the area of gene-environment interactions that may lead to the development of these autoantibodies is a fertile ground for investigations in the pathogenesis of RA.

ANIMAL STUDIES LINKING ENVIRONMENTAL FACTORS TO DEVELOPMENT OF AUTOANTIBODIES

Emerging data from animal models of disease that have explored the role of environmental factors such as smoking in the pathogenesis of IA may provide insight into specific mechanism(s) by which environmental exposures may trigger RA-related auto-immunity. In particular, in a murine model of collagen-induced arthritis, Okamoto and colleagues[199] induced IA by exposing mice nasally to cigarette-smoke condensate. However, other studies have shown that exposure to cigarette smoke delayed collagen-induced arthritis in mice, perhaps because of immunosuppressive constituents of cigarette smoke.[200] Therefore, additional work is needed to develop models that can help explain the pathophysiologic mechanisms by which exposure to environmental risk factors such as cigarette smoke may trigger RA. Regarding potential infectious triggers of RA, multiple animal models of collagen-induced arthritis have shown more severe arthritis in the setting of environments where organisms are present.[201,202] Furthermore, Kinloch and colleagues[203] reported in an *HLA DR4*-transgenic murine model of arthritis that immunization with both citrullinated and uncitrullinated forms of enolase from *P gingivalis* led to autoantibodies to the citrullinated mammalian form of this enzyme as well as arthritis. This latter discovery needs further work to determine its direct applicability to human disease; however, it does support a hypothesis that bacterial factors may be an important part of the development of RA.

REMAINING QUESTIONS AND FUTURE DIRECTIONS

The identification of autoantibodies and cytokines that are present many years before RA onset and the association of many environmental factors with RA development provide an exciting opportunity to intervene during the preclinical phase to prevent the development of symptomatic RA. However, it is critical to understand the key exposure windows to design interventions, especially if such interventions are to include modification of environmental exposures. Further research into the environment and gene-environment and epigenetic determinants of RA risk will provide important data for individualized studies to target potentially toxic therapy at individuals of highest risk, with such data preferably obtained through detailed, prospective studies of the natural history of RA so that we can understand the precise temporal as well as mechanistic relationships between genetic and environmental factors and the development of RA-related autoimmunity. The concept that RA is initiated at some mucosal site distal to the joints, potentially in relationship with environmental factors such as smoking, alcohol, or infection, is fascinating and may lead to a significant breakthrough in our understanding of how this disease develops, and needs additional study.

The ability to accurately predict an individual's risk of developing clinical RA would be an enormous advance in this area, enabling risk-factor modification and earlier introduction of effective therapies to abrogate the destruction and disability of this disease. Thus, predictive modeling incorporating RA genetic susceptibility alleles, hormonal, environmental, and behavioral risk factors, and their interactions is a key step in the progress toward a clinical trial of RA prevention.

REFERENCES

1. Majka DS, Deane KD, Parrish LA, et al. Duration of preclinical rheumatoid arthritis-related autoantibody positivity increases in subjects with older age at time of disease diagnosis. Ann Rheum Dis 2008;67:801–7.
2. Deane KD, O'Donnell CI, Hueber W, et al. The number of elevated cytokines and chemokines in preclinical seropositive rheumatoid arthritis predicts time to diagnosis in an age-dependent manner. Arthritis Rheum 2010;62:3161–72.
3. Rantapaa-Dahlqvist S, de Jong BA, Berglin E, et al. Antibodies against cyclic citrullinated peptide and IgA rheumatoid factor predict the development of rheumatoid arthritis. Arthritis Rheum 2003;48:2741–9.

4. Nielen MM, van Schaardenburg D, Reesink HW, et al. Specific autoantibodies precede the symptoms of rheumatoid arthritis: a study of serial measurements in blood donors. Arthritis Rheum 2004;50:380–6.

5. Chibnik LB, Mandl LA, Costenbader KH, et al. Comparison of threshold cutpoints and continuous measures of anti-cyclic citrullinated peptide antibodies in predicting future rheumatoid arthritis. J Rheumatol 2009;36:706–11.

6. Kokkonen H, Mullazehi M, Berglin E, et al. Antibodies of IgG, IgA and IgM isotypes against cyclic citrullinated peptide precede the development of rheumatoid arthritis. Arthritis Res Ther 2010;13:R13.

7. Kokkonen H, Soderstrom I, Rocklov J, et al. Up-regulation of cytokines and chemokines predates the onset of rheumatoid arthritis. Arthritis Rheum 2010; 62:383–91.

8. Jorgensen KT, Wiik A, Pedersen M, et al. Cytokines, autoantibodies and viral antibodies in premorbid and postdiagnostic sera from patients with rheumatoid arthritis: case-control study nested in a cohort of Norwegian blood donors. Ann Rheum Dis 2008;67:860–6.

9. Arnett FC, Edworthy SM, Bloch DA, et al. The American Rheumatism Association 1987 revised criteria for the classification of rheumatoid arthritis. Arthritis Rheum 1988;31:315–24.

10. Aletaha D, Neogi T, Silman AJ, et al. Rheumatoid arthritis classification criteria: an American College of Rheumatology/European League Against Rheumatism collaborative initiative. Arthritis Rheum 2010;62:2569–81.

11. Leslie D, Lipsky P, Notkins AL. Autoantibodies as predictors of disease. J Clin Invest 2001;108:1417–22.

12. Arbuckle MR, McClain MT, Rubertone MV, et al. Development of autoantibodies before the clinical onset of systemic lupus erythematosus. N Engl J Med 2003; 349:1526–33.

13. Klareskog L, Stolt P, Lundberg K, et al. A new model for an etiology of rheumatoid arthritis: smoking may trigger HLA-DR (shared epitope)-restricted immune reactions to autoantigens modified by citrullination. Arthritis Rheum 2006;54: 38–46.

14. Vessey MP, Villard-Mackintosh L, Yeates D. Oral contraceptives, cigarette smoking and other factors in relation to arthritis. Contraception 1987;35:457–64.

15. Hernandez-Avila M, Liang MH, Willett WC, et al. Reproductive factors, smoking, and the risk for rheumatoid arthritis. Epidemiology 1990;1:285–91.

16. Hernandez-Avila M, Liang MH, Willett WC, et al. Exogenous sex hormones and the risk of rheumatoid arthritis. Arthritis Rheum 1990;33:947–53.

17. Hazes JM, Dijkmans BA, Vandenbroucke JP, et al. Lifestyle and the risk of rheumatoid arthritis: cigarette smoking and alcohol consumption. Ann Rheum Dis 1990;49:980–2.

18. Heliovaara M, Aho K, Aromaa A, et al. Smoking and risk of rheumatoid arthritis. J Rheumatol 1993;20:1830–5.

19. Voigt LF, Koepsell TD, Nelson JL, et al. Smoking, obesity, alcohol consumption, and the risk of rheumatoid arthritis. Epidemiology 1994;5:525–32.

20. Symmons DP, Bankhead CR, Harrison BJ, et al. Blood transfusion, smoking, and obesity as risk factors for the development of rheumatoid arthritis: results from a primary care-based incident case-control study in Norfolk, England. Arthritis Rheum 1997;40:1955–61.

21. Karlson EW, Lee IM, Cook NR, et al. A retrospective cohort study of cigarette smoking and risk of rheumatoid arthritis in female health professionals. Arthritis Rheum 1999;42:910–7.

22. Uhlig T, Hagen KB, Kvien TK. Current tobacco smoking, formal education, and the risk of rheumatoid arthritis. J Rheumatol 1999;26:47–54.
23. Kallberg H, Ding B, Padyukov L, et al. Smoking is a major preventable risk factor for rheumatoid arthritis: estimations of risks after various exposures to cigarette smoke. Ann Rheum Dis 2011;70:508–11.
24. Criswell LA, Merlino LA, Cerhan JR, et al. Cigarette smoking and the risk of rheumatoid arthritis among postmenopausal women: results from the Iowa Women's Health Study. Am J Med 2002;112:465–71.
25. Krishnan E, Sokka T, Hannonen P. Smoking-gender interaction and risk for rheumatoid arthritis. Arthritis Res Ther 2003;5:R158–62.
26. Stolt P, Bengtsson C, Nordmark B, et al. Quantification of the influence of cigarette smoking on rheumatoid arthritis: results from a population based case-control study, using incident cases. Ann Rheum Dis 2003;62:835–41.
27. Costenbader KH, Feskanich D, Mandl LA, et al. Smoking intensity, duration, and cessation, and the risk of rheumatoid arthritis in women. Am J Med 2006;119:503–11.
28. Doran MF, Crowson CS, O'Fallon WM, et al. The effect of oral contraceptives and estrogen replacement therapy on the risk of rheumatoid arthritis: a population based study. J Rheumatol 2004;31:207–13.
29. Spector TD, Roman E, Silman AJ. The pill, parity, and rheumatoid arthritis. Arthritis Rheum 1990;33:782–9.
30. Brennan P, Bankhead C, Silman A, et al. Oral contraceptives and rheumatoid arthritis: results from a primary care-based incident case-control study. Semin Arthritis Rheum 1997;26:817–23.
31. Hazes JM, Dijkmans BC, Vandenbroucke JP, et al. Reduction of the risk of rheumatoid arthritis among women who take oral contraceptives. Arthritis Rheum 1990;33:173–9.
32. Jorgensen C, Picot MC, Bologna C, et al. Oral contraception, parity, breast feeding, and severity of rheumatoid arthritis. Ann Rheum Dis 1996;55:94–8.
33. Vandenbroucke JP, Valkenburg HA, Boersma JW, et al. Oral contraceptives and rheumatoid arthritis: further evidence for a preventive effect. Lancet 1982;2:839–42.
34. Vandenbroucke JP, Witteman JC, Valkenburg HA, et al. Noncontraceptive hormones and rheumatoid arthritis in perimenopausal and postmenopausal women. JAMA 1986;255:1299–303.
35. Wingrave SJ, Kay CR. Reduction in incidence of rheumatoid arthritis associated with oral contraceptives. Lancet 1978;1:569–71.
36. Walitt B, Pettinger M, Weinstein A, et al. Effects of postmenopausal hormone therapy on rheumatoid arthritis: the women's health initiative randomized controlled trials. Arthritis Rheum 2008;59:302–10.
37. Merlino LA, Cerhan JR, Criswell LA, et al. Estrogen and other woman reproductive risk factors are not strongly associated with the development of rheumatoid arthritis in elderly women. Semin Arthritis Rheum 2003;33:72–82.
38. Karlson EW, Mandl LA, Hankinson SE, et al. Do breast-feeding and other reproductive factors influence future risk of rheumatoid arthritis? Results from the Nurses' Health Study. Arthritis Rheum 2004;50:3458–67.
39. Pikwer M, Bergstrom U, Nilsson JA, et al. Breast feeding, but not use of oral contraceptives, is associated with a reduced risk of rheumatoid arthritis. Ann Rheum Dis 2009;68:526–30.
40. Berglin E, Kokkonen H, Einarsdottir E, et al. Influence of female hormonal factors, in relation to autoantibodies and genetic markers, on the development

of rheumatoid arthritis in northern Sweden: a case-control study. Scand J Rheumatol 2010;39:454–60.

41. Pikwer M, Bergstrom U, Nilsson JA, et al. Early menopause is an independent predictor of rheumatoid arthritis. Ann Rheum Dis 2012;71:378–81.

42. Stolt P, Kallberg H, Lundberg I, et al. Silica exposure is associated with increased risk of developing rheumatoid arthritis: results from the Swedish EIRA study. Ann Rheum Dis 2005;64:582–6.

43. Sluis-Cremer GK, Hessel PA, Hnizdo E, et al. Relationship between silicosis and rheumatoid arthritis. Thorax 1986;41:596–601.

44. Turner S, Cherry N. Rheumatoid arthritis in workers exposed to silica in the pottery industry. Occup Environ Med 2000;57:443–7.

45. Klockars M, Koskela RS, Jarvinen E, et al. Silica exposure and rheumatoid arthritis: a follow up study of granite workers 1940-81. Br Med J (Clin Res Ed) 1987;294:997–1000.

46. Steenland K, Sanderson W, Calvert GM. Kidney disease and arthritis in a cohort study of workers exposed to silica. Epidemiology 2001;12:405–12.

47. Hart JE, Laden F, Puett RC, et al. Exposure to traffic pollution and increased risk of rheumatoid arthritis. Environ Health Perspect 2009;117:1065–9.

48. de Pablo P, Chapple IL, Buckley CD, et al. Periodontitis in systemic rheumatic diseases. Nat Rev Rheumatol 2009;5:218–24.

49. Kallberg H, Jacobsen S, Bengtsson C, et al. Alcohol consumption is associated with decreased risk of rheumatoid arthritis: results from two Scandinavian case-control studies. Ann Rheum Dis 2009;68:222–7.

50. Pedersen M, Jacobsen S, Klarlund M, et al. Environmental risk factors differ between rheumatoid arthritis with and without auto-antibodies against cyclic citrullinated peptides. Arthritis Res Ther 2006;8:R133.

51. Jacobsson LT, Jacobsson ME, Askling J, et al. Perinatal characteristics and risk of rheumatoid arthritis. BMJ 2003;326:1068–9.

52. Mandl LA, Costenbader KH, Simard JF, et al. Is birthweight associated with risk of rheumatoid arthritis? Data from a large cohort study. Ann Rheum Dis 2009;68:514–8.

53. Hemminki K, Li X, Sundquist J, et al. Familial associations of rheumatoid arthritis with autoimmune diseases and related conditions. Arthritis Rheum 2009;60:661–8.

54. Stahl EA, Raychaudhuri S, Remmers EF, et al. Genome-wide association study meta-analysis identifies seven new rheumatoid arthritis risk loci. Nat Genet 2010;42:508–14.

55. Costenbader KH, Chang SC, De Vivo I, et al. Genetic polymorphisms in PTPN22, PADI-4, and CTLA-4 and risk for rheumatoid arthritis in two longitudinal cohort studies: evidence of gene-environment interactions with heavy cigarette smoking. Arthritis Res Ther 2008;10:R52.

56. Karlson EW, Chang SC, Cui J, et al. Gene-environment interaction between HLA-DRB1 shared epitope and heavy cigarette smoking in predicting incident rheumatoid arthritis. Ann Rheum Dis 2010;69:54–60.

57. Mahdi H, Fisher BA, Kallberg H, et al. Specific interaction between genotype, smoking and autoimmunity to citrullinated alpha-enolase in the etiology of rheumatoid arthritis. Nat Genet 2009;41:1319–24.

58. Karlson EW, Chibnik LB, Kraft P, et al. Cumulative association of 22 genetic variants with seropositive rheumatoid arthritis risk. Ann Rheum Dis 2010;69:1077–85.

59. del Puente A, Knowler WC, Pettitt DJ, et al. The incidence of rheumatoid arthritis is predicted by rheumatoid factor titer in a longitudinal population study. Arthritis Rheum 1988;31:1239–44.

60. Del Puente A, Knowler WC, Pettitt DJ, et al. High incidence and prevalence of rheumatoid arthritis in Pima Indians. Am J Epidemiol 1989;129:1170–8.
61. Silman AJ, Hennessy E, Ollier B. Incidence of rheumatoid arthritis in a genetically predisposed population. Br J Rheumatol 1992;31:365–8.
62. Aho K, Heliovaara M, Maatela J, et al. Rheumatoid factors antedating clinical rheumatoid arthritis. J Rheumatol 1991;18:1282–4.
63. Aho K, Palusuo T, Kurki P. Marker antibodies of rheumatoid arthritis: diagnostic and pathogenetic implications. Semin Arthritis Rheum 1994;23: 379–87.
64. Aho K, Palosuo T, Heliovaara M, et al. Antifilaggrin antibodies within "normal" range predict rheumatoid arthritis in a linear fashion. J Rheumatol 2000;27: 2743–6.
65. Berglin E, Padyukov L, Sundin U, et al. A combination of autoantibodies to cyclic citrullinated peptide (CCP) and HLA-DRB1 locus antigens is strongly associated with future onset of rheumatoid arthritis. Arthritis Res Ther 2004;6:R303–8.
66. Nielen MM, van Schaardenburg D, Reesink HW, et al. Simultaneous development of acute phase response and autoantibodies in preclinical rheumatoid arthritis. Ann Rheum Dis 2006;65:535–7.
67. Rantapaa-Dahlqvist S, Boman K, Tarkowski A, et al. Up regulation of monocyte chemoattractant protein-1 expression in anti-citrulline antibody and immunoglobulin M rheumatoid factor positive subjects precedes onset of inflammatory response and development of overt rheumatoid arthritis. Ann Rheum Dis 2007; 66:121–3.
68. Bos WH, Ursum J, de Vries N, et al. The role of the shared epitope in arthralgia with anti-cyclic citrullinated peptide antibodies (anti-CCP), and its effect on anti-CCP levels. Ann Rheum Dis 2008;67:1347–50.
69. Bos WH, Wolbink GJ, Boers M, et al. Arthritis development in patients with arthralgia is strongly associated with anti-citrullinated protein antibody status: a prospective cohort study. Ann Rheum Dis 2010;69:490–4.
70. Majka DS, Holers VM. Can we accurately predict the development of rheumatoid arthritis in the preclinical phase? Arthritis Rheum 2003;48:2701–5.
71. Deane KD, Norris JM, Holers VM. Preclinical rheumatoid arthritis: identification, evaluation, and future directions for investigation. Rheum Dis Clin North Am 2010;36:213–41.
72. Chouinard E, Walter S. Recall bias in case-control studies: an empirical analysis and theoretical framework. J Clin Epidemiol 1995;48:245–54.
73. Merlino LA, Curtis J, Mikuls TR, et al. Vitamin D intake is inversely associated with rheumatoid arthritis: results from the Iowa Women's Health Study. Arthritis Rheum 2004;50:72–7.
74. Symmons DP, Silman AJ. The Norfolk Arthritis Register (NOAR). Clin Exp Rheumatol 2003;21:S94–9.
75. Kolfenbach JR, Deane KD, Derber LA, et al. A prospective approach to investigating the natural history of preclinical rheumatoid arthritis (RA) using first-degree relatives of probands with RA. Arthritis Rheum 2009;61:1735–42.
76. El-Gabalawy HS, Robinson DB, Hart D, et al. Immunogenetic risks of anti-cyclical citrullinated peptide antibodies in a North American Native population with rheumatoid arthritis and their first-degree relatives. J Rheumatol 2009;36: 1130–5.
77. Padyukov L, Silva C, Stolt P, et al. A gene-environment interaction between smoking and shared epitope genes in HLA-DR provides a high risk of seropositive rheumatoid arthritis. Arthritis Rheum 2004;50:3085–92.

78. Stolt P, Yahya A, Bengtsson C, et al. Silica exposure among male current smokers is associated with a high risk of developing ACPA-positive rheumatoid arthritis. Ann Rheum Dis 2010;69:1072–6.

79. Makrygiannakis D, Hermansson M, Ulfgren AK, et al. Smoking increases peptidylarginine deiminase 2 enzyme expression in human lungs and increases citrullination in BAL cells. Ann Rheum Dis 2008;67:1488–92.

80. Verpoort KN, Cheung K, Ioan-Facsinay A, et al. Fine specificity of the anti-citrullinated protein antibody response is influenced by the shared epitope alleles. Arthritis Rheum 2007;56:3949–52.

81. Snir O, Widhe M, von Spee C, et al. Multiple antibody reactivities to citrullinated antigens in sera from patients with rheumatoid arthritis: association with HLA-DRB1 alleles. Ann Rheum Dis 2009;68:736–43.

82. Feitsma AL, van der Voort EI, Franken KL, et al. Identification of citrullinated vimentin peptides as T cell epitopes in HLA-DR4-positive patients with rheumatoid arthritis. Arthritis Rheum 2010;62:117–25.

83. Bhatia SS, Majka DS, Kittelson JM, et al. Rheumatoid factor seropositivity is inversely associated with oral contraceptive use in women without rheumatoid arthritis. Ann Rheum Dis 2007;66:267–9.

84. Hughes DA, Haslam PL, Townsend PJ, et al. Numerical and functional alterations in circulatory lymphocytes in cigarette smokers. Clin Exp Immunol 1985;61:459–66.

85. Robbins CS, Dawe DE, Goncharova SI, et al. Cigarette smoke decreases pulmonary dendritic cells and impacts antiviral immune responsiveness. Am J Respir Cell Mol Biol 2004;30:202–11.

86. Moszczynski P, Zabinski Z, Moszczynski P Jr, et al. Immunological findings in cigarette smokers. Toxicol Lett 2001;118:121–7.

87. Burton RC. Smoking, immunity, and cancer. Med J Aust 1983;2:411–2.

88. Bermudez EA, Ridker PM. C-reactive protein, statins, and the primary prevention of atherosclerotic cardiovascular disease. Prev Cardiol 2002;5:42–6.

89. Tracy RP, Psaty BM, Macy E, et al. Lifetime smoking exposure affects the association of C-reactive protein with cardiovascular disease risk factors and subclinical disease in healthy elderly subjects. Arterioscler Thromb Vasc Biol 1997;17:2167–76.

90. Tuomi T, Heliovaara M, Palosuo T, et al. Smoking, lung function, and rheumatoid factors. Ann Rheum Dis 1990;49:753–6.

91. Abhishek A, Butt S, Gadsby K, et al. Anti-TNF-alpha agents are less effective for the treatment of rheumatoid arthritis in current smokers. J Clin Rheumatol 2010;16:15–8.

92. Saevarsdottir S, Wedren S, Seddighzadeh M, et al. Patients with early rheumatoid arthritis who smoke are less likely to respond to treatment with methotrexate and tumor necrosis factor inhibitors: observations from the Epidemiological Investigation of Rheumatoid Arthritis and the Swedish Rheumatology Register cohorts. Arthritis Rheum 2011;63:26–36.

93. Sverdrup B, Kallberg H, Bengtsson C, et al. Association between occupational exposure to mineral oil and rheumatoid arthritis: results from the Swedish EIRA case-control study. Arthritis Res Ther 2005;7:R1296–303.

94. Kleinau S, Erlandsson H, Holmdahl R, et al. Adjuvant oils induce arthritis in the DA rat. I. Characterization of the disease and evidence for an immunological involvement. J Autoimmun 1991;4:871–80.

95. Cannon GW, Woods ML, Clayton F, et al. Induction of arthritis in DA rats by incomplete Freund's adjuvant. J Rheumatol 1993;20:7–11.

96. Lundberg I, Alfredsson L, Plato N, et al. Occupation, occupational exposure to chemicals and rheumatological disease. A register based cohort study. Scand J Rheumatol 1994;23:305–10.

97. Linos A, Worthington JW, O'Fallon WM, et al. The epidemiology of rheumatoid arthritis in Rochester, Minnesota: a study of incidence, prevalence, and mortality. Am J Epidemiol 1980;111:87–98.

98. Symmons DP, Barrett EM, Bankhead CR, et al. The incidence of rheumatoid arthritis in the United Kingdom: results from the Norfolk Arthritis Register. Br J Rheumatol 1994;33:735–9.

99. Goemaere S, Ackerman C, Goethals K, et al. Onset of symptoms of rheumatoid arthritis in relation to age, sex and menopausal transition. J Rheumatol 1990;17: 1620–2.

100. Silman A, Kay A, Brennan P. Timing of pregnancy in relation to the onset of rheumatoid arthritis. Arthritis Rheum 1992;35:152–5.

101. Wilder RL. Adrenal and gonadal steroid hormone deficiency in the pathogenesis of rheumatoid arthritis. J Rheumatol Suppl 1996;44:10–2.

102. Wilder RL, Elenkov IJ. Hormonal regulation of tumor necrosis factor-alpha, interleukin-12 and interleukin-10 production by activated macrophages. A disease-modifying mechanism in rheumatoid arthritis and systemic lupus erythematosus? [review]. Ann N Y Acad Sci 1999;876:14–31.

103. Allebeck P, Ahlbom A, Ljungstrom K, et al. Do oral contraceptives reduce the incidence of rheumatoid arthritis? A pilot study using the Stockholm County medical information system. Scand J Rheumatol 1984;13:140–6.

104. Linos A, Worthington JW, O'Fallon WM, et al. Case-control study of rheumatoid arthritis and prior use of oral contraceptives. Lancet 1983;1:1299–300.

105. Del Junco DJ, Annegers JF, Luthra HS, et al. Do oral contraceptives prevent rheumatoid arthritis? JAMA 1985;254:1938–41.

106. Hannaford PC, Kay CR, Hirsch S. Oral contraceptives and rheumatoid arthritis: new data from the Royal College of General Practitioners' oral contraception study. Ann Rheum Dis 1990;49:744–6.

107. Deighton CM, Sykes H, Walker DJ. Rheumatoid arthritis, HLA identity, and age at menarche. Ann Rheum Dis 1993;52:322–6.

108. Brun JG, Nilssen S, Kvale G. Breast feeding, other reproductive factors and rheumatoid arthritis. A prospective study. Br J Rheumatol 1995;34: 542–6.

109. Dugowson CE, Koepsell TD, Voigt LF, et al. Rheumatoid arthritis in women. Incidence rates in group health cooperative, Seattle, Washington, 1987-1989. Arthritis Rheum 1991;34:1502–7.

110. Doran MF, Pond GR, Crowson CS, et al. Trends in incidence and mortality in rheumatoid arthritis in Rochester, Minnesota, over a forty-year period. Arthritis Rheum 2002;46:625–31.

111. van de Sande MG, de Hair MJ, van der Leij C, et al. Different stages of rheumatoid arthritis: features of the synovium in the preclinical phase. Ann Rheum Dis 2011;70:772–7.

112. Lundberg K, Kinloch A, Fisher BA, et al. Antibodies to citrullinated alpha-enolase peptide 1 are specific for rheumatoid arthritis and cross-react with bacterial enolase. Arthritis Rheum 2008;58:3009–19.

113. Lundberg K, Wegner N, Yucel-Lindberg T, et al. Periodontitis in RA—the citrullinated enolase connection. Nature Rev 2010;6:727–30.

114. Mikuls TR. Help stop tooth decay. And prevent RA? J Rheumatol 2010;37: 1083–5.

115. Mikuls TR, Payne JB, Reinhardt RA, et al. Antibody responses to *Porphyromonas gingivalis* (*P. gingivalis*) in subjects with rheumatoid arthritis and periodontitis. Int Immunopharmacol 2009;9:38–42.
116. Wegner N, Wait R, Sroka A, et al. Peptidylarginine deiminase from *Porphyromonas gingivalis* citrullinates human fibrinogen and alpha-enolase: implications for autoimmunity in rheumatoid arthritis. Arthritis Rheum 2010;62:2662–72.
117. Ramirez AS, Rosas A, Hernandez-Beriain JA, et al. Relationship between rheumatoid arthritis and *Mycoplasma pneumoniae*: a case-control study. Rheumatology (Oxford) 2005;44:912–4.
118. Silman AJ, Pearson JE. Epidemiology and genetics of rheumatoid arthritis. Arthritis Res 2002;4(Suppl 3):S265–72.
119. Demoruelle MK, Weisman MH, Simonian PL, et al. Airways abnormalities and rheumatoid arthritis-related autoantibodies in subjects without arthritis: early injury or initiating site of autoimmunity? Arthritis Rheum 2012;64(6):1756–61.
120. Gizinski AM, Mascolo M, Loucks JL, et al. Rheumatoid arthritis (RA)-specific autoantibodies in patients with interstitial lung disease and absence of clinically apparent articular RA. Clin Rheumatol 2009;28:611–3.
121. Scher JU, Abramson SB. The microbiome and rheumatoid arthritis. Nat Rev Rheumatol 2011;7:569–78.
122. Blankenberg-Sprenkels SH, Fielder M, Feltkamp TE, et al. Antibodies to *Klebsiella pneumoniae* in Dutch patients with ankylosing spondylitis and acute anterior uveitis and to Proteus mirabilis in rheumatoid arthritis. J Rheumatol 1998;25:743–7.
123. Ebringer A, Rashid T, Wilson C. Rheumatoid arthritis, Proteus, anti-CCP antibodies and Karl Popper. Autoimmun Rev 2010;9:216–23.
124. Vaahtovuo J, Toivanen P, Eerola E. Bacterial composition of murine fecal microflora is indigenous and genetically guided. FEMS Microbiol Ecol 2003;44:131–6.
125. Edwards CJ. Commensal gut bacteria and the etiopathogenesis of rheumatoid arthritis. J Rheumatol 2008;35:1477–97.
126. Linos A, Kaklamani VG, Kaklamani E, et al. Dietary factors in relation to rheumatoid arthritis: a role for olive oil and cooked vegetables? Am J Clin Nutr 1999;70:1077–82.
127. Linos A, Kaklamanis E, Kontomerkos A, et al. The effect of olive oil and fish consumption on rheumatoid arthritis—a case control study. Scand J Rheumatol 1991;20:419–26.
128. Shapiro JA, Koepsell TD, Voigt LF, et al. Diet and rheumatoid arthritis in women: a possible protective effect of fish consumption. Epidemiology 1996;7:256–63.
129. Cerhan JR, Saag KG, Merlino LA, et al. Antioxidant micronutrients and risk of rheumatoid arthritis in a cohort of older women. Am J Epidemiol 2003;157:345–54.
130. Pattison DJ, Silman AJ, Goodson NJ, et al. Vitamin C and the risk of developing inflammatory polyarthritis: prospective nested case-control study. Ann Rheum Dis 2004;63:843–7.
131. Pattison DJ, Symmons DP, Lunt M, et al. Dietary beta-cryptoxanthin and inflammatory polyarthritis: results from a population-based prospective study. Am J Clin Nutr 2005;82:451–5.
132. Pattison DJ, Symmons DP, Lunt M, et al. Dietary risk factors for the development of inflammatory polyarthritis: evidence for a role of high level of red meat consumption. Arthritis Rheum 2004;50:3804–12.

133. Pedersen M, Stripp C, Klarlund M, et al. Diet and risk of rheumatoid arthritis in a prospective cohort. J Rheumatol 2005;32:1249–52.
134. Benito-Garcia E, Feskanich D, Hu FB, et al. Protein, iron, and meat consumption and risk for rheumatoid arthritis: a prospective cohort study. Arthritis Res Ther 2007;9:R16.
135. Karlson EW, Shadick NA, Cook NR, et al. Vitamin E in the primary prevention of rheumatoid arthritis: the Women's Health Study. Arthritis Rheum 2008;59: 1589–95.
136. Costenbader KH, Feskanich D, Holmes M, et al. Vitamin D intake and risks of systemic lupus erythematosus and rheumatoid arthritis in women. Ann Rheum Dis 2008;67:530–5.
137. Costenbader KH, Kang JH, Karlson EW. Antioxidant intake and risks of rheumatoid arthritis and systemic lupus erythematosus in women. Am J Epidemiol 2010;172:205–16.
138. Munger KL, Levin LI, Hollis BW, et al. Serum 25-hydroxyvitamin D levels and risk of multiple sclerosis. JAMA 2006;296:2832–8.
139. Hernan MA, Olek MJ, Ascherio A. Geographic variation of MS incidence in two prospective studies of US women. Neurology 1999;53:1711–8.
140. Arnson Y, Amital H, Shoenfeld Y. Vitamin D and autoimmunity: new aetiological and therapeutic considerations. Ann Rheum Dis 2007;66:1137–42.
141. Kamen DL, Cooper GS, Bouali H, et al. Vitamin D deficiency in systemic lupus erythematosus. Autoimmun Rev 2006;5:114–7.
142. Canning MO, Grotenhuis K, de Wit H, et al. 1-alpha,25-dihydroxyvitamin D3 (1,25(OH)(2)D(3)) hampers the maturation of fully active immature dendritic cells from monocytes. Eur J Endocrinol 2001;145:351–7.
143. Cantorna MT, Hayes CE, DeLuca HF. 1,25-Dihydroxycholecalciferol inhibits the progression of arthritis in murine models of human arthritis. J Nutr 1998;128:68–72.
144. Feser M, Derber LA, Deane KD, et al. Plasma 25,OH vitamin D concentrations are not associated with rheumatoid arthritis (RA)-related autoantibodies in individuals at elevated risk for RA. J Rheumatol 2009;36:943–6.
145. Patel S, Farragher T, Berry J, et al. Association between serum vitamin D metabolite levels and disease activity in patients with early inflammatory polyarthritis. Arthritis Rheum 2007;56:2143–9.
146. Andjelkovic Z, Vojinovic J, Pejnovic N, et al. Disease modifying and immunomodulatory effects of high dose 1 alpha (OH) D3 in rheumatoid arthritis patients. Clin Exp Rheumatol 1999;17:453–6.
147. James MJ, Gibson RA, Cleland LG. Dietary polyunsaturated fatty acids and inflammatory mediator production. Am J Clin Nutr 2000;71:343S–8S.
148. Rosell M, Wesley AM, Rydin K, et al. Dietary fish and fish oil and the risk of rheumatoid arthritis. Epidemiology 2009;20:896–901.
149. Stamp LK, James MJ, Cleland LG. Diet and rheumatoid arthritis: a review of the literature. Semin Arthritis Rheum 2005;35:77–94.
150. Simopoulos AP. Omega-3 fatty acids in inflammation and autoimmune diseases. J Am Coll Nutr 2002;21:495–505.
151. Heliovaara M, Knekt P, Aho K, et al. Serum antioxidants and risk of rheumatoid arthritis. Ann Rheum Dis 1994;53:51–3.
152. Knekt P, Heliovaara M, Aho K, et al. Serum selenium, serum alpha-tocopherol, and the risk of rheumatoid arthritis. Epidemiology 2000;11:402–5.
153. Comstock GW, Burke AE, Hoffman SC, et al. Serum concentrations of alpha tocopherol, beta carotene, and retinol preceding the diagnosis of rheumatoid arthritis and systemic lupus erythematosus. Ann Rheum Dis 1997;56:323–5.

154. Nissen MJ, Gabay C, Scherer A, et al. The effect of alcohol on radiographic progression in rheumatoid arthritis. Arthritis Rheum 2010;62:1265–72.
155. Maxwell JR, Gowers IR, Moore DJ, et al. Alcohol consumption is inversely associated with risk and severity of rheumatoid arthritis. Rheumatology (Oxford) 2010;49:2140–6.
156. Cerhan JR, Saag KG, Criswell LA, et al. Blood transfusion, alcohol use, and anthropometric risk factors for rheumatoid arthritis in older women. J Rheumatol 2002;29:246–54.
157. Lu B, Solomon DH, Costenbader KH, et al. Alcohol consumption and markers of inflammation in women with preclinical rheumatoid arthritis. Arthritis Rheum 2011;62:3554–9.
158. Imhof A, Froehlich M, Brenner H, et al. Effect of alcohol consumption on systemic markers of inflammation. Lancet 2001;357:763–7.
159. Cooper CL, Cameron DW. Effect of alcohol use and highly active antiretroviral therapy on plasma levels of hepatitis C virus (HCV) in patients coinfected with HIV and HCV. Clin Infect Dis 2005;41(Suppl 1):S105–9.
160. Boe DM, Nelson S, Zhang P, et al. Alcohol-induced suppression of lung chemokine production and the host defense response to Streptococcus pneumoniae. Alcohol Clin Exp Res 2003;27:1838–45.
161. Nelson S, Bagby GJ, Bainton BG, et al. The effects of acute and chronic alcoholism on tumor necrosis factor and the inflammatory response. J Infect Dis 1989;160:422–9.
162. Szabo G, Mandrekar P, Catalano D. Inhibition of superantigen-induced T cell proliferation and monocyte IL-1 beta, TNF-alpha, and IL-6 production by acute ethanol treatment. J Leukoc Biol 1995;58:342–50.
163. Thould AK, Thould BT. Arthritis in Roman Britain. Br Med J (Clin Res Ed) 1983; 287:1909–11.
164. Rothschild BM, Turner KR, DeLuca MA. Symmetrical erosive peripheral polyarthritis in the Late Archaic Period of Alabama. Science 1988;241:1498–501.
165. Fischer KM. Hypothesis: tobacco use is a risk factor in rheumatoid arthritis. Med Hypotheses 1991;34:116–7.
166. Bengtsson C, Nordmark B, Klareskog L, et al. Socioeconomic status and the risk of developing rheumatoid arthritis: results from the Swedish EIRA study. Ann Rheum Dis 2005;64:1588–94.
167. Neidell MJ. Air pollution, health, and socio-economic status: the effect of outdoor air quality on childhood asthma. J Health Econ 2004;23:1209–36.
168. Apelberg BJ, Buckley TJ, White RH. Socioeconomic and racial disparities in cancer risk from air toxics in Maryland. Environ Health Perspect 2005;113:693–9.
169. Penard-Morand C, Charpin D, Raherison C, et al. Long-term exposure to background air pollution related to respiratory and allergic health in schoolchildren. Clin Exp Allergy 2005;35:1279–87.
170. Sunyer J. Urban air pollution and chronic obstructive pulmonary disease: a review. Eur Respir J 2001;17:1024–33.
171. Karakatsani A, Andreadaki S, Katsouyanni K, et al. Air pollution in relation to manifestations of chronic pulmonary disease: a nested case-control study in Athens, Greece. Eur J Epidemiol 2003;18:45–53.
172. Dockery DW, Pope CA 3rd, Xu X, et al. An association between air pollution and mortality in six U.S. cities. N Engl J Med 1993;329:1753–9.
173. van Eeden SF, Yeung A, Quinlam K, et al. Systemic response to ambient particulate matter: relevance to chronic obstructive pulmonary disease. Proc Am Thorac Soc 2005;2:61–7.

174. Kunzli N, Jerrett M, Mack WJ, et al. Ambient air pollution and atherosclerosis in Los Angeles. Environ Health Perspect 2005;113:201–6.
175. Pope CA 3rd, Burnett RT, Thun MJ, et al. Lung cancer, cardiopulmonary mortality, and long-term exposure to fine particulate air pollution. JAMA 2002; 287:1132–41.
176. Nafstad P, Haheim LL, Oftedal B, et al. Lung cancer and air pollution: a 27 year follow up of 16 209 Norwegian men. Thorax 2003;58:1071–6.
177. Pereira FA, de Assuncao JV, Saldiva PH, et al. Influence of air pollution on the incidence of respiratory tract neoplasm. J Air Waste Manag Assoc 2005;55: 83–7.
178. Schwartz J, Dockery DW, Neas LM. Is daily mortality associated specifically with fine particles? J Air Waste Manag Assoc 1996;46:927–39.
179. Schwartz J, Laden F, Zanobetti A. The concentration-response relation between PM(2.5) and daily deaths. Environ Health Perspect 2002;110:1025–9.
180. Laden F, Neas LM, Dockery DW, et al. Association of fine particulate matter from different sources with daily mortality in six U.S. cities. Environ Health Perspect 2000;108:941–7.
181. Costenbader KH, Chang SC, Laden F, et al. Geographic variation in rheumatoid arthritis incidence among women in the United States. Arch Intern Med 2008; 168:1664–70.
182. Vieira VM, Hart JE, Webster TF, et al. Association between residences in U.S. northern latitudes and rheumatoid arthritis: a spatial analysis of the Nurses' Health Study. Environ Health Perspect 2010;118:957–61.
183. Silman AJ, MacGregor AJ, Thomson W, et al. Twin concordance rates for rheumatoid arthritis: results from a nationwide study. Br J Rheumatol 1993;32:903–7.
184. Linn-Rasker SP, van der Helm-van Mil AH, van Gaalen FA, et al. Smoking is a risk factor for anti-CCP antibodies only in rheumatoid arthritis patients who carry HLA-DRB1 shared epitope alleles. Ann Rheum Dis 2006;65:366–71.
185. Lee HS, Irigoyen P, Kern M, et al. Interaction between smoking, the shared epitope, and anti-cyclic citrullinated peptide: a mixed picture in three large North American rheumatoid arthritis cohorts. Arthritis Rheum 2007;56:1745–53.
186. Keenan BT, Chibnik LB, Cui J, et al. Effect of interactions of glutathione S-transferase T1, M1, and P1 and HMOX1 gene promoter polymorphisms with heavy smoking on the risk of rheumatoid arthritis. Arthritis Rheum 2010;62:3196–210.
187. Criswell LA, Saag KG, Mikuls TR, et al. Smoking interacts with genetic risk factors in the development of rheumatoid arthritis among older Caucasian women. Ann Rheum Dis 2006;65:1163–7.
188. Mikuls TR, Gould KA, Bynote KK, et al. Anticitrullinated protein antibody (ACPA) in rheumatoid arthritis: influence of an interaction between HLA-DRB1 shared epitope and a deletion polymorphism in glutathione S-transferase in a cross-sectional study. Arthritis Res Ther 2010;12:R213.
189. Mikuls TR, Levan T, Gould KA, et al. Impact of interactions of cigarette smoking with NAT2 polymorphisms on rheumatoid arthritis risk in African Americans. Arthritis Rheum 2012;64:655–64.
190. Hill JA, Southwood S, Sette A, et al. Cutting edge: the conversion of arginine to citrulline allows for a high-affinity peptide interaction with the rheumatoid arthritis-associated HLA-DRB1*0401 MHC class II molecule. J Immunol 2003; 171:538–41.
191. Karlson EW, Chibnik LB, Kraft P, et al. Cumulative association of 22 genetic variants with seropositive rheumatoid arthritis risk. Ann Rheum Dis 2010;69: 1077–85.

192. Demoruelle MK, Deane K. Antibodies to citrullinated protein antigens (ACPAs): clinical and pathophysiologic significance. Curr Rheumatol Rep 2011;13(5): 421–30.

193. Cooles FA, Isaacs JD. Pathophysiology of rheumatoid arthritis. Curr Opin Rheumatol 2011;23:233–40.

194. Kakumanu P, Sobel ES, Narain S, et al. Citrulline dependence of anti-cyclic citrullinated peptide antibodies in systemic lupus erythematosus as a marker of deforming/erosive arthritis. J Rheumatol 2009;36:2682–90.

195. Alenius GM, Berglin E, Rantapaa-Dahlqvist S. Antibodies against cyclic citrullinated peptide (CCP) in psoriatic patients with or without joint inflammation. Ann Rheum Dis 2006;65:398–400.

196. Kuhn KA, Kulik L, Tomooka B, et al. Antibodies against citrullinated proteins enhance tissue injury in experimental autoimmune arthritis. J Clin Invest 2006; 116:961–73.

197. Sokolove J, Zhao X, Chandra PE, et al. Immune complexes containing citrullinated fibrinogen costimulate macrophages via Toll-like receptor 4 and Fcgamma receptor. Arthritis Rheum 2011;63:53–62.

198. Zhao X, Okeke NL, Sharpe O, et al. Circulating immune complexes contain citrullinated fibrinogen in rheumatoid arthritis. Arthritis Res Ther 2008;10:R94.

199. Okamoto S, Adachi M, Chujo S, et al. Etiological role of cigarette smoking in rheumatoid arthritis: nasal exposure to cigarette smoke condensate extracts augments the development of collagen-induced arthritis in mice. Biochem Biophys Res Commun 2011;404:1088–92.

200. Lindblad SS, Mydel P, Jonsson IM, et al. Smoking and nicotine exposure delay development of collagen-induced arthritis in mice. Arthritis Res Ther 2009;11:R88.

201. Breban MA, Moreau MC, Fournier C, et al. Influence of the bacterial flora on collagen-induced arthritis in susceptible and resistant strains of rats. Clin Exp Rheumatol 1993;11:61–4.

202. Moudgil KD, Kim E, Yun OJ, et al. Environmental modulation of autoimmune arthritis involves the spontaneous microbial induction of T cell responses to regulatory determinants within heat shock protein 65. J Immunol 2001;166: 4237–43.

203. Kinloch AJ, Alzabin S, Brintnell W, et al. Immunization with *Porphyromonas gingivalis* enolase induces autoimmunity to mammalian alpha-enolase and arthritis in DR4-IE-transgenic mice. Arthritis Rheum 2011;63:3818–23.

Epilogue: How Will We Care for Patients with Early Arthritis?

Richard S. Panush, MD[a],*,
Francisco P. Quismorio Jr, MD, MACR[a], David A. Fox, MD[b]

KEYWORDS

• Early arthritis • Care • Rheumatoid arthritis • Prevention

> *Knowing is not enough; we must apply.*
> *Willing is not enough; we must do.*
> *—Goethe[1]*

Caring optimally for patients with early arthritis is one of the exciting challenges of contemporary rheumatology. Indeed we perceive this to be an urgent societal imperative.[2]

The superb contributions to this timely issue of *Rheumatic Disease Clinics* frame many of the pertinent issues. These articles inform us and permit us to identify the key questions, and provide an elegant state-of-the-art summary of potential predictors/triggers of inflammatory arthritis, sophisticated imaging (and serologic) methods to establish early/preclinical disease, and principles to guide the therapy for these patients to maximize their opportunity for favorable outcomes.

Several important questions remain unanswered. When does disease begin? This is a critical issue. The autoimmune diathesis that generates disease, when specific enough, is arguably a point of disease onset, and could be more amenable to treatment, even cure, perhaps with different approaches than we use in established disease. Considering that statins are increasingly used in primary and not just secondary prevention of vascular disease, we need not be too timid about considering treatment at this stage.

When should therapeutic intervention occur? What are needed are biomarkers that can guide treatment for both disease subsets and disease severity. In the not too distant future individual genetic profiles, even complete genomic sequences, may contribute not only to risk assessment but also to early diagnosis. It seems likely

[a] Division of Rheumatology, Department of Medicine, Keck School of Medicine at the University of Southern California, USC Medical Center, IRD 427, 2010 Zonal Avenue, Los Angeles, CA 90033, USA; [b] Division of Rheumatology, Department of Medicine, University of Michigan School of Medicine, Ann Arbor, MI 48109-5358, USA
* Corresponding author.
E-mail address: panush@usc.edu

Rheum Dis Clin N Am 38 (2012) 427–429
doi:10.1016/j.rdc.2012.04.003
0889-857X/12/$ – see front matter © 2012 Elsevier Inc. All rights reserved.

rheumatic.theclinics.com

that our current definitions and subclassifications of rheumatic diseases will change substantially and become more sharply focused with better insight into pathogenesis, and combined use of genetic, epigenetic, immunologic, inflammatory, and tissue-related biomarkers.

In rheumatoid arthritis (RA), have the new disease classification criteria made our task harder because, in an effort to capture patients with earlier RA, a much greater number of patients end up misclassified as RA who actually have a self-limited syndrome?

What are the incremental consequences of delayed therapy, particularly for preclinical illness?

Are there not disease subsets, certainly for RA, which perhaps merit differing approaches?

But most compelling to us is the challenge of assuring that all patients with early arthritis are provided optimal care. Only 41% of RA patients in Canada[3] were started on therapy within 6 months of presumed onset of disease; 78% of the delay was attributable to processes/events occurring before patients saw a rheumatologist. And these data were only for patients who were referred to and seen by rheumatologists. How many never get to rheumatologists or even primary care physicians? While some might view these data as reasonably salutary, we do not; we suspect the experience is worse in the United States and possibly other and underdeveloped countries. For example, at Los Angeles County + University of Southern California medical center there are approximately 1000 patients who will wait around 6 to 12 months for rheumatologic evaluation. We certainly respect the care this (and similar) system(s) will bring to an otherwise underserved, indeed neglected, population.[4] We understand the inherent problems and limitations. But we must not be complacent. We must not settle for less than the best possible care now available.

How, then, will we care for these patients? Someone once suggested that good questions are more important than answers; answers change, good questions do not. However, this query, we believe, demands response. We suggest it will require paradigmatic changes in how health care is provided. Surely there are not enough rheumatologists. Nor is it likely there will be any time soon. Training more is not the solution. In part rheumatologists will have to accept that other health care professionals will need to be a part of any plan to approach this issue; in the past, we have been reluctant to concede that others had the ability or ought to have a prerogative of caring for our patients.[5] But there are probably not enough primary care physicians either, although that may never be known. This means that nonphysicians (nurse practitioners, physician assistants, and/or new, specially trained rheumatology/musculoskeletal disease professionals)[6,7] will have to assume a prominent role if all patients with early arthritis are to be reached. These caregivers will need to use new approaches, including immediate-access clinics,[8] group visits, algorithms, and communication with patients by telephone and other electronic means, using new applications that are disease-specific and even patient-specific. Supervisory mechanisms will need to be devised, and referrals to rheumatologists will need to be selective.

The Institute of Medicine promulgated goals for health care for this century: care that is safe, timely, patient-centered/personalized, equitable, efficient, and effective (which we would infer includes humanistic and of high quality).[1] The expositions in this issue emphasize the value of prompt, aggressive treatment for early arthritis. It is tempting to reflect on the progress of rheumatology in but a few short years.[9] But we cannot be satisfied until we bring the benefits of our advances to all of our patients. It is our individual and societal responsibility to identify these patients and assure that they have opportunities to receive effective and affordable therapy.

Limitations to this are no longer our current art nor our science, but rather our communal resources and will.

Comprehensive medical economic analyses are needed of how to treat RA most effectively and with the least toxicity in the general population. We need to understand the trade-off between the cost and toxicity (and cost of toxicity) of early widespread use of biologics versus the economic benefits of preventing disability. Would it be economically more beneficial to give antimalarials to all patients with a positive anti-CCP antibody rather than very aggressive treatment of clinical RA? Some of these approaches could end up being tested in countries that cannot afford biologics. Do our current clinical measures of disease activity and radiographic anatomy optimally predict disability? Why do we assess structural changes in RA entirely by radiographic measurement of cartilage loss and erosions, some of which are very small, without also considering soft-tissue damage and deformities that are functionally significant? What about the cardiac and pulmonary aspects of rheumatic disease, for which our current so-called disease-modifying antirheumatic drugs, biologic and nonbiologic, may not be working so well?

Even better than remission or cure, of course, would be prevention. At the least we could begin with an organized approach to smoking cessation for individuals who have a family history of RA or who carry the MHC shared epitope.

It should be possible to do much, if not all of this, or certainly do better. We owe it to our patients.

REFERENCES

1. Crossing the quality chasm: a new health system for the 21st century. Committee on Quality of Healthcare in America, Institute of Medicine. Washington, DC: National Academy Press; 2001.
2. Ortiz EC, Torralba KD, O'Dell JR, et al. Later comes earlier, nowadays [editorial]. J Rheumatol 2011;38:2287–9.
3. Tavares R, Pope J, Tremblay JL, et al. Time to disease modifying anti-rheumatic drug treatment in rheumatoid arthritis and its predictors: a national, multi-center, retrospective cohort. J Rheumatol, in press.
4. Panush RS. Rheum with a view. Heroes. The Rheumatologist 2011;12.
5. Panush RS, Kaplan H. Who will care for our patients? [invited editorial]. J Rheumatol 1995;22:2197–8.
6. van Eijk-Hustings Y, van Tubergen A, Boström C, et al. EULAR recommendations for the role of the nurse in the management of chronic inflammatory arthritis. Ann Rheum Dis 2012;71:13–9.
7. Kroese ME, Severens JL, Schulpen GJ, et al. Specialized rheumatology nurse substitutes for rheumatologists in the diagnostic process of fibromyalgia: a cost-consequence analysis and a randomized controlled trial. J Rheumatol 2011;38: 1413–22.
8. Gartner M, Fabrizii JP, Koban E, et al. Immediate access rheumatology clinic: efficiency and outcomes. Ann Rheum Dis 2012;71:363–8.
9. Panush RS. What we don't know about rheumatoid arthritis and its therapy. In: Goodwin JS, editor. Mediguide for inflammatory diseases, vol. 9. New York: Lawrence Dellacorte Publications; 1990. p. 1–3.

Index

Note: Page numbers of article titles are in **boldface** type.

Rheum Dis Clin N Am 38 (2012) 431–439
doi:10.1016/S0889-857X(12)00052-X
0889-857X/12/$ – see front matter © 2012 Elsevier Inc. All rights reserved.

rheumatic.theclinics.com

Moving?

Make sure your subscription moves with you!

To notify us of your new address, find your **Clinics Account Number** (located on your mailing label above your name), and contact customer service at:

Email: journalscustomerservice-usa@elsevier.com

800-654-2452 (subscribers in the U.S. & Canada)
314-447-8871 (subscribers outside of the U.S. & Canada)

Fax number: 314-447-8029

Elsevier Health Sciences Division
Subscription Customer Service
3251 Riverport Lane
Maryland Heights, MO 63043

*To ensure uninterrupted delivery of your subscription, please notify us at least 4 weeks in advance of move.

Printed and bound by CPI Group (UK) Ltd, Croydon, CR0 4YY

03/10/2024

01040460-0001